Supportive Care of the Cancer Patient

JOHN W SWEETENHAM BSc DM FRCP
Senior Lecturer in Medical Oncology
CRC Wessex Medical Oncology Unit
University of Southampton, Southampton General Hospital,
Southampton, UK

CHRIS WILLIAMS DM FRCP
Co-ordinator,
Cochrane Cancer Network,
Institute of Health Sciences, Headington,
Oxford, UK

A member of the Hodder Headline Group
LONDON • SYDNEY • AUCKLAND
Co-published in the USA by
Oxford University Press, Inc., New York

First published in Great Britain 1997 by
Arnold, a member of the Hodder Headline Group,
338 Euston Road, London NW1 3BH

Co-published in the United States of America by
Oxford University Press, Inc.,
198 Madison Avenue, New York, NY10016
Oxford is a registered trademark of Oxford University Press

British Library Cataloguing in Publication Data
A catalogue record for this book is available from the British Library

Library of Congress Cataloging-in-Publication Data
A catalog record for this book is available from the Library of Congress

ISBN 0 340 56171 8

Typeset in 10/11 pt Times by J&L Composition Ltd, Filey, North Yorkshire
Printed and bound in Great Britian by JW Arrowsmith Ltd, Bristol and Hartnolls Ltd,
Bodmin, Cornwall

Contents

Part 5 Specific supportive problems

List of Contributors

Stephen J Birch BSc MB BS DMRD FRCR
Consultant Radiologist, Southampton University Hospital, Southampton, UK

Georg A Bjarnason MD FRCP(C)
Department of Medicine, University of Toronto, Division of Medical Oncology, Hematology and Clinical Pharmacology, Toronto-Sunnybrook Regional Cancer Centre, Sunnybrook Health Sciences Centre, Toronto, Ontario, Canada

Marcello De Cicco MD
Division of Anaesthesia, Centro di Riferimento Oncologico, Via Pedemontana Occidentale, Aviano, Italy

Richard E Clark MA(Cantab) MD(London) FRCP(UK) MRCPath
Senior Lecturer and Honorary Consultant Haematologist, University Department of Haematology, Royal Liverpool University Hospital, Liverpool, UK

Robert E Coleman FRCP(London and Edin) MD
Reader and Honorary Consultant Medical Oncologist, Weston Park Hospital, Sheffield, UK

Carol L Davis MA MRCP
Senior Lecturer in Palliative Medicine, Countess Mountbatten House, Moorgreen Hospital, Southampton, UK

Sander JH van Deventer MD PhD
Academic Medical Centre, University of Amsterdam, Laboratory of Experimental Internal Medicine, Amsterdam, The Netherlands

John L Francis PhD FRCPath
Walt Disney Memorial Cancer Institute at Florida Hospital, Altamonte Springs, Florida, USA

Alison G Freifeld MD
Senior Clinical Investigator and Head, Infectious Diseases Service, National Cancer Institute, Bethesda, Maryland, USA

Angela Hall BSc
Senior Research Fellow, CRC Communication and Counselling Research Centre, Department of Oncology, University College London Medical School, London, UK

William JM Hrushesky
Professor of Medicine and Microbiology/Immunology, Albany Medical College of Union University. Adjunct Professor of Chemical Engineering, Rensselaer Polytechnic Institute. Senior Attending Oncologist, Albany Veterans Administration Medical Center, Albany, New York, USA

Thérèse Loughlin MB BCh BAO NUI
Department of Clinical Oncology, Royal South Hants Hospital, Southampton, UK

Edith A Perez MD
Associate Professor of Medicine, Division of Hematology/Oncology, Mayo Clinic Jacksonville, Jacksonville, Florida, USA

Philip A Pizzo MD
Thomas Morgan Rotch Professor and Chair, Department of Pediatrics, Harvard Medical School. Physician-in-Chief and Chair, Department of Medicine, Children's Hospital, Boston, Massachusetts, USA

Tom van der Poll MD PhD
Academic Medical Centre, University of Amsterdam, Laboratory of Experimental Internal Medicine, Amsterdam, The Netherlands

Stuart Roath MD FRCPath FIBiol
Walt Disney Memorial Cancer Institute at Florida Hospital, Altamonte Springs, Florida, USA

Philip S Schein MD FRCP FRCP(Glasg)
Chairman and CEO, US Bioscience Inc., West Conshohocken, USA

John W Sweetenham BSc DM FRCP
LRF Senior Lecturer in Medical Oncology, CRC Wessex Medical Oncology Unit, University of Southampton, Southampton General Hospital, Southampton, UK

David S Tarver
Consultant, Poole Hospital, Dorset, UK

Richard D Thomas
Consultant, Royal Devon and Exeter Hospital, UK

Umberto Tirelli MD
Division of Medical Oncology and AIDS, Centro di Riferimento Oncologico, Aviano, Italy

Stephen R Veach MD
Memorial Sloan Kettering Cancer Center, New York, New York, USA

Rostislav Vyzula MD
Albany Veterans Administration Medical Center, Albany, New York, USA

Preface

There is little doubt that the role of supportive care in the management of patients with cancer is expanding. This is in part a reflection of the trend towards increasingly intensive cancer treatment, but it is also due to the availability of new supportive treatment and techniques, and an increasing realisation of the importance of the psychological and emotional support of these patients. Furthermore, there is increased awareness of the supportive needs of specific groups, such as the elderly, patients with malignant disease in association with HIV infection, and the carers of cancer patients.

In this book, we have sought to provide information on several aspects of supportive care, and have included some subjects which would perhaps not normally be regarded as strictly 'supportive' but which represent new approaches to improving quality of life for these patients. The inclusion of chapters on chronopharmacology and interventional radiology are good examples.

We hope that this book will provide valuable information for all health care professionals involved in the management of cancer patients. We extend our thanks to all of the contributors for their hard work and patience.

John Sweetenham
Chris Williams

To Stuart Roath

Supportive therapy

PART 1

Supportive therapy

CHAPTER 1

Bone marrow effects of anticancer therapy

RICHARD E CLARK

INTRODUCTION

Experienced oncologists and haematologists will be familiar with the effects of anticancer therapy on the peripheral blood (PB) cell count. The mean red blood cell lifespan is about 120 days,[1] whereas the half-life of platelets in the circulation is 5–7 days, and that of neutrophils is about 6 hours.[2] Following a single dose of a cytotoxic agent, the PB neutrophil count will fall over the next 7–10 days. If a sufficiently large dose has been given, the platelet count may also fall, typically a few days later than the neutrophil fall.[3] Conversely, a fall in the haemoglobin concentration is not usually apparent for several weeks, and is rarely seen after a single dose of a cytotoxic drug. This is because if the bone marrow suppression is temporary, then red blood cell production will have returned to normal before any fall in haemoglobin concentration is apparent. If the therapy is intensive enough to cause total bone marrow failure then (unless blood product support is given) the patient will have died of infection or haemorrhage before anaemia occurs.

The nadir of these cytopenias will vary depending on the agent and dose used, other concurrent and previous therapy, and the underlying disease. For example, oral chlorambucil given as therapy for chronic lymphocytic leukaemia (CLL) at a dose of 0.1 mg/kg/day causes minimal PB cytopenia, and is easily managed in the outpatient clinic.[4] Conversely the intensive chemotherapy schedules used in the treatment of acute leukaemia cause severe haematological toxicity, though marrow recovery will gradually occur over several weeks. The most intensive bone marrow suppressive therapy used is the very high dose chemotherapy and total body irradiation schedules used in conditioning for bone marrow transplantation (BMT).

This article reviews the basic physiology of haemopoiesis, emphasizing the importance of the haemopoietic microenvironment, and discusses how the bone marrow is affected by anticancer therapy, with special reference to the very high doses of therapy used in conditioning for BMT. The consequences of bone marrow suppression, and exploitation of this for therapeutic gain are discussed, focusing on chemotherapy-induced PB stem cell mobilization and *ex vivo* culture for bone marrow purging. The clinical use of haemopoietic growth factors

(HGFs) to accelerate bone marrow recovery, and the general management of infection in the neutropenic patient are the subjects of separate chapters and are not discussed in detail here. Since it appears likely that at least some secondary leukaemias in long-term survivors of malignant disease are therapy-related, a section is included on therapy-related leukaemia.

EFFECTS OF ANTICANCER THERAPY ON HAEMOPOIESIS

Bone marrow stromal cells and the microenvironments that they form may modulate the regulatory signals they produce in response to changing conditions, for example supporting lymphopoiesis under different culture conditions.[5] These modulations in turn can affect the overall pattern of haemopoiesis. This flexibility of stromal function may be important following chemoradiotherapy, which itself causes an inflammatory response and increases the risk of sepsis because of the resultant neutropenia. Thus, chemoradiotherapy may produce a stromal respose promoting neutrophil production, mediated through the action on stromal cells of several other cytokines. Tumour necrosis factor (TNF), interleukin-1 (IL-1) and bacterial endotoxin are all produced during an inflammatory response, and serum TNF levels rise following radiotherapy.[6] Bone marrow sinusoidal stromal cells can be stimulated to secrete IL-1, as well as HGFs.[7–9] Bone marrow stromal cells with receptors for IL-1, TNF and platelet-derived growth factor[10,11] can be stimulated to secrete factors that include the various HGFs and IL-6. These tissue, endothelial and stromal contributions may then act synergistically to promote myeloid differentiation.

Effects of radiotherapy

The dose–survival curves for the effects of irradiation on various haemopoietic cells are summarized in Fig. 1.1. Though there are species differences in the degree of radiosensitivity of haemopoietic progenitors and stem cells, in all species studied these cells are more radiosensitive than the stromal fibroblast progenitor CFU-F. The dose–survival curves for haemopoietic progenitors show little or no evidence of a shoulder at low dosage, whereas this is seen for CFU-F.[13] Clinical data from BMT recipients support the notion that stromal cells are less radiosensitive than haemopoietic cells. Most reports have found that the bone marrow stroma remains recipient in origin following allogeneic BMT,[14–16] though Keating et al.[17] reported that donor stromal engraftment may occur several months following the procedure. The report by Agematsu and Nakahori[18] using a Y-chromosome-specific cDNA probe suggests that following standard (cyclophosphamide–total body irradiation) conditioning for allogeneic BMT, the stroma remains host-derived for up to 1200 days.

The effects of radiation on the haemopoietic microenvironment have been extensively studied in *in vitro* culture and in experimental animals (mostly mice).[12,19] Most stromal cells are in G_0 at any given time, and can repair irradiation-induced damage whilst in this state.[20] Stromal proliferation is severely impaired in long-term bone marrow culture established from mice

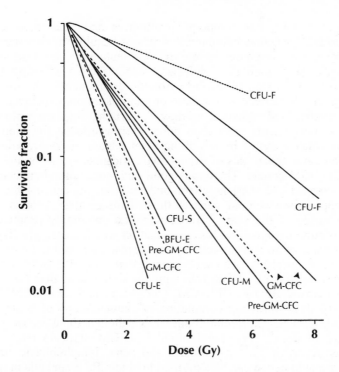

Fig. 1.1. Survival of haemopoietic and stromal progenitor cells to acute doses of low linear energy transfer radiation. Solid line: mouse; broken line: human; dotted line: dog. (Data from ref. 12.)

irradiated with 5–10 Gy. This impairment persists for several months, though gradually improves with time.[20] It is not clear whether this recovery is due to proliferation of comparatively undamaged stromal cells, which gradually repopulate the bone marrow, or whether the radiation-induced damage is gradually repaired. Irradiation upregulates the gene for TNF,[6] which may explain the familiar side-effects of clinical radiotherapy.

Effects of chemotherapy

The myelosuppressive effects of cytotoxic drugs can be assessed by changes in PB cell counts (mainly neutropenia and thrombocytopenia) and bone marrow cellularity. The extent and timing of cytopenias vary from drug to drug, and similar initial changes in the peripheral blood count may be followed by quite different patterns of cytopenia.[21] Vincristine and L-asparaginase have little effect on the PB count, whereas anthracyclines and alkylating agents have profound and predictable effects, often necessitating prophylactic measures to minimize the risk of infection. Drugs within the same class of cytotoxics may vary in myelosuppressive properties; vinblastine is more myelosuppressive than vincristine, yet they are closely related vinca alkaloids, which both act via effects on tubulin. Hydroxyurea produces rapid decreases in circulating neutrophils within 2–3 days, but complete quantitative and qualitative stem cell recovery is usual,[22] whereas comparable doses of busulphan, also widely used in the therapy of chronic-phase chronic myeloid leukaemia, can lead to permanent quantitative and qualitative defects.[23] Other factors affecting the time course of myelosuppression following cytotoxic drugs include the total cumulative dose given, the schedule and route of administration, concurrent therapy and prior cytotoxic and radiation therapy.[24] Certain drugs may produce PB cytopenias by mechanisms other than bone marrow effects; for example cisplatinum may cause anaemia by inhibiting renal release of erythropoietin.

Marsh[25] compared the effects of twenty-two anticancer agents on the PB with concurrent CFU-GM counts. There was good rank correlation between neutropenia and decreased CFU-GM numbers, and those agents causing the greatest CFU-GM suppression were in general those with greatest *in vivo* efficacy. Successive courses of the same cytotoxic regime commonly produce longer and more profound cytopenias. Dosage reduction was increasingly likely with successive courses of an Adriamycin–cyclophosphamide regime given as adjuvant therapy of metastatic breast cancer, and in that study, PB and bone marrow CFU-GM numbers were also lower following the sixth course than following the first.[26] Bone marrow BFU-E, CFU-GM, CFU-Mega and CFU-GEMM are all decreased 5–10 days following completion of chemotherapy of acute myeloid leukaemia (AML) with daunorubicin and ara-C, though some recovery is seen over the next 10 days.[27] Peripheral blood CFU-GM numbers rise following chemotherapy for AML,[28,29] myeloma[30] and acute lymphoblastic leukaemia (ALL).[29] This phenomenon can be exploited to obtain PB stem cells in sufficient numbers to support haemopoietic reconstitution (see below).[31,32]

Cytotoxic agents may also damage the haemopoietic microenvironment. Stromal cells treated *in vitro* with Adriamycin demonstrated vacuolization of the cell membrane, swollen mitochondria and altered growth following explant to culture.[33] Cisplatinum, ara-C[34] and busulphan[35] all similarly cause ultrastructural damage to stromal cells *in vitro*. In a series of elegant experiments in mice, high doses of cyclophosphamide and busulphan impaired the ability of stroma to support *in vivo* haemopoiesis, and busulphan also caused CFU-S damage. The cyclophosphamide-induced stromal damage gradually improved over several weeks and eventually achieved pretreatment values, whereas busulphan-induced damage did not.[36]

In comparison with radiation, less is known about the long-term effects of chemotherapy on the bone marrow stroma in humans. Treatment of preformed normal stroma with the nitrosourea 1,3-bis-(2-chloroethyl)-1-nitrosourea (BCNU) impairs its ability to support haemopoiesis, though this effect is reversible over 7 days.[37] Both stromal and haemopoietic progenitor cell compartments are defective in long-term bone marrow culture established from long-term survivors of AML,[38] ALL[39] and Hodgkin's disease.[40]

Therapy-related leukaemia

In recent years, leukaemia has become recognized as the most serious long-term complication of therapy for a previous unrelated malignancy. Patients surviving for some years after otherwise successful treatment for Hodgkin's disease,[41] non-Hodgkin lymphoma (NHL),[42] multiple myeloma,[43] testicular and ovarian cancer[44] and certain childhood cancers[45] are at increased risk of developing AML. Several studies also report an increased incidence of myelodysplastic syndrome (MDS) in these patients. Many studies have correlated the risk of secondary leukaemia with previous treatment details, especially for Hodgkin's disease. In that condition, cases treated initially by radiotherapy, and subsequently by salvage chemotherapy at relapse are at greatest risk (cumulative risk of 9.9 +/− 2.9 per cent at 9 years).[46] Though less information is available, the risk in NHL appears similar; the Copenhagen group reports an 8 per cent incidence of AML/MDS at 9 years.[47] Studies in Hodgkin's disease suggest a maximum incidence of AML 3–9 years after initial chemotherapy.[48] Some conditioning regimes may be more leukaemogenic than others,[43,49,50] and some reports have related the incidence of leukaemias to dosage of alkylating agents[51] or epipodophyllotoxins.[45]

Ras oncogene mutations have been identified in PB white cells in approximately 15 per cent of patients treated successfully for lymphoma some years previously,[52] and similar findings have been reported for the *fms* oncogene, which encodes the M-CSF receptor.[53] These patients also showed an excess of random chromosomal aberrations when compared to an age-matched control population.[54] It is suggested that radiotherapy/chemotherapy may lead to genetic damage in haemopoietic stem cells. In a minority of patients, this damage may cause a mutation in a critical area of the genome such as a proto-oncogene, and thus confer a survival advantage for that cell. If the damage is not lethal, over a latent interval (probably many years), expansion in this affected clone eventually permits the detection of the mutation in PB white cells derived from affected stem cells. It is not known whether these mutations alone are sufficient to cause secondary MDS/AML, or whether additional genetic change is necessary for leukaemogenesis.

BONE MARROW TRANSPLANTATION AND HAEMOPOIESIS

Leucocytes begin to reappear in the PB 2–3 weeks following BMT. The initial reappearance of PB neutrophils after BMT may be due to differentiation of infused progenitor cells already committed to myeloid differentiation, but durable engraftment may depend on proliferation and differentiation of more primitive stem cells.[55,56] The kinetics of reappearance of total leucocytes, neutrophils, monocytes, lymphocytes, platelets and reticulocytes is shown in Fig. 1.2. Recovery is slower if methotrexate or T-cell depletion is used, and bone marrow cellularity is decreased for several months following BMT. Although PB neutrophil and platelet numbers have returned to normal by 3–6 months, several studies have demonstrated long-term reductions in bone marrow CFU-GM and BFU-E for up to 48 months following allogeneic BMT.[58–60] Following autologous BMT, the decrease in bone marrow CFU-GM may be more profound and of longer duration.[61] Slower rates of PB recovery after autologous BMT when compared to allograft recipients may be due to lower progenitor cell numbers in the graft because of previous cytotoxic therapy. An alternative explanation is that the cryopreservation causes significant loss of progenitor cells, thus delaying

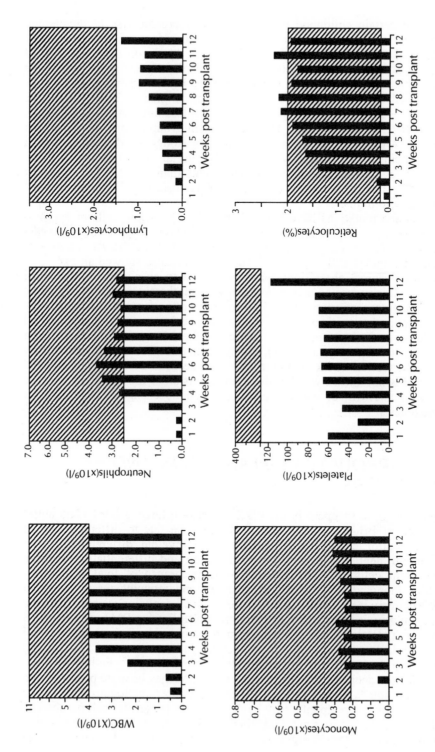

Fig. 1.2. Reconstitution of leucocytes (WBC), neutrophils, lymphocytes, monocytes, platelets and reticulocytes in 79 recipients of unmanipulated marrow transplantation from HLA-identical siblings, performed for haematological malignancy. Conditioning was with cyclophosphamide 120 mg/kg and fractionated total body irradiation 12–14 Gy; post-transplant immunosuppression was with cyclosporin. (Data from ref. 57.)

engraftment in the autograft recipients.[62] Circulating levels of GM-CSF,[63] G-CSF[64] and M-CSF[65] all rise following BMT, and return to basal levels as the PB cell counts recover.

One of the aims of BMT conditioning therapy is to eradicate the host's immune system, to minimize rejection of the incoming graft. BMT (unlike radiotherapy or chemotherapy in standard dosage) therefore causes severe and prolonged damage to the host immune system. T- and B-cell function takes many months to return to normal after BMT.[57] This is due to the time required for lymphocyte development to occur; there is less functional thymic tissue available in the adult for T-cell education. Following allogeneic BMT, the host and/or graft may be deliberately T-cell-depleted to minimize the risk of graft-versus-host disease (GVHD), and post-transplant T-cell immunosuppression with cyclosporin A/methotrexate is usual. Finally, GVHD selects the lymphoid system (as well as the skin, gut and liver) as a target organ; BMT recipients who develop significant chronic GVHD may never regain normal T- and B-cell function.

An acquired severe combined immune deficiency therefore consistently occurs after BMT, similar to that seen in AIDS. CD8+ ('cytotoxic suppressor') T cells return to the normal range within 12 weeks, and may remain elevated, whereas CD4+ ('helper') T cells remain low for long periods.[66] This leads to inversion of the normal CD4-to-CD8 (T4-to-T8) ratio of 2, to values less than 1, and is seen after allogeneic, autologous and syngeneic BMT. The proportion of both CD8+ and CD4+ cells expressing markers of activation (HLA-DR antigens and OKT 10) increases.[67] CD16+ natural killer cells rise rapidly after both allogeneic and autologous BMT,[67] though not after conventional cytotoxic chemotherapy.[68]

Serum IgG and IgM return to normal by about 9 months post-BMT.[69] In contrast, both serum and secretory IgA levels are deficient for several years post-BMT, especially in patients who develop chronic GVHD.[70] *In vivo* antibody production to neoantigens is severely impaired in the first 3 months in both allogeneic and syngeneic recipients; this returns to normal in healthy long-term survivors but not in those cases with significant chronic GVHD.[71]

The bone marrow stroma is also affected by the high doses of chemotherapy and radiotherapy used as conditioning. Histological abnormalities are seen 3 weeks after BMT; before this time the bone marrow is too hypocellular for evaluation.[72] The formation of a confluent stromal layer is poor in long-term bone marrow culture established from BMT recipients,[73,74] but gradually improves with increasing time from transplant.[74] Bone marrow CFU-F growth is decreased 21 days following allogeneic BMT though later recovers to normal levels.[75] The cellular composition of the stromal layer formed after BMT has not been widely studied; one report suggests that it may be abnormal in patients with poor graft function.[76] Stromal cells from BMT recipients grown in long-term bone marrow culture under serum-deprived conditions will produce GM-CSF, but only stromal cells from patients with good graft function also produced G-CSF.[76] It is not known whether this defect of G-CSF production is a consequence or a cause of graft failure. The effect of BMT conditioning therapy on the composition of the bone marrow extracellular matrix is unknown.

Chemotherapy-induced stem cell mobilization

The post-chemotherapy rise in circulating stem and progenitor cells can be exploited to obtain large numbers of stem cells from the PB by leukapheresis, following mobilization with high doses of chemotherapy.[31,32] There is considerable current interest in the use of PB stem cells obtained in this way (or after mobilization with HGFs) to facilitate the recovery of bone marrow function following high-dose chemoradiotherapy.[77,78] The approach has the advantage of improving PB cell counts approximately a week earlier than would be expected with autologous BMT,[79] and also can be used on patients with bone marrow involvement by disease or who are unharvestable because of previous pelvic radiotherapy. PB stem cell infusions have been used both alone[80] and also with conventional autologous bone marrow infusion.[81] The minimum necessary dose of CFU-GM is unclear because of interlaboratory variations in assay techniques.

An interesting development in PB stem cell transplantation for solid tumours is the use of positive selection for CD34-positive cells. This antigen is expressed on 1–4 per cent of human bone marrow cells, and is expressed on virtually all CFU (unipotent and multipotent CFU, blast CFU and precursors of CFU detectable in long-term bone marrow culture). The number of circulating CD34+ cells is greatly increased following chemotherapy or HGF-induced mobilization.[85] Small numbers of CD34+ cells will completely reconstitute haemopoiesis in experimental animals.[86] Since this antigen is not expressed on a variety of solid tumours (e.g. breast carcinoma, neuroblastoma), PB stem cell transplants which have been positively selected for CD34 expression should theoretically offer an effective way of purging potential contaminating tumour cells.[86]

SUMMARY

Many agents used as therapy for cancer cause unwanted effects on the bone marrow. The net results of these agents are immune defects and PB cytopenias, and these are seen in their most extreme form following the very high doses of therapy given as conditioning for bone marrow transplantation. Damage occurs not only to haemopoietic progenitor and stem cells, but also to the marrow microenvironment. The marrow has considerable capacity for recovery, and this can be exploited to therapeutic gain by using chemotherapy (with or without myeloid growth factors) to mobilize early haemopoietic cells into the peripheral blood; these can then be used as rescue following further high-dose therapy. Therapy-induced microenvironmental damage may underlie the long-term cytopenias commonly seen in heavily pretreated cancer patients. It is suggested that damage to haemopoietic stem cells may be related to the subsequent development of secondary leukaemia.

REFERENCES

1. Cavill I, Ricketts C, Napier JAF, Jacobs A. Ferrokinetics and erythropoiesis in man: red cell production and destruction in normal and anaemic subjects. *British Journal of Haematology* 1977; **35**: 33–40.

2. Buckner CD, Clift RA. Prophylaxis and treatment of infection of the immunocompromised host by granulocyte transfusions. *Clinics in Haematology* 1984; **13**: 557–72.
3. Spiegel RJ. The acute toxicities of chemotherapy. *Cancer Treatment Reviews* 1981; **8**: 197–208.
4. French Cooperative Group on Chronic Lymphocytic Leukaemia. Effects of chlorambucil and therapeutic decision in initial forms of chronic lymphocytic leukaemia (Stage A): Results of a randomised clinical trial on 612 patients. *Blood* 1990; **75**: 1414–21.
5. Whitlock CA, Witte ON. Long-term culture of B-lymphocytes and their precursors from murine bone marrow. *Proceedings of the National Academy of Sciences, USA* 1982; **79**: 3608–12.
6. Hallahan DE, Spriggs DR, Beckett MA, Kufe DW, Weichselbaum RR. Increased tumor necrosis factor alpha mRNA after cellular exposure to ionizing radiation. *Proceedings of the National Academy of Sciences, USA* 1989; **86**: 10104.
7. Bagby GC, McCall E, Bergstrom KA, Burger D. A monokine regulates colony-stimulating activity production by vascular endothelial cells. *Blood* 1983; **62**: 663–8.
8. Broudy VC, Kaushansky K, Segal GM, Harlan JM, Adamson JW. Tumor necrosis factor type alpha stimulates human endothelial cells to produce granulocyte/macrophage colony-stimulating factor. *Proceedings of the National Academy of Sciences, USA* 1986; **83**: 7467–71.
9. Seelentag WK, Mermod J-J, Montesano R, Vassali P. Additive effects of interleukin-1 and tumour necrosis factor on the accumulation of three granulocyte and macrophage colony-stimulating factor mRNAs in human endothelial cells. *EMBO Journal* 1987; **6**: 2261–5.
10. Pietrangeli CE, Hayashi SI, Kincade PW. Stromal cell lines which support lymphocyte growth: Characterisation, sensitivity to radiation and responsiveness to growth factors. *European Journal of Immunology* 1988; **18**: 863–72.
11. Rosenfeld M, Keating A, Bowen-Pope DF, Singer JW, Ross R. Responsiveness of the *in vitro* haemopoietic microenvironment to platelet-derived growth factor. *Leukaemia Research* 1985; **9**: 427–34.
12. Hendry JH. The cellular basis of long-term bone marrow injury after irradiation. *Radiotherapy and Oncology* 1985; **3**: 331–8.
13. Fitzgerald TJ, Rothstein L, Kase K, Greenberger JS. Radiosensitivity of human bone marrow granulocyte-macrophage progenitor and stromal colony forming cells: effect of dose rate on purified target cell populations. *Radiation Research* 1986; **107**: 205.
14. Gordon MY. The origin of stromal cells in patients treated by bone marrow transplantation. *Bone Marrow Transplantation* 1988; **3**: 247–51.
15. Simmons PJ, Przepiorka D, Thomas ED, Torok-Storb B. Host origin of marrow stromal cells following allogeneic bone marrow transplantation. *Nature* 1987; **328**: 429.
16. Laver J, Jhanwar SC, O'Reilly RJ, Castro-Malaspina H. Host origin of the human hematropoietic microenvironment following allogeneic bone marrow transplantation. *Blood* 1987; **70**: 1966–8.
17. Keating A, Singer JW, Killen PD et al. Donor origin of the in vitro haemopoiesis microenvironment after marrow transplantation in Man. *Nature* 1982; **298**: 280.
18. Agematsu K, Nakahori Y. Recipient origin of bone marrow-derived fibroblastic stromal cells during all periods following bone marrow transplantation in humans. *British Journal of Haematology* 1991; **79**: 359–65.
19. Greenberger JS. Toxic effects on the haemopoietic microenvironment. *Experimental Haematology* 1991; **19**: 1101–9.
20. Anklesaria P, Fitzgerald TJ, Kase K, Ohara A, Bentley S, Greenberger JS. Improved hematopoiesis in anemic SL/Sl^d mice by therapeutic transplantation of a hematopoietic microenvironment. *Blood* 1989; **74**: 1144–51.

21. Schofield R. Assessment of cytotoxic injury to bone marrow. *British Journal of Cancer* 1986; **53** (Suppl. VII): 115–25.
22. Ross EAM, Anderson N, Micklem HS. Serial depletion and regeneration of the murine haematopoietic system. *Journal of Experimental Medicine* 1982; **155**: 432.
23. Morley A, Trainor K. An animal model of chronic aplastic marrow failure after busulphan. *Blood* 1974; **44**: 49.
24. Gale RP. Antineoplastic Chemotherapy myelosuppression: Mechanisms and new approaches. *Experimental Haematology* 1985; **13** (Suppl. 16): 3–7.
25. Marsh JC. Correlation of hematologic toxicity of antineoplastic agents with their effects on bone marrow stem cells: interspecies studies using an in vivo assay. *Experimental Haematology* 1985 **13** (Suppl. 16): 16–22.
26. Schreml W, Lohrmann H-P, Anger B. Stem cell defects after cytoreductive therapy in man. *Experimental Haematology* 1985; **13** (Suppl. 16): 31–42.
27. Beyer GS, Bruno E, Hoffman R. *In vitro* hematopoiesis following induction chemotherapy for acute leukaemia. *Cancer Research* 1985; **45**: 5921–5.
28. To LB, Haylock DN, Kimber RJ, Juttner CA. High levels of circulating haemato-poietic stem cells in very early remission from acute non-lymphoblastic leukaemia and their collection and cryopreservation. *British Journal of Haematology* 1984; **58**: 399–410.
29. Reid CDL, Kirk A, Muir J, Chanarin I. The recovery of circulating progenitor cells after chemotherapy in AML and ALL and its relation to the rate of bone marrow regeneration after aplasia. *British Journal of Haematology* 1989; **72**: 21–7.
30. Henon P, Beck G, Debecker A, Eisenmann SC, Lepers M, Kandel G. Autografting using peripheral blood stem cells collected after high dose melphalan in high risk multiple myeloma. *British Journal of Haematology* 1988; **70**: 254–5.
31. Siena S, Bregni M, Brando B, Ravajnani F, Bonadonna G, Gianni AM. Circulation of CD34+ hematopoietic stem cells in the peripheral blood of high dose cyclophos-phamide-treated patients; enhancement by intravenous recombinant human granulo-cyte-macrophage colony stimulating factor. *Blood* 1989; **74**: 1905–14.
32. To LB, Shepperd KM, Haylock DN *et al.* Single high doses of cyclophosphamide enable the collection of high numbers of hemopoietic stem cells from the peripheral blood. *Experimental Haematology* 1990; **18**: 442.
33. Cavazzana M, Calvo F, Facchin B *et al.* Use of liquid culture and cell cycle analysis to compare drug damage following in vitro treatment of normal human bone marrow cells with Adriamycin, arabinosyl-cytosine, and etoposide. *Experimental Haematology* 1988; **16**: 876.
34. Gringeri A, Keng PC, Borch RF. Diethylthiocarbamate inhibition of murine bone marrow toxicity caused by cisdiamminedichloroplatinum (II) or diammine-(1,1-cyclobutanedicarboxylato) platinum (II). *Cancer Research* 1988; **48**: 5708.
35. Wathen LM, DeGowin RL, Gibson DP, Knapp SA. Residual injury to the haemo-poietic microenvironment following sequential radiation and busulfan. *International Journal of Radiation Oncology Biology, Physics* 1982; **8**: 1315.
36. Fried W, Adler S. Late effects of chemotherapy on hematopoietic progenitor cells. *Experimental Haematology* 1985; **13** (Suppl. 16): 49–56.
37. Uhlman DL, Verfaillie C, Jones RB, Likart SD. BCNU treatment of marrow stromal monolayers reversibly alters haematopoiesis. *British Journal of Haematology* 1991; **78**: 304–9.
38. Chang J, Geary CG, Testa NG. Long-term bone marrow damage after chemotherapy for acute myeloid leukaemia does not improve with time. *British Journal of Hae-matology* 1990; **75**: 68–72.
39. Bhavnani M, Morris-Jones PH, Testa NG. Children in long-term remission after treatment for acute lymphoblastic leukaemia show persisting haemopoietic injury in clonal and long-term cultures. *British Journal of Haematology* 1989; **71**: 37–41.
40. Radford JA, Testa NG, Crowther D. The long term effects of MVPP chemotherapy

for Hodgkins disease on bone marrow function. *British Journal of Cancer* 1990; **62**: 127–32.

41. Kaldor JM, Day NE, Clarke EA *et al.* Leukemia following Hodgkins disease. *New England Journal of Medicine* 1990; **322**: 7–13.
42. Levine EG, Bloomfield CD. Secondary myelodysplastic syndromes and leukaemias. *Clinics in Haematology* 1986; **15**: 1037–80.
43. Cuzick J, Erskine S, Edelman D, Galton DAG. A comparison of the incidence of the myelodysplastic syndrome and acute myeloid leukaemia following melphalan and cyclophosphamide treatment for myelomatosis. *British Journal of Cancer* 1987; **55**: 523–9.
44. Kaldor JM, Day NE, Band P *et al.* Second malignancies following testicular cancer, ovarian cancer and Hodgkins disease: an international collaborative study among cancer registries. *International Journal of Cancer* 1987; **39**: 571–85.
45. Hawkins MM, Kinnier Wilson LM *et al.* Epipodophyllotoxins, alkylating agents, and radiation and risk of secondary leukaemia after childhood cancer. *British Medical Journal* 1992; **304**: 951–8.
46. Pedersen-Bjergaard J, Larsen SO. Incidence of acute non-lymphocytic leukemia, preleukemia and acute myeloproliferative syndrome up to 10 years after treatment of Hodgkins disease. *New England Journal of Medicine* 1982; **307**: 965–71.
47. Pedersen-Bjergaard J, Ersboll J, Sorensen HM *et al.* Risk of acute non-lymphocytic leukaemia and preleukaemia in patients treated with cyclophosphamide for non-Hodgkin lymphoma. *Annals of Internal Medicine* 1985; **103**: 195–200.
48. Blayney DW, Longo DL, Young RC *et al.* Decreasing risk of leukaemia with prolonged follow-up after chemotherapy and radiotherapy for Hodgkins disease. *New England Journal of Medicine.* 1987; **316**: 710–14.
49. Kaldor JM, Day NE, Hemminki K. Quantifying the carcinogenicity of antineoplastic drugs. *European Journal of Cancer and Clinical Oncology* 1988; **24**: 703–11.
50. Greene MH, Harris EL, Gershenson DM *et al.* Melphalan may be a more potent leukemogen than cyclophosphamide. *Annals of Internal Medicine* 1986; **105**: 360–7.
51. Pedersen-Bjergaard J, Larsen SO, *et al.* Risk of therapy-related leukaemia and preleukaemia after Hodgkins disease. *Lancet* 1987; **ii**: 83–8.
52. Carter G, Hughes DC, Clark RE *et al. Ras* mutations in patients following cytotoxic therapy for lymphoma. *Oncogene* 1990; **5**: 411–16.
53. Cachia PG, Ridge SA, Carter G *et al. Fms* and *ras* mutations following cytotoxic therapy for lymphoma. *British Journal of Haematology* 1990; **74** (Suppl. 1): 12.
54. White AD, Jones BM, Clark RE, Jacobs A. Chromosome aberrations following cytotoxic therapy in patients in complete remission from lymphoma. *Carcinogenesis* 1992; **13**: 1095–99.
55 Demuynck H, Pettengell R, De Campos E, Dexter TM, Testa NG. The capacity of peripheral blood stem cells mobilised with chemotherapy plus G-CSF to repopulate irradiated marrow stroma in vitro is similar to that of bone marrow. *European Journal of Cancer* 1992; **28**: 381–6.
56. Lopez M, Mortel O, Pouillart P *et al.* Acceleration of hemopoietic recovery after autologous bone marrow transplantation by low doses of peripheral blood stem cells. *Bone Marrow Transplantation* 1991; **7**: 173–81.
57. Atkinson K. Reconstruction of the haemopoietic and immune systems after marrow transplantation. *Bone Marrow Transplantation* 1990; **5**: 209–226.
58. Arnold R, Schmeiser T, Heit W. Hemopoietic reconstitution after bone marrow transplantation. *Experimental Haematology* 1986; **14**: 271–7.
59. Barrett AJ, Adams J. A proliferative defect of human bone marrow after transplantation. *British Journal of Haematology* 1981; **49**: 159–64.
60. Li S, Champlin R, Fitchen JH, Gale P. Abnormalities of myeloid progenitor cells after 'successful' bone marrow transplantation. *Journal of Clinical Investigation* 1985; **75**: 234–41.

61. Vellenga E, Sizoo W, Hagenbeek A, Loewenberg B. Different repopulation kinetics of erythroid (BFU-E), myeloid (CFU-GM) and T lymphocyte (TL-CFU) progenitor cells after autologous and allogeneic bone marrow transplantation. *British Journal of Haematology* 1987; **65**: 137–42.

62. Gorin NC, Donay L, David R, Stachowiak J, Duhamel G. Delayed kinetics of recovery of haemopoiesis following autologous bone marrow transplantation. The role of excessively rapid marrow freezing rates after the release of fusion. *European Journal of Cancer and Clinical Oncology* 1983; **10** 485–91.

63. Yamasaki K, Solberg LA, Jamal N *et al.* Hemopoietic colony growth-promoting activities in the plasma of bone marrow transplant recipients. *Journal of Clinical Investigation* 1988; **82**: 255.

64. Watari K, Asano S, Shirafuji N *et al.* Serum granulocyte colony-stimulating factor levels in healthy volunteers and patients with various disorders as estimated by enzyme immunoassay. *Blood* 1988; **72** (Suppl. 1): 138a.

65. Shadduck RK, Waheed A, Rosenfeld CS. Serum and urine colony stimulating factor-1 levels in patients undergoing bone marrow transplantation. *Blood* 1988; **72** (Suppl. 1): 134a.

66. Elfenbein GJ, Ashkenazi YJ, Bath KC. Further phenotypic characterisation of T cells after human allogeneic bone marrow transplantation. *Transplantation* 1985; **39**: 97–102.

67. Ault KE, Antin JH, Ginsburg D *et al.* Phenotype of recovering lymphoid cell populations after marrow transplantation. *Journal of Experimental Medicine* 1985; **161**: 1483–502.

68. Reittie JE, Gottlieb D, Heslop HE *et al.* Endogenously generated activated killer cells circulate after autologous and allogeneic marrow transplantation but not after chemotherapy. *Blood* 1989; **73**: 1351–8.

69. Noel DR, Witherspoon RP, Storb R *et al.* Does graft versus host disease influence the tempo of immunologic recovery after allogeneic human marrow transplantation? An observation on long term survivors. *Blood* 1978; **51**: 1087–105.

70. Izutsu KT, Sullivan KM, Schubert MM *et al.* Disordered salivary immunoglobulin secretion and sodium transport in human chronic graft-versus-host disease. *Transplantation* 1983; **35**: 441–6.

71. Witherspoon RP, Matthews D, Storb R *et al.* Recovery of in vivo cellular immunity after human marrow grafting. Influence of time post-grafting and the influence of acute graft-versus-host disease. *Transplantation* 1981; **58**: 360–8.

72. van den Berg H, Kluin PM, Vossen JM. Early reconstitution of haematopoiesis after allogeneic bone marrow transplantation: a prospective histopathological study of bone marrow biopsy specimens. *Journal of Clinical Pathology* 1990; **43**: 365–9.

73. Rice A, Reiffers J, Bernard P *et al.* Long-term marrow cultures after allogeneic bone marrow transplantation. *Blood* 1990; **75**: 266–7.

74. Treweeke A, Hampson J, Clark RE. Long term bone marrow cultures established from bone marrow transplant recipients. *Leukaemia and Lymphema* 1993; **12**: 117–22.

75. Da WM, Ma DDF, Biggs JC. Studies of hemopoietic stromal fibroblastic colonies in patients undergoing bone marrow transplantation. *Experimental Haematology* 1986; **14**: 266–70.

76. Migliaccio AR, Migliaccio G, Johnson G, Adamson JW, Torok-Storb B. Comparative analysis of hematopoietic growth factors released by stromal cells from normal donors or transplanted patients. *Blood* 1990; **75**: 305–12.

77. Kessinger A, Armitage JO. The evolving role of autologous peripheral stem cell transplantation following high-dose therapy for malignancies. *Blood* 1991; **77**: 211–13.

78. Kotasek D, Shepherd KM, Sage RE *et al.* Factors affecting blood stem cell collection

following high dose cyclophosphamide mobilization in lymphoma, myeloma and solid tumours. *Bone Marrow Transplantation* 1992; **9**: 11–17.

79. Kessinger A, Armitage JO, Smith DM, Landmark JD, Bierman PJ, Weisenburger DD. High-dose therapy and autologous peripheral blood stem cell transplantation for patients with lymphoma. *Blood* 1989; **74**: 1260.

80. Kessinger A, Bierman PJ, Vose JM, Armitage JO. High-dose cyclophosphamide, carmustine and etoposide followed by autologous peripheral stem cell transplantation for patients with relapsed Hodgkins disease. *Blood* 1991; **77**: 2322–5.

81. Sheridan WP, Begley CG, Juttner CA *et al.* Effect of peripheral blood progenitor cells mobilised by filgrastim (G-CSF) on platelet recovery after high-dose chemotherapy. *Lancet* 1992; **339**: 640–4.

82. Civin CI, Strauss LC, Brovall C, Fackler MJ, Schwartz JF, Shaper JH. Antigenic analysis of hematopoiesis. III. A hematopoietic progenitor cell surface antigen defined by a monoclonal antibody raised against KG-1a cells. *Journal of Immunology* 1984; **133**: 157.

83. Andrews RG, Singer JW, Bernstein ID. Monoclonal antibody 12.8 recognises a 115-kD molecule present on both unipotent and multipotent hematopoietic colony-forming cells and their precursors. *Blood* 1986; **67**: 842.

84. Leary AG, Ogawa M. Blast cell colony assay for umbilical cord blood and adult bone marrow progenitors. *Blood* 1987; **69**: 953.

85. Siena S, Bregni M, Brando B *et al.* Flow cytometry for clinical estimation of circulating hematopoietic progenitors for autologous transplantation in cancer patients. *Blood* 1991; **77**: 400–9.

86. Berenson RJ, Andrews RG, Bensinger WI *et al.* Antigen CD34+ marrow cells engraft lethally irradiated baboons. *Journal of Clinical Investigation* 1988; **81**: 951.

CHAPTER 2

Antimicrobial therapy of infectious complications in the patient with cancer

ALISON G FREIFELD AND PHILIP A PIZZO————————————————

INTRODUCTION

The management of infections in cancer patients has evolved both conceptually and practically over the past 30 years. With the introduction of cytotoxic chemotherapy in the 1960s came the prospect of controlling and even curing certain malignancies. However, the periods of bone marrow suppression resulting from such therapies predictably left the patient open to serious and often life-threatening infectious complications. Observations by Bodey *et al.* revealed that the degree and duration of neutropenia were primary risk factors for the occurrence of serious bacterial infections.[1] These observations led to the basic premise that broad-spectrum empirical antibiotic therapy should be initiated promptly when a neutropenic cancer patient presents with fever, even in the absence of localizing signs of infection. While this concept deviated from the traditional dictum of directing antibiotics toward a specifically identified infection, it nonetheless dramatically improved survival as well as quality of life in patients undergoing cytotoxic chemotherapy. Indeed, the concept of empirical antibiotic therapy has been the single most important advance in the management of the febrile neutropenic cancer patients over the last three decades, and it is now the standard of care.

Since the 1960s there have been substantial changes in the armamentarium of antimicrobial agents used routinely to bridge the gap of immunologic vulnerability in cancer patients. Indeed, the development of newer antibacterials, as well as the introduction of other classes of antimicrobial drugs such as antivirals and antifungals, have further improved the outlook for immunosuppressed patients. An understanding of the appropriate use of these new agents, as well as a knowledge of the preventive measures which are most efficacious for protecting cancer patients from infectious complications, are both essential adjuncts to the practice of oncology.

ANTIBIOTICS

Historical perspective

The vast majority of pathogens associated with new fevers in neutropenic cancer patients are bacteria.[2] In the late 1960s through the 1970s, aerobic Gram-negative bacteria were the predominant organisms identified. Other Enterobacteriaceae as well as Gram-positive organisms (e.g. *Staphylococcus aureus*, streptococcal species) were also noted to cause infections in neutropenic patients. Given the broad array of organisms repsonsible for disease, it was clear to early investigators that any empirical regimen designed to prevent early infectious morbidity and mortality, would itself need to be broad in its spectrum of activity. The limitations of antibiotics available at the time (e.g. first-generation cephalosporins, carboxypenicillins and the aminoglycosides) made combination antibiotic therapy essential in order to provide additive or synergistic therapy, as well as to overcome the development of resistance when drugs like carbenicillin or ticarcillin were used alone, or to prevent the treatment failures observed with aminoglycosides used as single agents in neutropenic patients.[3] With prompt initiation of two or three drug regimens which included both a β-lactam and an aminoglycoside, however, survival rates for febrile neuturopenic patients improved.[4,5] Double β-lactam combinations were also shown to be efficacious.[6] Indeed, a number of different regimens have been employed, which provide broad-spectrum activity and bactericidal levels against most of the important pathogens, as well as relatively little toxicity. Nonetheless, no specific combination of agents has proved to be clearly superior to the others.

Over the last 15 years the development of several new classes of antibiotics, including the third-generation cephalosporins, monobactams, carbapenems and the quinolones has provided a broader range of antibiotic choices. The expansion of our antibiotic armamentarium with these agents has resulted in increased simplicity, safety and efficacy in the empirical as well as the therapeutic treatment of febrile neutropenic patients.

Third-generation cephalosporins

The cephalosporins are structurally and functionally related to the penicillins, and their antimicrobial activity is similarly based upon interference with bacterial cell wall biosynthesis and activation of bacterial autolysis. The three generations of cephalosporins are defined by their antimicrobial activity, with the third-generation drugs being most active against aerobic Gram-negative organisms. Although their activity against most Gram-positive cocci is adequate, it is less potent than that of the first-generation cephalosporins and the 'anti-staphylococcal' penicillins. Notably, the available third-generation cephalosporins have virtually no activity against anaerobic organisms, they are inactive against enterococci, methicillin-resistant staphylococci and *Listeria*, and they have suboptimal activity against coagulase-negative staphylococci. Nonetheless, the third-generation cephalosporins possess potent bactericidal activity against the Gram-negative organisms which cause most serious infections in neutropenic patients, making them attractive agents for empirical coverage in the setting of fever and neutropenia. Ceftazidime and cefoperazone, specifically, have excellent activity against *Pseudomonas aeruginosa*, an organism which is notoriously virulent in neutropenic patients, leading to rapid death if untreated or inadequately treated.[7] Although the incidence of *Pseudomonas* infections appears to have decreased in recent years, good antipseudomonal activity remains an essential quality of empirical antibiotic therapy. Accordingly, most studies evaluating the third-generation cephalosporins for the treatment of febrile neutropenia have focused on ceftazidime. Cefoperazone use is often hampered by the development of a coagulation defect, such that it is rarely employed.[8]

Ceftazidime, in combination with a second β-lactam drug or with an aminoglycoside, is effective empirical therapy for fever in neutropenic patients.[9,10] However, multidrug combination regimes present a number of potential problems, including aminoglycoside oto- and renal toxicity, the potential for β-lactamase induction with the double β-lactam regimens, as well as the added expense, extra work and possibility of error related to the preparation and administration of multiple antibiotics. These concerns have paved the way for consideration of single-agent antibiotic therapy as initial treatment for a new fever in neutropenic patients. The third-generation cephalosporins, and ceftazidime in particular, possess greater antibacterial potency and breadth of spectrum than many of the earlier agents such as the aminoglycosides and carboxy- or ureidopenicillins, and have thus offered the unique potential for successful monotherapy.

Ceftazidime monotherapy for febrile neutropenia has been studied extensively with quite favorable results, although initial studies were fraught with the difficulties of having small numbers of patients or of being non-randomized.[9-15] A large, prospectively randomized trial comparing ceftazidime, as a single agent, to the combination of carbenicillin, cephalothin and gentamicin was performed in the early 1980s at the National Cancer Institute.[16] The results of this study, based upon 550 patient episodes, confirmed the safety and efficacy of ceftazidime monotherapy for the initial empirical treatment of fever in neutropenic patients. Survival in both the combination therapy and the monotherapy groups was equally high at 72 hours and at the overall time points, with approximately 90 per cent overall survival in patients with documented infections and 98 per cent overall survival in those presenting with fever of undetermined origin. Of the small number of deaths occurring on study, none were attributable to a specific deficiency in one regimen that was not present in the other. In addition, the average time to defervescence of fever was equivalent for those receiving monotherapy and those treated with combination antibiotics

Among neutropenic episodes complicated by unexplained fever, nearly 80 per cent in both study groups (e.g. ceftazidime monotherapy and combination antibiotic therapy) were successfully treated without requiring any changes in the initial anitibiotic regimen. However, patients who presented with a documented source of infection, and those with prolonged neutropenia (>1 week) appeared to more frequently require modifications of their initial antibiotic regimen in order to survive the neutropenic period. Specifically, two-thirds of patients with documented infections required antibiotic additions or modifications for a successful outcome. Such modifications were not considered a failure of either regimen, *per se*, but were felt to be reflective of the limitations of any antibiotic regimen used to treat patients who are at high risk for multiple serious infections. This standard of evaluation is based upon the notion that the goal of empirical antibiotics is to prevent the early morbidity and mortality associated with untreated or inadequately treated infections, rather than to 'single-handedly' and definitively treat every potential pathogen that might arise during neutropenia. Modifications of initial therapy should be accepted as a consequence of constant and careful clinical evaluation during the course of neutropenia in patients who are susceptible to a myriad of infectious complications while their granulocyte counts are low.

In summary, ceftazidime monotherapy is an acceptable alternative to multi-drug antibiotic regimens for the empirical treatment of fever in a neutropenic host. However, the choice of an antibiotic regimen should always be based upon individual patient and institutional experience, taking into account the status of the patient on presentation, the nature of certain documented infections (e.g. coagulase-negative staphylococcus, anaerobes, etc.) that might require specific antibiotic additions, such as vancomycin or metronidazole to broaden the scope of initial therapy. It is also critical to tailor empirical antibiotic regimens to the patterns of microbial epidemiology within a given hospital (e.g. high incidence of infection with methicillin-resistant *S. aureus*). One important area for concern is the potential for certain organisms to develop resistance to ceftazidime and related drugs, during the course of therapy. *Enterobacter* spp., *Serratia* spp. and *Citrobacter* spp. are most notorious for their inducible β-lactamases that inhibit the activity of β-lactam antibiotics to which these organisms may initially appear to be sensitive.[17,18] Thus, it is recommended that an aminoglycoside be added to ceftazidime or other third-generation cephalosporins used for the treatment of these organisms, in order to prevent the emergence of resistance.[19] More recently, one group has suggested that the third-generation cephalosporins should be avoided completely for the treatment of serious *Enterobacter* spp. infections, due to the frequency of developing resistance to those agents during the course of therapy.[20] Such considerations underscore the appropriateness of maintaining a flexible approach with regard to the selection of the initial empirical regimen, and recognizing the potential need for modification of that regimen during the course of neutropenia.

Imipenem

Imipenem is a member of a class of β-lactam compounds, the carbapenems. Since it is readily degraded by a dihydropeptidase enzyme located in the renal tubular brush border, imipenem must be administered in a fixed combination with cilastatin, an inhibitor of that enzyme. Like other β-lactam drugs, imipenem exerts its bactericidal effect by inhibiting bacterial cell wall synthesis, but it is unique in its breadth of spectrum. Imipenem is highly effective against the aerobic Gram-negative organisms, including *P. aeruginosa*, *Serratia* spp., *Enterobacter* spp. and the Enterobacteriaceae. It also has potent activity against most Gram-positive organisms such as staphylococci and streptococci, as well as *Listeria* and many group D streptococci (enterococci). Finally, imipenem possesses excellent anti-anaerobic activity. Among the few limitations of imipenem are its lack of activity against non-*aeruginosa Pseudomonas* species, methicillin-resistant *S. aureus*, and many coagulase-negative staphylococci.[21] In addition, although it may be sensitive initially, *P. aeruginosa* can rapidly become resistant to imipenem during the therapy, and it has been recommended that serious infections due to this organism should be treated with the combination of imipenem plus an aminoglycoside.[22,23]

Owing to its broad spectrum and potent bactericidal activity against many important pathogens, imipenem is also an attractive candidate for use as monotherapy in the management of febrile neutropenic patients. Several non-comparative trials have indicated that imipenem is effective as a single agent, but interestingly, two randomized studies have not shown it to be superior to combination therapy.[24–27] Theoretically, the increased coverage provided by imipenem over ceftazidime might make it an even more reliable agent for empirical treatment of fever and neutropenia. However, a randomized trial comparing ceftazidime to imipenem monotherapy has recently been completed, with preliminary results indicating that the two drugs are comparably efficacious.[28] Patients with fever of unknown etiology who received ceftazidime did require significantly more modifications of therapy in order to achieve a successful outcome as compared to those who were initially treated with imipenem. Nonetheless, the overall survival of patients in both groups was equally high.

Several drawbacks to the use of imipenem have been encountered. These include the potential of the drug to decrease the seizure threshold in elderly patients or in those with central nervous system pathology, and the fairly frequent occurrence of nausea and vomiting in patients receiving imipenem.[21,29] In the NCI trial, approximately one-third of patients on imipenem reported significant nausea, with about one-third of those requiring discontinuation of the drug. Thus, while imipenem monotherapy is yet another alternative treatment for febrile neutropenia, its toxicities may preclude general use. Imipenem may be best utilized as initial antibiotic coverage in those neutropenic patients who present with a potential anaerobic source of infection, such as a perirectal infection or necrotizing gingivitis, thereby avoiding the need for a multiple antibiotic regimen at the outset.

Aztreonam

Aztreonam is a monobactam antibiotic, differing from the traditional β-lactam drugs structurally in that is has a single ring nucleus. Its antimicrobial spectrum is similar to that of the aminoglycosides, being limited to Gram-negative organisms and including the Enterobacteriaceae, many strains of *Pseudomonas aeruginosa*, *Serratia*, and *Enterobacter*. Unlike aminoglycosides, however, aztreonam is not synergistic with other β-lactam antibiotics against Gram-negative organisms or enterococci.[30,31]

Due to its lack of Gram-positive or anaerobic coverage, aztreonam cannot be considered an appropriate empirical monotherapeutic agent for fever and neutropenia, or for any infectious process in which a variety of organisms might be involved. However, since aztreonam does not cross-react antigenically with other β-lactam antibiotics, it has proved to be particularly useful for patients with significant β-lactam allergy in whom Gram-negative antibiotic activity is required.[32,33] In this regard, the combination of aztreonam with vancomycin appears to be effective empirical treatment for febrile neutropenia. Aztreonam alone, or in concert with an aminoglycoside, has been used successfully for the treatment of serious *P. aeruginosa* infections.[34,35]

Fluoroquinolones

The fluoroquinolones are a group of synthetic antibiotics with a broad spectrum of activity and a unique mechanism of antimicrobial activity. These agents are rapidly bactericidal, primarily by inhibiting the bacterial DNA gyrase enzyme which mediates changes in DNA structure during replication. This mechanism is not shared by any other class of antibiotic, such that cross-resistance between the fluoroquinolones and other commonly employed agents is rare. Thus, organisms which may be multiply resistant, such as *Pseudomonas aeruginosa, Serratia, Enterobacter*, and *Klebsiella*, will often maintain susceptibility to a fluoroquinolone. Many coagulase-negative staphylococci as well as most *Staphylococcus aureus* isolates are sensitive to the fluoroquinolones, including some that are resistant to methicillin. However, certain of the fluoroquinolones, notably ciprofloxacin, possess inadequate activity against streptococcal species. Nonetheless, of the available fluoroquinolones, ciprofloxacin is the most potent against Gram-negative organisms and particularly against *P. aeruginosa*, making it the most logical choice for use in immunocompromised patients.[36,37]

Intravenous ciprofloxacin has anecdotally demonstrated efficacy as a single agent for the treatment of certain severe, multidrug resistant Gram-negative infections in neutropenic patients.[38,39] As empirical therapy for fever and neutropenia, however, ciprofloxacin alone or in combination with an aminoglycoside, has proved to be inadequate due to a high incidence of breakthrough infections, often due to streptococci.[40,41] The combination of ciprofloxacin with vancomycin or a penicillin appears to have eliminated this problem in several small non-randomized trials.[42,43] Such combinations are comparable to traditional β-lactam plus aminoglycoside regimens with regard to patient defervescence within 72 hours of initial therapy, and in the eradication of microbiologically documented infections.

The high bioavailability, excellent tolerability and broad spectrum of the oral quinolones have made them attractive agents for infection prophylaxis in neutropenic patients. Oral ciprofloxacin, norfloxacin and ofloxacin used prophylactically have all been shown to be more effective than traditional regimens such as trimethoprim–sulfamethoxazole with or without colistin, or the combination of vancomycin with polymixin B, in preventing Gram-negative infections in neutropenic patients.[44–48] Fluoroquinolone prophylaxis has also been associated with a decrease in the overall incidence of fever and in the requirement for empirical antibiotics in several studies. [46–48a] A comparison of norfloxacin with trimethoprim–sulfamethoxazole found that although fewer Gram-negative infections occurred in the norfloxacin group, there were more Gram-positive infections documented in patients receiving the quinolone.[44] A recent randomized study of norfloxacin versus ciprofloxacin prophylaxis indicated that patients receiving the latter had a significant overall decrease in the incidence of fever, the number of febrile episodes and duration of empirical antibiotic therapy, and in the incidence of documented Gram-negative infections, compared with those who took norfloxacin.[49] However, a multivariate analysis showed that the advantageous effects of ciprofloxacin prophylaxis occurred only in patients with relatively short neutropenias (<100 cells/mm for less than 7 days), a group in whom there is probably no need to use any antibiotic prophylaxis since they are at relatively low risk for serious infection. Current consensus of expert opinion states that antibiotic prophylaxis should be considered only for afebrile patients with profound neutropenia expected to last for a period of more than 7 days, although this is by no means a standard of care for such patients.[50] Even in this setting, the decision to use antibiotic prophylaxis must be balanced by the recognition that this intervention has never been shown to decrease mortality in neutropenic patients, and that prophylaxis with fluoroquinolones and other agents has been associated with gastrointestinal colonization as well as systemic infections due to resistant bacterial species.[45,51-53]

Several studies have focused on the use of oral ciprofloxacin to complete a course of empirical antibiotics begun intravenously for febrile neutropenia.[28,42,54] Results suggest that this may be a viable approach for patients who have defervesced on initial intravenous drugs, but breakthrough fevers as well as several documented bacteremias with *viridans* streptococci and *Fusobacterium* spp. occurred in a small proportion of those receiving oral ciprofloxacin, underscoring the weaknesses in the antimicrobial spectrum of the drug. Such superinfections might easily be avoided by the addition of a penicillin or clindamycin to the oral ciprofloxacin 'switch' regimen. If such a regimen can prove successful in suppressing recrudescent fever and infection in neutropenic patients, it will clearly simplify the medical management of those patients, and potentially shorten the duration of their hospitalization.

The excellent bioavailability and broad spectrum of the oral fluoroquinolones, particularly ciprofloxacin and ofloxacin, make them attractive for use in the management of low risk patients with fever and neutropenia. Low-risk patients may be defined as those who have fever in the setting of an anticipated short duration of neutropenia (e.g. less than 10 days) and no medical comorbid conditions (e.g. hypotension, abdominal pain, vomiting, mental status changes, respiratory compromise) on presentation. To explore the use of oral antibiotic therapy. Rubenstein *et al.* randomized 83 episodes of low risk febrile neutropenia to treatment with either oral ciprofloxacin plus clindamycin or intravenous therapy consisting of aztreonam plus clindamycin, with both regimens administered in an outpatient setting.[55] Overall responses were good in both groups, with no mortality. All therapy was accomplished in the outpatient setting, following a 24–36 hour initial treatment and observation period in the clinic. However, six patients in the oral regimen cohort were readmitted for persistent fever or for nephrotoxicity that appeared to be associated with ciprofloxacin use in dehydrated patients. This study was relatively small and did not include a comparison to inpatient management, but it does suggest that outpatient therapy is a feasible alternative for low-risk patients with febrile neutropenia.

In a larger study performed in Pakistan (*n*=122 patients), Malik *et al.* found that ofloxacin monotherapy given orally at 400 mg every 12 hours, also appears to be comparable in efficacy to combination parental antibiotics for management of low-risk fever and neutropenia in adults. There were no differences in rates of successful therapy, either with or without modifications of the initial regimen, between the two treatment groups. Overall sucess for patients in each cohort was approximately 75%.[56] Significantly lower response rates were seen in both groups for patients with prolonged and profound neutropenia, and for those with documented infections compared to those with fever of unknown etiology. Two *P. aeruginosa* bacteremias were treated with ofloxacin in this trial, although the outcomes are not specifically reported. As the antimicrobial activity of ofloxacin is less potent than that of ciprofloxacin against *P. aeurginosa*, it is theoretically less reliable for empirical therapy in cancer centers where this organism is more prevalent. However, ofloxacin may be more potent than ciprofloxacin against *Staphylococcus aureus* and less prone to breakthrough drug resistant isolates. These features may amount to an overall benefit as Gram-positive organisms are increasingly isolated in the setting of febrile neutropenia. The same investigators recently reported a prospective, randomized trial comparing inpatient and outpatient management of low-risk fever and neutropenia with oral ofloxacin.[57] There were no differences in overall outcome and most patients were treated without modifications of the empirically employed oral fluoroquinolone. However, 21% of those assigned originally to outpatient therapy required readmission for persistent fever or unresolved infection. Mortality was very low and was comparable in both groups (2% vs 4% for inpatients vs outpatients). However, a single early death in an outpatient who developed vomiting and difficulty with oral intake, and subsequent refusal to be admitted to hospital, emphasizes the need for good patient compliance as well as close patient contact and strict vigilance by health-care workers when treating even low-risk patients outside of the hospital setting.

The importance of these studies was the demonstration of efficacy, excellent tolerability, relative decreased expense and low toxicity of oral fluoroquinolone therapy compared with parental combination antibiotics, for the management of fever and neutropenia in low-risk patients. At the NCI, we have paired oral ciprofloxacin with amoxicillin/clavulanate in a double blind randomized comparison of this oral combination to IV ceftazidime monotherapy among low-risk febrile neutropenic inpatients. As data accrues in this and similar studies, the use of oral empirical antibiotic therapy in the outpatient setting may become a more acceptable alternative for low-risk patients.

Significant interference with oral fluoroquinolone absorption occurs with the co-administration of oral antacids or sucralfate, and these agents should be strictly avoided during a course of antibiotic therapy. Concerns regarding the potential for arthropathies to occur in children receiving ciprofloxacin are waning as more clinical experience with the drug is acquired in populations of immunocompromised children. A recent evaluation of this experience indicated that less than 1 per cent of children taking ciprofloxacin developed transient, reversible arthralgias without radiographic evidence of joint abnormalities.[58]

ANTIVIRALS

Acyclovir

As early empirical antibiotic therapy has overcome many of the acute problems associated with bacterial infections, non-bacterial agents such as viruses and fungi have assumed a more significant role as pathogens in immunocompromised patients. Herpes virus infections represent a major problem, particularly in bone marrow and solid organ transplant patients. Acyclovir is the drug of choice for both prophylaxis and treatment of herpes simplex types 1 and 2 (HSV) infections in these patients. Either oral (200 mg five times daily) or intravenous (250 mg every 8 hours) acyclovir is effective in ameliorating the course of established mucocutaneous HSV infections in bone marrow transplant patients, with decreases in duration of symptoms, length of viral shedding and time to healing.[59,60] Oral and intravenous acyclovir (oral doses of 1–2 g daily) also provides effective prophylaxis against reactivation of HSV in seropositive patients undergoing intensive chemotherapy, and the drug is used routinely for this purpose in allogeneic bone marrow transplant patients and in those with leukemia undergoing intensive chemotherapy.[61–64]

Varicella-zoster virus (VZV) is approximately 10-fold less sensitive than HSV to the antiviral effects of acyclovir, and the drug is not highly bioavailable, such that even high doses of oral acyclovir therapy may result in serum drug levels that are subinhibitory for VZV. Thus, although oral acyclovir at 600–800 mg five times daily has been shown to modestly improve the course of chickenpox and herpes zoster in normal individuals, there is not yet sufficient data to support its routine use in immunocompromised patients.[65–68] Intravenous acyclovir, however, has clearly been shown to decrease the incidence of zoster dissemination and its mortality, making it the current choice for dermatomal zoster in patients with moderate to severe immune impairment.[69] In mildly compromised patients with single dermatome zoster it may be appropriate to withhold antiviral therapy, since dissemination is less common and there is some evidence to suggest that intravenous acyclovir initiated promptly at the time of cutaneous dissemintion will successfully limit the infection.[70]

Acyclovir-resistant isolates of HSV and VZV have been reported with increasing frequency in recent years, particularly in patients with HIV infection and less often in patients undergoing intensive chemotherapy.[71–75] Most of these isolates appear to possess mutations in the viral thymidine kinase which phosphorylates acyclovir to its active triphosphate form. Lesions due to acyclovir-resistant HSV tend to be chronic, progressive ulcerations which do not resolve during long courses of acyclovir. Indeed, the development of HSV resistance appears to be promoted by the administration of multiple courses of low-dose oral acyclovir in the setting of immune suppression. Varicella-zoster resistance to acyclovir has been reported under similar circumstances, albeit less frequently. Resistant VZV often results in non-healing dry, papular skin lesions persisting after a bout of chickenpox or zoster in an immunocompromised patient.[74,75] Foscarnet, which directly inhibits the viral DNA polymerase without requiring phosphorylation, has been used to successfully clear the lesions associated with resistant HSV and VZV.[75–78] Recurrences following foscarnet treatment may be due to acyclovir-sensitive virus.[78]

Ganciclovir

Ganciclovir, like acyclovir, inhibits the DNA polymerase enzyme of most of the human herpesviruses, but it is 30-fold more active against cytomegalovirus (CMV) than is acyclovir *in vitro*.[79] In patients with AIDS, ganciclovir is effective for initial treatment of CMV retinitis, often arresting sight-threatening hemorrhage and exudate within several days. However, patients will inevitably relapse when therapy is discontinued, and most will experience progressive retinal disease even while on therapy. Similarly, CMV colitis will respond initially to ganciclovir but long durability of such response is rare in AIDS patients. Nonetheless, for CMV retinitis or colitis in AIDS patients, lifelong maintenance antiviral therapy on ganciclovir or foscarnet or both is the current standard of care.[80]

In bone marrow transplant patients, CMV pneumonia has historically been associated with greater than 80 per cent rate of mortality.[81] Ganciclovir alone is ineffective in altering the course of this disease.[82] However, several small uncontrolled studies have shown that the combination of ganciclovir with intravenous immunoglobulin (polyclonal or CMV-specific) can dramatically improve the outcome of CMV pneumonia in these patients, increasing their survival to nearly 60 per cent.[83,84] It is hypothesized that the immunoglobulin blocks CMV antigens expressed on infected pulmonary cells and thereby interferes with the targets of cytotoxic T-cell mediated lung destruction, while ganciclovir limits CMV replication.[85] Clearly the combined effects of both agents are required for improvement in survival, since neither one alone impacts upon the course of CMV pneumonitis. Despite the uncontrolled nature of the studies demonstrating the efficacy of immunoglobulin and ganciclovir, the marked survival advantage conferred by this combination has made it a standard therapy in bone marrow transplant patients.[81]

Schmidt *et al.* have explored the 'pre-emptive' use of ganciclovir for prophylaxis against CMV disease in bone marrow recipients who have a positive CMV culture from throat, urine, blood, or bronchial lavage fluid obtained routinely at day 35 post-transplant.[86] Ganciclovir prophylaxis significantly reduced the incidence of CMV pneumonia from 65 per cent in patients who did not receive ganciclovir for positive CMV surveillance cultures, to 15 per cent in ganciclovir recipients. Similar results were obtained by Goodrich *et al.* who conducted a double-blind, placebo-controlled study in which ganciclovir therapy was begun when CMV was first recovered from the throat, urine, or blood or from the day 35 bronchoalveolar lavage fluid of bone marrow allograft recipients.[87] A 93 per cent reduction in severe CMV disease was reported in this study, with a decrease in both pneumonitis and gastrointestinal disease. Additionally, a significant decrease in mortality at both 100 and 180 days post-transplant was noted in those who received early 'pre-emptive' ganciclovir treatment. The notion of directing prophylaxis to patients who are found to be culture-positive for CMV, rather than to those who are simply seropositive, may help to limit the use of ganciclovir to those who are at highest risk for serious CMV disease at a time when therapy would be maximally beneficial. Neutropenia is the most important dose-limiting effect of ganciclovir, occurring in approximately 30 per cent of patients.[80] Therefore, it is critical to identify precisely which patients will benefit from ganciclovir prophylaxis, despite its significant bone marrow suppressive effects.

Foscarnet

Foscarnet is a pyrophosphate analog which directly inhibits herpesvirus DNA polymerases without requiring phosphorylation to become active. As noted, foscarnet has found a unique function as a useful agent for the treatment of acyclovir-resistant HSV and VZV infections. Foscarnet is also a potent inhibitor of the CMV DNA polymerase, and it has some intrinsic antiretroviral activity.[88] Favorable responses to foscarnet have been documented in bone marrow transplant patients with CMV infections, in several small uncontrolled trials, although no dramatic improvements in survival have been reported.[89–91] In AIDS patients with CMV retinitis, foscarnet appears to be as effective as ganciclovir in inducing and maintaining disease remissions, and it seems to confer a slight survival advantage to patients with symptomatic AIDS, possibly due to its antiretroviral activity.[92] Foscarnet is best administered by central venous catheter and its primary adverse effect is renal toxicity, which occurs in the majority of patients. These drawbacks have limited the use of foscarnet to the most urgent indications, i.e. life- or sight-threatening CMV disease or debilitating ulcerative disease due to acyclovir-resistant HSV.[93]

ANTIFUNGALS

Azoles

Until recently, amphotericin B was the only available treatment for presumed or documented mycoses. While it is effective against most *Candida* species which commonly cause invasive disease in immunocompromised patients, the efficacy of amphotericin B against a number of other fungi, such as *Aspergillus* spp., *Fusarium*, *Pseudoallescheria* (which mimics *Aspergillus* infections in the compromised host) and *Trichosporin* has been suboptimal. In addition, amphotericin B therapy is fraught with numerous toxicities, most commonly fever and chills during infusion, and renal toxicity with chronic administration. The development of the antifungal azoles has enabled us to treat and potentially prophylax against fungal disease with less toxic, often orally available, and perhaps more potent agents.[94]

The antifungal azoles act by blocking fungal enzymes required to synthesize ergosterol, the principal sterol component of the cell membranes of most fungi. The earliest azoles, clotrimazole and ketoconazole, were relatively limited in their antifungal spectrum to *Candida* species and other amphotericin-sensitive fungi. Clotrimazole is poorly absorbed but is useful for the topical treatment of non-invasive oropharyngeal or esophageal candidiasis in cancer patients. Ketoconazole has a slightly broader spectrum of activity and is orally bioavailable, although its absorption can be erratic in patients receiving chemotherapy and is significantly inhibited by co-administration of antiacids or H_2 blockers. Thus, while ketoconazole may be useful for teatment of mucosal candidiasis, it is not reliably so.[94] Ketoconazole prophylaxis in neutropenic patients has not been shown to decrease the incidence of systemic candidiasis or the requirement for empirical amphotericin B.[95–97] Furthermore, ketoconazole used as an empirical antifungal therapy for persistent fever during neutropenia, was less effective than amphotericin B in preventing progressive invasive fungal disease.[98]

Fluconazole is a triazole antifungal drug that is more water soluble than the earlier compounds, rendering it highly bioavailable when given orally and endowing it with a particularly long half-life so that once or twice daily dosing is rational. In addition, fluconazole lacks the suppressive effect on steroid hormone synthesis which is commonly associated with high-dose ketoconazole therapy, and it has the advantage of being available both in oral and intra-venous forms.[99] In AIDS patients with cryptococcal meningitis of mild severity, fluconazole appears to be as effective as amphotericin B for initial therapy, although conversion of spinal fluid from positive to negative for cryptococcus appears to be significantly slower in those treated with fluconazole (42 days versus 64 days to culture negativity).[100] For patients with more pronounced symptoms, such as lethargy or mental status changes, neither fluconazole nor amphotericin B is very effective. Nonetheless, until there are further data, it is most prudent to employ the standard agent, amphotericin B, in this setting. In AIDS patients who have recovered from the acute phase of cryptococcal meningitis, maintenance suppressive antifungal therapy is an essential component of treatment and daily fluconazole (usually 200 mg/day orally) has proven to be effective for long-term suppression.[101–103] Oropharyngeal and esophageal candidiasis in immunocompromised patients, including those with AIDS, are readily treated with oral fluconazole at doses of 50–100 mg per day, although it is probably no more effective than its less expensive predecessor, ketoconazole.[104–106]

There is some evidence to suggest that fluconazole is effective therapy for hepatosplenic candidiasis deemed unresponsive to prior amphotericin B, although many of the reported amphotericin failures in these series might be attributed to an inadequate total dose of amphotericin therapy.[107,108] Alternatively, fluconazole may be a useful maintenance therapy for chronic disseminated candidiasis, following an initial course of amphotericin B, although there are currently no available data to support its routine use as such. For candidemia or other serious mycoses, including cryptococcal and coccidioidal disease, there is only anecdotal success with fluconazole therapy.[109–111] *Aspergillus* infections are generally unresponsive to fluconazole. Thus, fluconazole cannot currently be regarded as a routine substitute for amphotericin B therapy for life-threatening fungal infections in immunocompromised patients, unless they have clearly failed to respond or cannot tolerate treatment with conventional therapy. A recent double-blind, randomized, placebo-controlled trial indicated that fluconazole can provide effective prophylaxis against superficial or disseminated fungal infections in patients with prolonged neutropenia.[112] Breakthrough infections due to the relatively azole-resistant species *Candida kruzei* have been reported in patients receiving prophylactic fluconazole, however, and these breakthroughs represent a potential hazard of antimicrobial prophylaxis.[112,113]

Itraconazole is a more recently developed orally available triazole antifungal with improved activity against *Aspergillus*. It is undergoing clinical evaluation to determine whether it might provide more effective prophylaxis than the other azoles, and less toxic therapy than amphotericin B, for *Aspergillus* infections. However, the erratic absorption of itraconazole into the gastrointestinal tract in cancer patients yields inconsistent serum drug levels, thereby limiting its utility.

Liposomal amphotericin

The recent introduction of lipid formulations has been an important therapeutic advance in improving the therapeutic index of amphotericin B. As toxicity is the major dose-limiting factor of amphotericin B, lipid formulations of amphotericin B have been developed to reduce toxicity and permit larger doses to be administered. While classically considered as 'liposomal' formulations of amphotericin B, there are actually several different structural configurations of amphotericin B in association with lipid. Liposomes, defined as phospholipid bilayers of one or more closed concentric structures, as well as other lipid formulations have been used as vehicles for amphotericin B with encouraging results. The lipid formulation may provide a selective diffusion gradient toward the fungal cell membrane and away from mammalian cell membrane, thereby reducing the toxic effects of amphotericin B for mammalian cells.

Three lipid formulations of amphotericin B have been approved in western Europe: a small unilamellar vesicle formulation (AmBisome) which is a true liposome consisting of a phospholipid bilayer in a closed concentric structure around the amphotericin B core; amphotericin B lipid complex (ABLC, Abelcet) in which amphotericin is intercalated between ribbon-like strands of lipid; and amphotericin B colloidal dispersion (ABCD; Amphocil)[114] based upon open label compassionate release and randomized studies.[115,116] Amphotericin B lipid complex in 228 cases treated under a compassionate release protocol was found to be active in treatment of immunocompromised patients with refractory mycoses or those with intolerance to conventional amphotericin B.[115] This study found little dose-limiting nephrotoxicity of ABLC. The randomized trial of ABLC versus amphotericin B in treatment of candidiasis showed equivalent antifungal efficacy but significantly reduced nephrotoxicity of ABLC.[116]

While associated with less nephrotoxicity, lipid formulations may confer their own patterns of toxicity. For example, the multilamellar lipid formulation of amphotericin B induced reversible hypoxemia, pulmonary hypertension, and depression of cardiac output during infusion. All of the lipid formulations of amphotericin B have been associated with elevated serum transaminases with a frequency that appears to be greater than that associated with conventional amphotericin B.

The most appropriate use for the lipid formulations of amphotericin B is for treatment of proven or suspected infections (empirical therapy) in profoundly immunocompromised patients. Further basic investigation of AmBisome and other lipid polyene formulations are leading to newer understanding of the mechanisms of antifungal activity of these compounds.

INFECTION PROPHYLAXIS

Infections in immunocompromised cancer patients arise primarily from endo-genous flora, with newly acquired organisms accounting for a smaller but still signficant proportion.[117] Since the range of pathogens include bacteria, fungi, viruses and/or parasites, and since they can affect different body sites, it is difficult to envision a single or simple method of preventing these multiple infectious etiologies. Numerous methods have been investigated over the past few decades, including suppression of the host's own microbial flora by use of various prophylactic antibiotics, reduction in the patient's acquisition of new organisms by the use of environmental manipulations and isolation techniques, and finally, by attempts to improve the host's own defenses by administration of intravenous immunoglobulin, white blood cell transfusions, and most recently, by the use of hematopoietic growth factors.

Total protected isolation

Early attempts to prevent infections in cancer patients were aimed at altering their internal and external microenvironments. Isolation rooms with laminar air flow that cleans incoming air by passage through HEPA (high-efficiency particulate air) filters, and disinfection of all physical surfaces as well as all objects transported into the room were the initial steps taken. Food and water were fully cooked or boiled to minimize microbial titers, and personnel entering the room were required to wear disposable gowns, masks, gloves and boots. Added to this structured setting was a vigorous decontamination regimen for skin surfaces, orifices and the gastrointestinal tract with topical and non-absorbable antibiotics. Several controlled studies demonstrated that the incidence of serious infection is reduced when neutropenic cancer patients remained in this so-called 'total protected environment', with particular benefit being shown for those with prolonged neutropenia due to very intensive chemotherapy or bone marrow transplantation.[118,119] Nonetheless, a study performed at the National Cancer Institute showed that despite a decrease in the number of documented infections, the incidence of unexplained fevers was unchanged between patients in a total protected environment and those receiving standard care, and most significantly, there was no difference in survival between the two groups. Furthermore, after 1–2 weeks in the protected setting, nearly half of the patients were unable to tolerate the daily routine of gastrointestinal decontamination, due to the unpalatability of non-absorbable antibiotics employed.[120]

Thus, despite the fact that treatment in a total protected environment can reduce the incidence of infections in certain patients, its excessive cost and impracticality, coupled with the significant improvements which have been made in the management of infections in cancer patients, have rendered this approach much less attractive. Indeed, many centers now perform bone marrow transplantation in a standard care setting. Modifications of the total protected environment, such as air filtration and laminar airflow, and limitation of fresh fruits and vegetables as well as non-processed dairy products (since these foods are naturally contaminated with Gram-negative bacteria) may be desirable in situations involving prolonged neutropenia (i.e. greater than 21 days). Most epidemiological studies indicate, however, that transmission of bacteria from inanimate sources requires a human vector.[121] Therefore, the simplest, most effective, and least expensive environmental manipulation to prevent infections in cancer patients is adherence to strict handwashing procedures.

Oral antibiotic prophylaxis

The use of oral antibiotics for infection prophylaxis has been largely based upon the concept of 'selective decontamination' of the gastrointestinal tract, in which aerobic organisms are suppressed but anaerobic flora remains intact. Experimental data suggest that preservation of the anaerobic gastrointestinal flora allows the host to resist colonization with more pathogenic aerobic and fungal organisms.[122,123] This 'colonization resistance' can be achieved with oral non-absorbable antibiotics (e.g. polymyxin, colistin and amphotericin B) as well as certain absorbable antibiotics (e.g. trimethoprim-sulfamethoxazole (TMP-SMX), nalidixic acid and the quinolones). Most of the non-absorbable antibiotics (e.g.

vancomycin, gentamicin or nystatin) are unpalatable and are poorly tolerated, making compliance a problem. Furthermore, the emergence of resistant isolates from patients receiving such drugs, and the failure to show their efficacy in reducing serious infections, has limited the prophylactic use of the non-absorbable antibiotics in neutropenic patients.[120] Although combinations of absorbable and non-absorbable agents (i.e. TMP-SMX, amphotericin B, polymyxin and nalidixic acid) were shown to significantly reduce the incidence of infections in recipients compared with controls in two small studies, no larger confirmatory studies exist to support their routine use.[124,125] Again, this approach is complicated by the issues of poor compliance and requirements for strict surveillance of patient microflora (stool samples particularly) for the emergence of bacterial species resistant to the prophylactic agents (and potentially to other antibiotics used for empirical therapy) and which are potentially serious pathogens in the neutropenic patient. Selective decontamination regimens are less commonly employed in the US due to the effort and cost associated with drug administration and microbial surveillance, the potential for microbial resistance, and the lack of consistently conclusive data demonstrating their efficacy.

Trimethoprim-sulfamethoxazole (TMP-SMX), as a single agent, has been evaluated for oral antibiotic prophylaxis in cancer patients, with early trials showing a marked reduction in infection rates. Later studies have yielded conflicting results, however, perhaps due to variations in study design and failure to monitor patient compliance, the latter being critical to the success of oral prophylaxis.[126–132] Although a few studies showed a decrease in bacterial infections, none have demonstrated a decrease in the frequency of fevers or in the requirement for parenteral antibiotics with TMP-SMX prophylaxis.[120] Furthermore, TMP-SMX prophylaxis has been associated with bone marrow suppression and prolongation of neutropenia, as well as the emergence of resistant isolates and breakthrough infections.[133] Thus, the use of TMP-SMX prophylaxis for neutropenic patients remains a controversial issue. The notable exception is, of course, the use of TMP-SMX for prophylaxis against *Pneumocystis carinii* pneumonia, for which there is clear evidence that the drug is highly effective, even when given on a twice or thrice weekly basis.[134]

The lack of fluoroquinolone activity against anaerobes offers a benefit in potentially preserving 'colonization resistance'. However, since the fluoroquinolones have a high volume of distribution, may achieve therapeutic serum levels, and provide very broad-spectrum coverage, they should be considered as systemic prophylaxis rather than as selective gut decontamination. In fact, it has been suggested that fluoroquinolone 'prophylaxis' should be regarded as early antibiotic treatment for latent infections.[120] As noted, early studies employing norfloxacin and ciprofloxacin prophylactically have shown reductions in the incidence of Gram-negative bacterial infections in neutropenic patients. Nonetheless, the overall incidence of fever and the requirement for antibiotic therapy have been unchanged by the use of fluoroquinolone prophylaxis in these studies, suggesting that the fluoroquinolones may simply convert latent Gram-negative infections into infections of undetermined origin. Furthermore, the risk of developing resistant bacterial isolates during fluoroquinolone prophylaxis is a concern and several outbreaks of resistant coagulase-negative staphylococci have occurred in cancer hospitals employing ciprofloxacin prophylaxis.[52,53] It is important to note that none of the studies examining fluoroquinolones, or any other prophylactic regimen, have demonstrated a reduction in infection-related mortality. Again, the use of prophylactic antibiotics remains a point of controversy.

Strategies to improve host defenses

A number of methods aimed at augmenting impaired host immune responses to offending pathogens have been investigated, including active immunization with bacterial component vaccines against *Pseudomonas aeruginosa* and *Streptococcus pneumoniae*, passive immunotherapy with specific immunoglobulin preparations directed against core antigens of the Gram-negative cell wall, and granulocyte transfusions given on a daily 'prophylactic' schedule or as an adjunct to antibiotic therapy for Gram-negative sepsis. While early clinical data for each of these interventions were encouraging, later results have not always confirmed their utility.

Vaccination trials exploring the efficacy of immunization against *P. aeruginosa*, *Hemophilus influenzae* or *S. pneumoniae* have indicated that immunosuppressed cancer patients often fail to mount a significant antibody response to the vaccine antigens and thus remain unprotected.[120,135] More recently, experience with the live attenuated varicella vaccine has shown it to be highly effective prophylaxis against severe chickenpox in children with leukemia, particularly if the vaccinations are given between cycles of chemotherapy, when the patient is in remission.[136]

Passive immunization with polyclonal antiserum prepared against the J5 mutant of *E. coli* was initially shown to significantly reverse shock and reduce mortality in a cohort of patients with Gram-negative bacteremia. However, J5 antiserum therapy did not affect survival in patients with cancer or neutropenia.[137] A prospective clinical trial showed that the HA1A monoclonal antibody, directed against the lipid A domain of endotoxin, could improve survival in non-neutropenic patients with documented Gram-negative sepsis, if it was administered within the first 6 hours of shock.[138] However, since Gram-negative sepsis accounts for only 40% of hypotensive shock episodes, the routine use of HA1A in all patients with shock would constitute a vast excess of therapy and expense.

Attempts to increase granulocyte counts in neutropenic cancer patients initially involved the use of granulocyte transfusions. As with the other interventions, early controlled trials yielded positive results, suggesting that granulocyte transfusions might improve survival in bacteremic patients.[139–142] However, a larger randomized study in patients with Gram-negative bacteremias did not show a difference in survival, even in patients with prolonged bone marrow suppression.[143] The technical difficulties in procuring granulocytes, and the potential toxicities associated with granulocyte infusions (pulmonary complications, CMV infection) further limited their routine use, both for therapy of documented infections and for infection prophylaxis in immunocompromised patients.[144,145] Recent improvements in granulocyte collection techniques and the administration of G-CSF to granulocyte donors prior to leukopheresis, have improved granulocyte yields significantly. With these advances, there is current interest in re-exploring the efficacy of granulocyte transfusions using much higher numbers of granulocyte colony-stimulating factor (G-CSF) stimulated granulocytes.

With the recent cloning and mass production of myeliod growth factors, particularly granulocyte colony-stimulating factor (G-CSF) and granulocyte-macrophage colony-stimulating factor (GM-CSF), we now have the potential to increase neutrophil numbers to levels that may abrogate the severity of neutropenia resulting from intensive regimens, thereby reducing the risk of infectious complications. Two sentinel randomized, prospective studies evaluated G-CSF prophylaxis in adult patients receiving standard chemotherapy for small-cell lung cancer.[146,147] In both trials, the use of G-CSF reduced the depth and duration of neutropenia as well as the number of patients requiring antibiotics through multiple cycles of chemotherapy. In the trial by Crawford *et al.*, in which patients were randomized for the entirety of their chemotherapy course to receive either G-CSF or placebo, treatment with G-CSF resulted in a statistically significant reduction in the incidence of at least one infectious event (fever and documented infections) over all cycles of therapy (76% in those receiving placebo versus 40% of those receiving G-CSF).[146] Analysis of the first cycle only, however, demonstrated a significant decrease in the incidence of hospitalization (69% versus 52%, $p = 0.032$) and the incidence of antibiotic usage (60% versus 38%, $p = 0.003$). Data from later cycles is not as compelling as in the initial cycle because of the small number of patients who completed all six cycles of randomized therapy (17% and 43% of patients randomized to placebo and G-CSF, respectively).

In a similar study by Pettengell *et al.*, beneficial effects of G-CSF administration, including reduction in febrile, neutropenic events and days on antibiotics, were evident in latter cycles, when compared with those receiving no cytokine.[147] However, this study failed to demonstrate a significant reduction in documented infections over all six cycles of chemotherapy for small-cell lung cancer in patients receiving G-CSF.

In a third randomized prospective study in adult patients treated for non-Hodgkins lymphoma, G-CSF prophylaxis resulted in a reduction of febrile, neutropenic events but it did not reduce hospitalization rates or antibiotic usage, in contrast to the results of the prior studies. However, G-CSF use was associated with a greater likelihood of administering chemotherapy on schedule.[148] The significance of the ability to deliver more chemotherapy with G-CSF support indicates that G-CSF can allow for increases in chemotherapy dose-intensity. Whether or not dose-intensity translates into increased survival could not be determined from this study, due to the very high rate of remission and the short-term follow-up.

Like G-CSF, GM-CSF has been used to abbreviate the course of neutropenia, primarily in the autologous bone marrow transplant population.[149,150] In those patients, GM-CSF has been shown to significantly decrease the number of days of neutropenia, the number of febrile, neutropenic days and the overall requirement for antibiotic coverage.[150] Similar findings have been reported in smaller studies with patients undergoing allogeneic bone marrow transplantation.[151,152] However, no study has demonstrated either a significant reduction in documented infections or improvement in survival post-transplant with the adjunctive employment of GM-CSF.

Although the myeloid growth factors do reduce the duration of neutropenia and the incidence of fever as well as documented infections in some instances, it is notable that increased survival, prolonged remission duration or increased cure rate have not been demonstrated with their use. Furthermore, their costliness is a major drawback. In an analysis provided by the American Society of Clinical Oncology, it is suggested that only those patients whose cancer chemotherapy regimens are anticipated to result in a greater than 40% incidence of febrile neutropenia should have adjunctive G- or GM-CSF treatment.[153] Use of these agents with less intensive chemotherapeutic regimens leads to gross overtreatment of patients who are unlikely to become febrile during neutropenia, and adds significantly to the overall cost of treatment. The importance of utilizing these costly agents rationally and judiciously cannot be overly emphasized.

REFERENCES

1. Bodey GP, Buckley M, Sathe Y *et al.* Quantitative relationships between circulating leukocytes and infection in patients with acute leukemia. *Annals of Internal Medicine* 1966; **64**: 328–40.
2. Pizzo P, Robichaud K, Wesley R, Commers J. Fever in the pediatric and young adult patient with cancer: a prospective study of 1001 episodes. *Medicine* 1982; **61**: 153–65.
3. Rubin MM, Hathorn JW, Pizzo PA, Controversies in the management of febrile neutropenic cancer patients. *Cancer Investigations* 1988; **6**: 167–84.
4. Schimpff S, Satterlee W, Young V, Serpick A. Empiric therapy with carbenicillin and gentamicin for febrile patients with cancer and granulocytopenia. *New England Journal of Medicine* 1971; **284**: 1061–5.
5. Love L, Schimpff S, Schiffer C *et al.* Improved prognosis for granulocytopenic patients with gram-negative bacteremia. *American Journal of Medicine* 1980; **68**: 1–10.
6. Dejace P, Klastersky J. Competitive review of combination therapy: two beta-lactam versus beta-lactam plus aminoglycoside. *American Journal of Medicine* 1986; **80**: 29–38.
7. Barriere S, Flaherty J. Third-generation cephalosporins: a critical evaluation. *Clinical Pharmacology* 1984; **3**: 351–73.
8. Sattler F, Colao D, Caputo G *et al.* Cefoperazone for empiric therapy in patients with impaired renal function. *American Journal of Medicine* 1986; **81**: 229–36.
9. Kramer B, Ramphal R, Rand K. Randomized comparison between two ceftazidime-containing regimens and cephalothin-gentamicin-carbenicillin in febrile granulocytopenic cancer patients. *Antimicrobial Agents and Chemotherapy* 1986; **30**: 64–8.
10. Fainstein V, Bodey GP, Bolivar R, Keating M, McCredie K, Valdivieso M. A randomized study of ceftazidime compared to ceftazidime and tobramycin for the treatment of infections in cancer patients. *Journal of Antimicrobial Chemotherapy* 1983; **12**: 101–10.
11. Darbyshire P, Williamson D, Pedler S, Speller D, Mott M, Oakhill A. Ceftazidime in the treatment of febrile immunosuppressed children. *Journal of Antimicrobial Chemotherapy* 1983; **12**: 357–60.
12. DePauw B, Kauw F, Muytjens H, Williams K, Bothof T. Randomized study of ceftazidime versus gentamicin plus cefotaxime for infections in severely granulocytopenic patients. *Journal of Antimicrobial Chemotherapy* 1983; **12**: 93–9.
13. Morgan G, Duerden B, Lilleyman J. Ceftazidime as a single agent in the management of children with fever and neutropenia. *Journal of Antimicrobial Chemotherapy* 1983; **12**: 347–51.
14. Ramphal R, Kramer B, Rand K, Weiner R, Shands JJ. Early results of a comparative trial of ceftazidime versus cephlothin, carbenicillin, and gentamicin in the

treatment of febrile granulocytopenic patients. *Journal of Antimicrobial Chemotherapy* 1983; **12**: 81–8.

15. Reilly J, Brada M, Bellingham A, Hart C, Bennet C. Ceftazidime compared to tobramycin and ticarcillin in immunocompromised haematological patients. *Journal of Antimicrobial Chemotherapy*. 1983; **12**: 89–92.

16. Pizzo P, Hathorn J, Hiemenz J *et al.* A randomized trial comparing ceftazidime alone with combination antibiotic therapy in cancer patients with fever and neutropenia *New England Journal of Medicine* 1986; **315**: 552–8.

17. Sykes R, Bush K. Interaction of new cephalosporins with beta-lactamases and beta lactamase-producing gram-negative bacilli. *Reviews of Infectious Diseases* 1983; **5** (Suppl. 5): S356–67.

18. Dworzack D, Pugsley M, Sanders C, Horowitz E. Emergence of resistance in gram-negative bacteria during therapy with expanded-spectrum cephalosporins. *European Journal of Clinical Microbiology* 1987; **6**: 456–9.

19. Milatovic D, Braveny I. Development of resistance during antibiotic therapy. *European Journal of Clinical Microbiology* 1987; **6**: 234–44.

20. Chow J, Fine M, Shlaes D *et al.* Enterobacter bacteremia: clinical features and emergence of antibiotic resistance during therapy. *Annals of Internal Medicine* 1991; **115**: 585–90.

21. Sobel J. Imipenem and aztreonam. *Infectious Disease Clinics of North America* 1989; **3**: 613–24.

22. Salata R, Gebhart R, Palmer D. Pneumonia treated with imipenem/cilastatin. *American Journal of Medicine* 1985; **78**: 104–9.

23. Acar J. Therapy for lower respiratory tract infections with imipenem/cilastatin: a review of worldwide experience. *Reviews of Infectious Diseases* 1985; **7**: 594–602.

24. Bodey G, Elting L, Jones P, Alvarea M, Rolston K, Fainstein V. Imipenem/cilastatin therapy of infections in cancer patients. *Cancer* 1987; **60**: 255–62.

25. Huijgens PC, Ossenkoppele GJ, Weijers TF *et al.* Imipenem-cilastatin for empirical therapy in neutropenic patients with fever: an open study in patients with hematologic malignancies. *European Journal of Haematology* 1991; **46**: 42–6.

26. Mortimer J, Miller S, Balck D, Kwok K, Kirby W. Comparison of cefoperazone and mezlocillin with imipenem as empiric therapy in febrile neutropenic cancer patients. *American Journal of Medicine* 1988; **85**: 17–20.

27. Norrby S, Vandercam B, Louie T *et al.* Imipenem-cilastatin versus amikacin plus piperacillin in the treatment of infections in neutropenic patients: a prospective randomized multi-clinic study. *Scandinavian Journal of Infectious Diseases* 1987; Suppl. **52**: 65–78.

28. Pizzo P. unpublished observations.

29. Calandra G, Lydick E, Carrigan J, Weiss L, Guess H. Factors predisposing to seizures in seriously ill infected patients receiving antibiotics: experiences with imipenem/cilastatin. *American Journal of Medicine* 1988; **84**: 911–18.

30. Sykes R, Bonner D. Aztreonam: the first monobactam. *American Journal of Medicine* 1985; **78**: 2–10.

31. Neu H. Aztreonam activity, pharmacology, and clinical uses. *American Journal of Medicine* 1990; **88**: 2S–6S.

32. Saxon A, Hassner A, Swabb E, Wheeler B, Adkinson NJ. Lack of cross-reactivity between aztreonam, a monobactam antibiotic, and penicillin in penicillin-allergic subjects. *Journal of Infectious Diseases* 1984; **149**: 16–22.

33. Adkinson NJ, Saxon A, Spence M, Swabb E. Cross-allergenicity and immunogenicity of aztreonam. *Review of Infectious Diseases* 1985; **7**: S613–21.

34. Scully B, Neu H. Use of aztreonam in the treatment of serious infections due to multiresistant gram-negative organisms, including *Pseudomonas aeruginosa*. *American Journal of Medicine* 1985; **78**: 251–61.

35. Jones, P, Rolston K, Fainstein V, Elting L, Walter R, Bodey G. Aztreonam therapy in neutropenic patients with cancer. *American Journal of Medicine* 1986; **81**: 243–8.
36. Hooper D, Wolfson J. Fluoroquinolone antimicrobial agents. *New England Journal of Medicine* 1991, **324**: 384–94.
37. Hooper D, Wolfson J, Ng E, Swartz M. Mechanisms of action of and resistance to ciprofloxacin. *American Journal of Medicine* 1987; **82**: 12–20.
38. Patton W, Smith G, Leyland M, Geddes A. Multiply resistant *Salmonella typhimurium* septicaemia in an immunocompromised patient successfully treated with ciprofloxacin. *Journal of Antimicrobial Chemotherapy* 1985; **16**: 667–9.
39. Wood M, Newland A. Intravenous ciprofloxacin in the treatment of infection in immunocompromised patients. *Journal of Antimicrobial Chemotherapy* 1986; **18**: 175–8.
40. Smith G, Leyland M, Farrell I, Geddes A. Preliminary evaluation of ciprofloxacin, a new 4-quinolone antibiotic, in the treatment of febrile granulocytopenic patients. *Journal of Antimicrobial Chemotherapy* 1986; **18**: 165–74.
41. Bayston KF, Want S, Cohen J. A prospective, randomized comparison of ceftazidime and ciprofloxacin as initial empiric therapy in neutropenic patients with fever. *American Journal of Medicine* 1989; **87**: S269–73.
42. Smith G, Leyland M, Farrell I, Geddes A. A clinical, microbiological and pharmakokinetic study of ciprofloxacin plus vancomycin as initial therapy of febrile episodes in neutropenic patients. *Journal of Antimicrobial Chemotherapy*, 1988; **21**: 647–55.
43. Chan C, Oppenheim B, Anderson H, Swindell R, Scarffe J. Randomized trial comparing ciprofloxacin plus netilmicin versus piperacillin plus netilmicin for empiric treatment of fever in neutropenic patients. *Antimicrobial Agents and Chemotherapy* 1989; **33**: 87–91.
44. Bow E, Raynor E, Louie T. Comparison of norfloxacin with cotrimoxazole for infection prophylaxis in acute leukemia. *American Journal of Medicine* 1988; **84**: 847–54.
45. Dekker A, Rozenberg-Arska M, Verhoef J. Infection prophylaxis in acute leukemia: a comparison of ciprofloxacin with trimethoprim-sulfamethoxazole and colistin. *Annals of Internal Medicine* 1987; **106**: 7–12.
46. Cruciani M, Concia E, Navarra A *et al.* Prophylactic co-trimoxazole versus norfloxacin in neutropenic children – prospective randomized study. *Infection* 1989; **17** 65–9.
47. Winston D, Ho W, Bruckner D, Gale R, Champlin R. Ofloxacin versus vancomycin/polymyxin for prevention of infections in granulocytopenic patients. *American Journal of Medicine* 1990; **88**: 36–42.
48. Liang R, Yung R, Chan T-K *et al.* Ofloxacin versus co-trimoxazole for prevention of infection in neutropenic patients following cytotoxic chemotherapy. *Antimicrobial Agents and Chemotherapy* 1990; **34**: 215–18.
48a. Lew MA, Kehoe K, Ritz J *et al.* Prophylaxis of bacterial infections with ciprofloxacin in patients undergoing bone marrow transplantation. *Transplantation* 1991; **51**: 630–6.
49. GIMEMA, program i. Prevention of bacterial infection in neutropenic patients with hematologic malignancies. *Annals of Internal Medicine* 1991; **115**: 7–12.
50. Hughes W, Armstrong D, Bodey G *et al.* Guidelines for the use of antimicrobial agents in neutropenic patients with unexplained fever. *Journal of Infectious Diseases* 1990; **161**: 381–96.
51. Rozenberg-Arska M, Dekker A, Verhoef J. Ciprofloxacin for selective decontamination of the alimentary tract in patients with acute leukemia during remission induction treatment: the effect on fecal flora. *Journal of Infectious Diseases* 1985; **152**: 104–7.
52. Kotilainen P, Nikoskelainen J, Huovinen P. Emergence of ciprofloxacin-resistant

coagulase-negative staphylococcal skin flora in immunocompromised patients receiving ciprofloxacin. *Journal of Infectious Diseases* 1990; **161**: 41–4.

53. Oppenheim BA, Hartley JW, Lee W, Burnie JP. Outbreak of coagulase negative staphylococcus highly resistant to ciprofloxacin in a leukaemia unit. *British Medical Journal* 1989; **229**: 294–7.

54. Flaherty JP, Waitley D, Edlin B *et al.* Multicenter, randomized trial of ciprofloxacin plus azlocillin versus ceftazidime plus amikacin for empiric treatment of febrile neutropenic patients. *American Journal of Medicine* 1989; **87**: 2785–825.

55. Rubenstein E, Rolston K, Benjamin R, *et al.* Outpatient treatment of febrile episodes in low-risk neutropenic patients with cancer. *Cancer* 1993; **71**: 3640–46.

56. Malik I. Randomised comparison of oral ofloxacin alone with combination of parenteral antibiotics in neutropenic febrile patients. *Lancet* 1992; **339**: 1092–6.

57. Malik I, Khan W, Karim M, *et al.* Feasibility of outpatient management of fever in cancer patients with low-risk neutropenia: results of a prospective randomized trial. *American Journal of Medicine* 1995; **98**: 224–31.

58. Chysky V, Kapila K, Hullmann R, Arcieri G, Schacht P, Echols R. Safety of ciprofloxacin in children: worldwide clinical experience based on compassionate use. Emphasis on joint evaluation. *Infection* 1991; **19**: 289–96.

59. Wade J, Newton B, McLaren C *et al.* Intravenous acyclovir to treat mucocutaneous herpes simplex virus infections after marrow transplantation. *Annals of Internal Medicine* 1982; **96**: 265–9.

60. Shepp D, Newton B, Dandliker P, Fluornoy N, Meyers J. Oral acyclovir therapy for mucocutaneous herpes simplex virus infections in immunocompromised marrow transplant recipients *Annals of Internal Medicine* 1985; **102**: 783–5.

61. Saral R, Burns W, Laskin O, Santos G, Leitman P. Acyclovir prophylaxis of herpes simplex virus infections. *New England Journal of Medicine* 1981; **305**: 63–7.

62. Saral R, Ambinder R, Burns W *et al.* Acyclovir prophylaxis against herpes simplex infection in patients with leukemia. A randomized double-blind, placebo-controlled study. *Annals of Internal Medicine* 1983; **99**: 773–6.

63. Wade J, Newton B, Fluornoy N, Meyers J. Oral acyclovir for prevention of herpes simplex virus reactivation after marrow transplantation. *Annals of Internal Medicine* 1984; **100**: 823–8.

64. Gluckman E, Lotsberg J, Devergie A *et al.* Prophylaxis of herpes infections after bone-marrow transplantation by oral acyclovir. *Lancet* 1983; **2**: 706–8.

65. Wassilew S, Reimlinger S, Nasemann T, Jones D. Oral acyclovir for herpes zoster: a double blind controlled trial in normal subjects. *British Journal of Dermatology* 1987; **117**: 495–501.

66. Huff J, Bean B, Balfour HH Jr *et al.* Therapy of herpes zoster with oral acyclovir *American Journal of Medicine* 1988; **85** (Suppl. 2A): 84–9.

67. Cobo M. Reduction of the ocular complications of herpes zoster ophthalmicus by oral acyclovir. *American Journal of Medicine* 1988; **85** (Suppl. 2A): 90–3.

68. Dunkle L, Arvin A, Whitley R *et al.* A controlled trial of acyclovir for chickenpox in normal children *New England Journal of Medicine* 1991; **325**: 1539–44.

69. Balfour H, Bean B, Laskin O *et al.* Acyclovir halts progression of herpes zoster in immunocompromised patients. *New England Journal of Medicine* 1983; **308**: 1448–53.

70. Whitley R, Liu C, Pollard R *et al.* Acyclovir versus vidarabine therapy of disseminated herpes zoster in the immunocompromised host. *30th Interscience Conference on Antimicrobial Agents and Chemotherapy, Atlanta, Georgia*, 1990: abstract no. 728.

71. Englund J, Zimmerman M, Swierkosz E, Goodman J, Scholl D, Balfour HJ. Herpes simplex virus resistant to acyclovir. *Annals of Internal Medicine* 1990; **112**: 416–22.

72. Sacks S, Wanklin R, Reese D, Hicks K, Tyler K, Coen D. Progressive esophagitis

from acyclovir-resistant herpes simplex. *Annals of Internal Medicine* 1989; **111**: 893–9.

73. Erlich K, Mills J, Chatis P *et al.* Acyclovir-resistant herpes simplex in patients with the acquired immunodeficiency syndrome. *New England Journal of Medicine* 1989; **320**: 293–6.

74. Pahwa G, Biron K, Lim W *et al.* Continuous varicella-zoster virus infection associated with acyclovir resistance in a child with AIDS. *Journal of the American Medical Association* 1988; **260**: 2879–82.

75. Jacobson M, Berger T, Fikrig S *et al.* Acyclovir-resistant varicella zoster virus infection after chronic oral acyclovir therapy in patients with the acquired immunodeficiency syndrome (AIDS). *Annals of Internal Medicine* 1990; **112**: 187–91.

76. Erlich K, Jacobson M, Koehler J *et al.* Foscarnet therapy for severe acyclovir-resistant herpes simplex virus type 2 infections in patients with the acquired immunodeficiency syndrome. *Annals of Internal Medicine* 1989; **110**: 187–91.

77. Chatis P, Miller C, Schrager L *et al.* Successful treatment with foscarnet of an acyclovir-resistant mucocutaneous infection with herpes simplex virus in a patient with acquired immunodeficiency syndrome. *New England Journal of Medicine* 1989; **320**: 297–300.

78. Safrin S, Berger T, Gilson I *et al.* Foscarnet therapy in five patients with AIDS and acyclovir-resistant varicella-zoster virus infection. *Annals of Internal Medicine* 1991; **115**: 19–21.

79. Cole N, Balfour H. *In vitro* susceptibility of cytomegalovirus isolates from immunocompromised patients to acyclovir and ganciclovir. *Diagnostic Microbiology and Infectious Disease* 1987; **6**: 255–61.

80. Balfour HJ. Management of cytomegalovirus disease with antiviral drugs. *Reviews of Infectious Diseases* 1990; **12**: S849–60.

81. Winston D, Ho WG, Baroni K *et al.* Ganciclovir therapy for cytomegalovirus infections in recipients of bone marrow transplants and other immunosuppressed patients. *Reviews of Infectious Diseases* 1988; **10**: S547–53.

82. Shepp D, Dandliker P, de Miranda P *et al.* Activity of 9-[2-hydroxy-1-(hydroxylmethyl)ethoxymethyl]guanine in the treatment of cytomegalovirus pneumonia. *Annals of Internal Medicine* 1985; **103**: 368–73.

83. Reed E, Bowden R, Dandliker P, Lilleby K, Meyers J. Treatment of cytomegalovirus pneumonia with ganciclovir and intravenous cytomegalovirus immunoglobulin in patients with bone marrow transplants. *Annals of Internal Medicine* 1988; **109** 783–8.

84. Emanuel D, Cunningham I, Jules-Elysee K *et al.* Cytomegalovirus penumonia after bone marrow transplantation successfully treated with the combination of ganciclovir and high dose intravenous immune globulin. *Annals of Internal Medicine* 1988; **109**: 777–82.

85. Grundy J, Shanley J, Griffiths P. Is cytomegalovirus interstitial pneumonia in transplant recipients an immunopathological condition? *Lancet* 1987; **ii**: 996–9.

86. Schmidt G, Horak D, Niland J, Duncan S, Formen S, Zaia J, Group CoH-S-SCS. A randomized, controlled trial of prophylactic ganciclovir for cytomegalovirus pulmonary infection in recipients of allogeneic bone marrow transplants. *New England Journal of Medicine* 1991; **324**: 1005–11.

87. Goodrich J, Mori M, Gleaves C *et al.* Early treatment with ganciclovir to prevent cytomegalovirus disease after allogeneic bone marrow transplantation. *New England Journal of Medicine* 1991; **325**: 1601–7.

88. Sandstrom E, Byington R, Kaplan J, Hirsch M. Inhibition of human T-cell lymphotropic virus type III *in vitro* by phosphonoformate. *Lancet* 1985; **i**: 1480–2.

89. Klintmalm G, Lonnqvist B, Ober B *et al.* Intravenous foscarnet for the treatment of severe cytomegalovirus infection in allograft recipients. *Scandinavian Journal of Infectious Disease* 1985; **17**: 157–63.

90. Ringden O, Wilczek H, Lonnqvist B, Gahrton G, Wahren B, Lernestedt J. Foscarnet for cytomegalovirus infections. *Lancet* 1985; i: 1503–4.
91. Apperley J, Marcu R, Goldman J, Wardle D, Gravett P, Chanas A. Foscarnet for cytomegalovirus pneumonia [letter]. *Lancet* 1985; i: 1151.
92. Studies of October Complications of AIDS Research Group (SOCA). Mortality in patients with the acquired immunodeficiency syndrome treated with either foscarnet or ganciclovir for cytomegalovirus retinitis. *New England Journal of Medicine.* 1992; **326**: 213–20.
93. Jacobson M, Crowe S, Levy J *et al.* Effect of foscarnet therapy on infection with human immunodeficiency virus in patients with AIDS. *Journal of Infectious Diseases* 1988; **158**: 862–5.
94. Walsh T, Pizzo P. Treatment of systemic fungal infections: recent progress and current problems. *European Journal of Clinical Microbiology and Infectious Diseases* 1988; **7**: 460–75.
95. Meunier-Carpentier F. Chemoprophylaxis of fungal infections. *American Journal of Medicine* 1984; **76**: 652–6.
96. Shepp D, Klosterman A, Siegel M, Meyers J. Comparative trial of ketoconazole and nystatin for prevention of fungal infection in neutropenic patients treated in a protective environment. *Journal of Infectious Diseases* 1985; **152**: 1257–63.
97. Tricot G, Joosten E, Boogaerts M, Vande Pitte J, Cauwenbergh G. Ketoconazole vs itraconazole for antifungal prophylaxis in patients with severe granulocytopenia: preliminary results of two nonrandomized studies. *Reviews of Infectious Diseases* 1987; **9**: 94–9.
98. Walsh T, Rubin M, Gress J *et al.* Amphotericin B vs high-dose ketoconazole for empirical antifungal therapy among febrile granulocytopenic cancer patients. *Archives of Internal Medicine* 1991; **151**: 765–70.
99. Brammer K, Farow P, Faulkener J. Pharmacokinetics and tissue penetration of fluconazole in humans. *Reviews of Infectious Diseases* 1990; **12**: S318–26.
100. Saag M, Powderly W, Cloud G *et al.* Comparison of amphotericin B with fluconazole in the treatment of acute AIDS-associated cryptococcal meningitis. *New England Journal of Medicine* 1992; **326**: 83–9.
101. Stern J, Hartman B, Sharkey P *et al.* Oral fluconazole therapy for patients with acquired immunodeficiency syndrome and cryptococcosis: experience with 22 patients. *American Journal of Medicine* 1988; **85**: 477–80.
102. Sugar A, Saunders C. Oral fluconazole as suppressive therapy of disseminated cryptococcosis in patients with acquired immunodeficiency syndrome. *American Journal of Medicine* 1988; **85**: 481–9.
103. Bozzette S, Larsen R, Chiu J *et al.* A placebo-controlled trial of maintenance therapy with fluconazole after treatment of crytococcal meningitis in the acquired immunodeficiency syndrome. *New England Journal of Medicine* 1991; **324**: 580–4.
104. DeWit S, Weerts D, Goossens H, Clumeck N. Comparison of fluconazole and ketoconazole for oropharyngeal candidiasis in AIDS. *Lancet* 1989; i: 746–8.
105. Dupont B, Drouhet E. Fluconazole for the treatment of fungal diseases in immunosuppressed patients. *Annals of the New York Academy of Sciences* 1988; **544**: 564–70.
106. Meunier F, Aoun M, Gerard M. Therapy for oropharyngeal candidiasis in the immunocompromised host: a randomized double-blind study of fluconazole vs. ketoconazole. *Reviews of Infectious Diseases* 1990; **12**(Suppl. 3): S364–8.
107. Kauffman C, Bradley S, Ross S, Weber D. Hepatosplenic candidiasis: successful treatment with fluconazole. *American Journal of Medicine* 1991; **91**: 137–41.
108. Anaisse E, Bodey G, Kantarjian H *et al.* Fluconazole therapy for chronic disseminated candidiasis in patients with leukemia and prior amphotericin B therapy. *American Journal of Medicine* 1991; **91**: 142–50.
109. Ikemoto H. A clinical study of fluconazole for the treatment of deep mycoses. *Diagnostic Microbiology and Infectious Disease* 1989; **12**(Suppl. 4): 239S–247S.

110. Robinson P, Knirsch A, Joseph J. Fluconazole for life-threatening fungal infections in patients who cannot be treated with conventional antifungal agents. *Reviews of Infectious Diseases* 1990; **12**: S349–55.
111. Viscoli C, Castagnola E, Fioredda F, Ciravegna B, Barigione G, Terragna A. Fluconazole in the treatment of candidiasis in immunocompromised children. *Antimicrobial Agents and Chemotherapy* 1991; **35**: 365–7.
112. Goodman J, Winston D, Greenfield R *et al.* A controlled trial of fluconazole to prevent fungal infections in patients undergoing bone marrow transplantation. *New England Journal of Medicine.* 1992; **326**: 845–51.
113. Wingard J, Merz W, Rinaldi M *et al.* Increase in *Candida krusei* infection among patients with bone marrow transplantation and neutropenia treated prophylactically with fluconazole. *New England Journal of Medicine.* 1991; **325**: 1274–7.
114. Walsh TJ, Gonzalez C, Lyman CA, Chanock S, and Pizzo PA. Recent advances in diagnosis and treatment of invasive fungal infections in children. *Advances in Pediatric Infectious Diseases* (in press).
115. Walsh TJ, Hiemenz JW, Seibel N, and Anaissie EJ. Amphotericin B lipid complex in the treatment of 228 cases of invasive mycosis. *Abstracts of the 34th Interscience Conference on Antimicrobial Agents and Chemotherapy* Orlando, Florida; October 4–7, 1994; p. 247; Abstr. M69.
116. Anaissie EJ, White M, Uzun O, *et al.* Amphotericin B lipid complex versus amphotericin B for treatment of hematogenous and invasive candidiasis: a prospective, randomized, multicenter trial. *Abstracts of the 35th Interscience Conference on Antimicrobial Agents and Chemotherapy* San Francisco, CA; September 17–20, 1995; p. 330; Abstr. LM21.
117. Schimpff S, Young V, Greene W, Vermeulen G, Moody M, Wiernick P. Origin of infection in acute nonlymphocytic leukemia. Significance of hospital acquisition of potential pathogens. *Annals of Internal Medicine* 1972; **77**: 707–14.
118. Pizzo P. Do the results justify the expense of protected environments? In: Wiernik P ed. *Controversies in Oncology.* New York: John Wiley & Sons, 1982: 267–77.
119. Pizzo P. Antibiotic prophylaxis in the immunosuppressed patient with cancer. In: Remington J, Swartz M eds. *Current clinical topics in infectious diseases.* New York: McGraw-Hill, 1983: 153–67.
120. Pizzo P. Considerations for the prevention of infectious complications in patients with cancer. *Reviews of Infectious Diseases* 1989; **11** (Suppl. 7): S1551–63.
121. Albert R, Condie F. Handwashing patterns in medical intensive care units. *New England Journal of Medicine* 1981; **304**: 1465–6.
122. Clasener H, Vollaard E, Saene Hv. Long-term prophylaxis of infection by selective decontamination in leukopenia and in mechanical ventilation. *Reviews of Infectious Diseases* 1987; **9**: 295–328.
123. van der Waaij D, deVries JB, van der Wees JL. Colonization resistance of the digestive tract in conventional and antibiotic-treated mice. *Journal of Hygiene (London)* 1971; **69**: 405–11.
124. Sleijfer D, Mulder N, Vries-Hospers Hd, Fidler V, Nieweg H, Waaij Dvd, Saene Hv. Infection prevention in granulocytopenic patients by selective decontamination of the digestive tract. *European Journal of Cancer* 1980; **16**: 859–69.
125. Guiot H, Boek Pvd, Meer Jvd, Furth Rv. Selective antimicrobial modulation of the intestinal flora of patients with acute nonlymphocytic leukemia. A double-blind, placebo-controlled study. *Journal of Infectious Diseases* 1983; **147**: 615–23.
126. Gurwith M, Brunton J, Lank B *et al.* A prospective controlled investigation of prophylactic trimethoprim/sulfamethoxazole in hospitalized granulocytopenic patients. *American Journal of Medicine* 1979; **66**: 248.
127. Pizzo P, Robichaud K, Edwards B, Schumaker C, Kramer B, Johnson A. Oral antibiotic prophylaxis in patients with cancer: a double-blind randomized placebo-controlled trial. *Journal of Pediatrics* 1983; **102**: 125–33.

128. Weiser B, Lang M, Fialk M *et al.* Prophylactic trimethoprim-sulfamethoxazole during consolidation chemotherapy for acute leukemia: a controlled trial. *Annals of Internal Medicine* 1981; **95**: 436–8.
129. Dekker A, Rozenberg-Arska M, Sixma J *et al.* Prevention of infection by trimethoprim–sulfamethoxazole plus amphotericin B in patients with acute nonlymphocytic leukemia. *Annals of Internal Medicine* 1981; **95** 555–9.
130. Gualtieri R, Donowitz G, Kaiser C *et al.* Double-blind randomized study of prophylactic trimethoprim-sulfamethoxazole in granulocytopenic patients with hematologic malignancies. *American Journal of Medicine* 1983; **74**: 934–40.
131. Wade J, de Jongh C, Newman K, Crowley J, Wiernik P, Schimpff S. Selective antimicrobial modulation as prophylaxis against infection during granulocytopenia: trimethoprim-sulfamethoxazole vs. nalidixic acid. *Journal of Infectious Diseases* 1983; **147**: 624–34.
132. EORTC, Group IATP. Trimethoprim-sulfamethoxazole in prevention of infection in neutropenic patients. *Journal of Infectious Diseases* 1984; **150**: 372–9.
133. Wilson J, Guinery D. Failure of oral trimethoprim-sulfamethoxazole prophylaxis in acute leukemia: isolation of resistant plasmids from strains of Enterobacteriaceae causing bacteremia. *New England Journal of Medicine*. 1982; **306**: 16.
134. Hughes W, Rivera G, Schell M, Thornton D, Lott L. Successful intermittent chemoprophylaxis for *Pneumocystis carinii* pneumonitis. *New England Journal of Medicine*. 1987; **316**: 1627–32.
135. Pizzo P. Empirical therapy and prevention of infection in the immunocompromised host. In: Mandell G, Douglas RJ, Bennett J eds. *Principles and practice of infectious diseases* 3rd edn. New York: Churchill Livingstone, 1990: 2303–12.
136. Gershon A. Live attenuated varicella vaccine. *Journal of Pediatrics*. 1987; **110**: 154–7.
137. Ziegler E, McCutchan J, Fierer J *et al.* Treatment of gram-negative bacteremia and shock with human antiserum to a mutant Escherichia coli. *New England Journal of Medicine* 1982; **307**: 1225–30.
138. Ziegler E, Fisher C, Sprung C. Treatment of gram-negative bacteremia and septic shock with HA-1A human monoclonal antibody against endotoxin. *New England Journal of Medicine*. 1991; **324**: 429–36.
139. Higby D, Yates J, Henderson E. Filtration leukopheresis for granulocyte transfusion therapy. *New England Journal of Medicine*. 1977; **292**: 761–6.
140. Herzig R, Herzig G, Graw R *et al.* Successful granulocyte transfusion therapy for gram-negative septicemia. *New England Journal of Medicine*. 1977; **296**: 701–5.
141. Alavi J, Root R, Djerassi I *et al.* A randomized clinical trial of granulocyte transfusions for infection in acute leukemia. *New England Journal of Medicine*. 1977; **296**: 706–11.
142. Vogler W, Winston E. A controlled study of the efficacy of granulocyte transfusions in patients with neutropenia. *American Journal of Medicine* 1977; **63**: 548–55.
143. Winston D, Ho W, Gale R. Therapeutic granulocyte transfusions for documented infections. A controlled trial in ninety-five infectious granulocytopenic episodes. *Annals of Internal Medicine*. 1982; **97**: 509–15.
144. Winston D, Ho W, Young L *et al.* Prophylactic granulocyte transfusions during human bone marrow transplantation. *American Journal of Medicine* 1980; **68**: 893–7.
145. Strauss R, Connett J, Gale R *et al.* A controlled trial of prophylactic granulocyte transfusions during initial induction of chemotherapy for acute myelogenous leukemia. *New England Journal of Medicine*. 1981; **305**: 597–603.
146. Crawford J, Ozer H, Stoller R *et al.* Reduction by granulocyte colony-stimulating factor of fever and neutropenia induced by chemotherapy in patients with small-cell lung cancer. *New England Journal of Medicine* 1991; **325**: 164–70.
147. Pettengell R, Gurney H, Radford JA *et al.* Granulocyte colony-stimulating factor to

prevent dose-limiting neutropenia in non-Hodgkin's lymphoma: a randomized controlled trial. *Blood* 1992; **80**: 1430–36.

148. Trillet-Lenoir V, Green J, Manegold C *et al*. Recombinant granulocyte colony stimulating factor reduces the infectious complications of cytotoxic chemotherapy. *European Journal of Cancer* 1993; **29**A: 319–24.

149. Miller AM. Hematopoietic growth factors in autologous bone marrow transplantation. *Seminars in Oncology* 1993; **20**: 88–95.

150. Neumanitis J, Rabinowe SN, Singer JW *et al*. Recombinant granulocyte-macrophage colony-stimulating factor after bone marrow transplanatation for lymphoid cancer. *New England Journal of Medicine* 1991; **324**: 1773–8.

151. Blazar BR, Kersy JH, McGlave PB *et al*. In vivo administration of recombinant human granulocyte macrophage factor in acute lymphoblastic leukemia patients receiving purged allografts. *Blood* 1989; **73**: 849–57.

152. Powles R, Smith C, Milan S *et al*. Human recombinant GM-CSF in allogeneic bone marrow transplantation: a placebo controlled trial. *Lancet* 1990; **336**: 1417–20.

153. ASCO. American Society of Clinical Oncology recommendations for the use of hematopoietic colony-stimulating factors: evidence-based clinical practice guidelines. *Journal of Clinical Oncology* 1994; **12**: 2471–508.

CHAPTER 3

Supportive care of non-hematologic complications of cytotoxic therapy

STEPHEN R VEACH AND PHILIP S SCHEIN————————————

INTRODUCTION

Since 1896 when EH Grubbe, a Chicago cancer researcher, first administered X-rays to a woman with breast cancer and 1942 when Gustave Lindskog at Yale University successfully used nitrogen mustard to treat a patient with malignant lymphoma,[1] the therapy for cancer has been plagued by concomitant toxic effects on normal tissue. Throughout this century patients with cancer have endured often harsh treatments with the hope that any adversity will have been worth the ultimate cure. Patients with cancer are highly motivated and able, and in fact willing, to accept radical treatments which may require considerable hardship.[2] It is only within the last decade that there has been any consistent use of compounds that may mollify in some way the unwanted effects on normal tissue while still maintaining the same therapeutic index.[3] The goal of this chapter is to make available information regarding the protection or amelioration of the non-hematologic complications of cytotoxic therapy in the treatment of cancer. The emphasis will be on chemotherapeutic modalities of treatment, and toxicities of cytotoxic therapy are perhaps most easily categorized by organ system. Rozencweig et al.[4] have grouped the life-threatening toxicities of cytoxic therapy according to the frequency the organ is affected: gastrointestinal (92 per cent including nausea and vomiting), hepatic (52 per cent), renal (40 per cent), cardiovascular (40 per cent), neurologic (28 per cent) and pulmonary (20 per cent). Additionally, endocrinologic and cutaneous effects of chemotherapy are common, even if not usually life-threatening. Therapeutic benefit, as well as toxicity, may be dependent on dose, route and schedule of chemotherapy and individual patient metabolic and genetic variability. Currently, as hematologic injury is assuaged by both protectors (e.g. amifostine) and stimulators (G-CSF, GM-CSF) the ability to achieve high dose intensity is confounded by the non-hematologic toxicities. By increasing the dose intensity of the currently existent chemotherapeutic regimens, higher response rates are evident in breast cancer,[5] small cell lung cancer,[6] colorectal cancer[7] ovarian cancer[8] and malignant lymphoma.[9] Dose and scheduling is critical in the analysis of acute toxicities in that high single bolus dosing often yields greater toxicity than the same dose spread over a prolonged period. In the case of the cardiac toxicity of anthracyclines[10] and gastrointestinal toxicities of 5-fluorouracil,[11] organ toxicity as well as the development of resistance is a major consideration for the development of combination drug regimens. Drugs are selected for their non-overlapping toxicities and mechanisms of action.

MANAGEMENT OF MUCOCUTANEOUS TOXICITY

Mucositis

Mucositis is a cytotoxic complication associated with many chemotherapeutic agents and radiation therapy. The most common agents implicated are methotrexate, bleomycin, cytarabine and the anthracyclines. Usually, the first symptoms include erythema and sensitivity of the mucosal surfaces within the first week of administration of the chemotherapeutic agents followed by ulcerations occurring in any part of the mouth or gastrointestinal mucosa. The degree of injury is related to dosage and frequency of adminstration of chemotherapy and/ or radiation, but in the case of chemotherapy healing usually begins within 3–5 days providing there is only a single dose. Often mucositis is mild and controlled with local therapies including systemic or topical analgesics, such as viscous xylocaine or oral rinses which include diphenhydramine hydrochloride and/or hydrocortisone. With repeated chemotherapeutic dosing, ulcerations develop resulting in the secondary infection of bacterial, viral and fungal etiology. Often oncology centers will utilize oral antibiotics and antifungals as a toxicity preventative in locally compounded and designed symptomatic treatments.[12]

Radiation therapy to the head and neck often results in significant decrease in the salivary gland function, resulting in dry mucous membranes of the mouth and pharynx which predispose to secondary infections.

Attempts to prevent oral and dental complications secondary to radiation treatment have included the use of fluoride 'carriers' to protect against dental caries. Topical and preventive oral rinsing with compounds such as folinic acid and hyaluronidase (which aids the transfer of folinic acid across mucous membranes) have been attempted to prevent the mucositis associated with methotrexate administration for head and neck cancers.[13] Folinic acid and hyaluronidase did not prevent oral mucosal toxicity nor did intravenous leucovorin in the 'high-dose' methotrexate regime for the treatment of sarcomas. Although topical folinic acid is still recommended by some clinicians as empiric therapy, and topical oral folinic acid can be absorbed through intact oral mucosa, the protective effect may be a systemic effect and not a local topical effect.[14] In the rat, salivary gland uptake of the radiation protector amifostine provides a dose-modifying factor of 1.7–2.5. Salivary glands in rats were well-protected from the effects of radiation therapy with amifostine as a pretreatment, and this could conceivably result in the protection of the salivary gland from the effects of head and neck radiation therapy.[15] Randomized clinical trials attempting to improve the degree of xerostomia resulting from the therapeutic radiation treatment of carcinoma of the maxillary antrum have shown significant improvement in dry mouth with the use of amifostine (52 per cent occurrence of xerostomia versus 73 per cent xerostomia with radiation alone.)[16] An additional double-blind study was carried out in head and neck cancer which also demonstrated protection of salivary gland function.[17] Oral absorption of amifostine has been increased through the use of carriers such as dimethyl sulfoxide (DMSO). Topical protection of rat skin with amifostine has been shown with the concomitant use of DMSO.[18] Radiation-induced skin reaction, especially in the intertriginous zones, has been alleviated by the use of *N*-acetylcysteine pretreatment,[19] but systemic use of thymidine[20] and asparaginase[21] have not significantly altered the mucocutaneous toxicity of methotrexate. However, methotrexate is known to have significant gastrointestinal mucosal toxicity which can be ameliorated with the use of leucovorin within 42 hours of methotrexate adminstration.[22]

5-Fluorouracil (5-FU) is implicated in mucocutaneous toxicity. Laboratory studies utilizing concomitant allopurinol[23] (which selects a different primary metabolic pathway or may affect the concentration ratios of 5-FU to allopurinol in normal cells) resulted in less clinical toxicity, but unfortunately this observation was not supported in clinical trials. Likewise uridine infusions have been attempted and have shown some protection of cells against 5-FU toxicity.[24] Clinically the uridine seems to have had a beneficial effect on protection of the myeloid precursors of the bone marrow; however, there was no evidence of mucocutaneous protection.[25] Inhibition of 5-FU stomatitis has been accomplished by the simple inexpensive maneuver of holding ice chips in the mouth during 5-FU infusion.

Anthracycline chemoprotectants have centered around the compound ICRF 187, concentrating primarily on the ability to reduce cardiac toxicity. ICRF 187 permits longer treatment with doxorubicin in women with breast cancer. A comparison of the stomatitis in the treated and non-treated patients found 20 per cent in both the ICRF-treated and chemotherapy alone arms.

Taxol-induced mucositis is characterized by dysphagia from oral and esophageal ulceration, but only symptomatic therapy has been tried to date.[26]

It is apparent, therefore, that the rapid rate of cell turnover in the oral mucosa, especially the non-keratinized epithelium, is responsible for the greater susceptibility to ulceration following chemotherapy and radiation. Immunosuppression additionally increases the possibilities for secondary infection and injury.

Extravasation

Due to the cytotoxic nature of chemotherapeutic agents used to treat both malignant disease and some immunologically mediated inflammatory diseases, cutaneous side-effects are, although rarely life-threatening, the cause of serious patient and treatment team concern. Toxic effects occur after direct contact with the skin. (There are other less direct effects which will not be the subject of this discussion, e.g. hypersensitivity reactions or cutaneous infections resulting from immunosuppression as a secondary result of the bone marrow suppression of cytotoxic chemotherapy.)

Many chemotherapeutic agents are vesicants (agents that cause tissue necrosis resulting in cutaneous ulceration upon direct contact). Table 3.1 lists the agents in current use that are the most likely to produce tissue necrosis upon inadvertent extravasation.

Table 3.1   Chemotherapy
agents associated with
tissue necrosis

Anthracycline type
Doxorubicin
Daunorubicin
Esorubicin
Epirubicin
Dactinomycin
Amsacrine

Mechlorethamine type
Nitrogen mustard
Mitomycin C
Vinca type
Vincristine
Vinblastine
Vindesine
Vinorelbine

Although all hospitals and clinics should have standard procedures for the administration of vesicant chemotherapeutic agents, the most dramatic innovation to date that has resulted in the reduction of extravasation has been the use of vascular access devices. Although these devices do not totally eliminate the possibility of extravasation, if they are utilized the risk is markedly reduced.

If extravasation occurs it has been shown that perhaps as few as a third of all vesicant extravasations will result in ulceration.[27] Any clinic administering vesicant type chemotherapy should have antidote kits and instructions readily available. The recognition that the extravasation has taken place and the immediate aspiration of any material that is still in the tissue is most important. After aspiration, it is necessary to leave the needle or catheter in place to facilitate the delivery of a local antidote. Pressure should *not* be used in that it may broaden the area affected. As soon as an antidote or treatment has been administered, elevation of the affected area is advisable to enhance normal absorption of extravasated fluids. Whether to apply either cooling or heating to an area of extravasation has been the subject of considerable investigation,[28] and in the anthracycline type extravasation, topical cooling does not reduce skin concentrations of doxorubicin but does appear to change the fluidity of the plasma membranes rendering cells insensitive to the toxicity. Thus, in anthracycline extravasation cooling probably is of significant benefit and should be routinely recommended. Warming is probably not indicated in any situation except for perhaps the vinca type extravasation in which Dorr and Alberts[29] have shown some benefit from warming of the skin over the extravasation site. Surgery is fortunately rarely indicated; however, persistent pain in the extravasated area for 5–7 days may help select those patients that may require surgical debridement.

Therapy for anthracycline type extravasation

The DNA intercalators, once in contact with tissue, produce free radicals of oxygen resulting in tissue injury. Alteration of the tissue pH using sodium bicarbonate infusion has shown little success.[30] Furthermore, sodium bicarbonate is itself a vesicant, and is thus not recommended. Although injection of hydrocortisone into the site has in some reports reduced the severity of ulceration,[31] hydrocortisone may be of more benefit for the doxorubicin-induced, venous flare reactions (evidenced by erythema and tenderness tracking along the vein) than for extravasation itself. Tissue perfusion with hydrocortisone is not recommended. Because the anthracyclines are producers of free radicals, the antioxidants such as α-tocopherol (vitamin E), butylated hydroxytoluene (BHT) and vitamin A could be of benefit. Perhaps the best results, in an experimental setting, have involved the combinations of antioxidants with dimethyl sulfoxide (DMSO). Ludwig *et al.*[32] have shown quite convincing evidence of reduction of toxicity in a human trial by applying a combination of 90 per cent DMSO and 10 per cent α-tocopherol over 2 days and no ulcers were observed in six patients with anthracycline extravasation. Convincing trials in Sprague–Dawley rats have shown efficacy for DMSO alone.[33] Numerous clinical trials have also corroborated DMSO's benefit in humans;[34,35] however, the difficulty in the US still remains that DMSO is not approved for this use and its current formulation is a 50 per cent solution in water. Probably a much higher concentration of a DMSO solution is necessary for its optimal action either alone or combined with an antioxidant. It is hypothetically possible that DMSO alone may be acting as an antioxidant or may have other effects which inhibit the toxicity of the anthracyclines. Newer formulations of the anthracyclines which are considerably less toxic when extravasated have been developed, most prominent being mitoxantrone. Newer techniques of encapsulating doxorubicin into liposomes (phosphatidylcholine:cholesterol unilamellar vesicles) have shown only minor skin reaction in a randomized trial.[36] Dactinomycin has not been shown to be as responsive to cooling or topical DMSO.[37,38]

Therapy for mechlorethamine type extravasation

Nitrogen mustard extravasation has been known to produce immediate pain, erythema, edema and thrombophlebitis. Hyperpigmentation of the vein after repeated use is common. Because nitrogen mustard is an alkylating agent whose cytotoxic reaction results from the generation of intracellular electrophiles which are bound and inactivated by thiols, sodium thiosulfate was considered to be an appropriate protective agent. Animal studies[39] and experience with human extravasations have shown that sodium thiosulfate may be antidotal, by direct chemical complexation with nitrogen mustard. Currently, a one-sixth molar sodium thiosulfate solution is recommended for emergency extravasation. Significant delay and reduced ratios of less than 200:1 (thiosulfate:HN_2)[40] have markedly diminished the effectiveness of thiosulfate injections.

Although mitomycin C is thought to produce DNA cross-linking it is also considered to produce free radicals; thus, soft tissue necrosis has been shown to be severe and surgical excision is often required. In addition to sodium thiosulfate, which has been shown to be effective for mitomycin C ulceration, DMSO has been effective experimentally.[41] α-Tocopherol has also been combined with DMSO in the setting of mitomycin C ulceration in a single case report;[42] no ulceration was seen. Although not known for producing a serious level of cutaneous toxicity, if a large amount of concentrated cisplatin solution is extravasated, sodium thiosulfate is known to inactivate cisplatin on contact. Thus the same prepared solution for nitrogen mustard type extravasation can be used for cisplatin.

Therapy for vinca type extravasation

Extravasation of the vinca alkaloids is characterized by erythema and immediate tissue edema followed by pain and skin vesicle formation. Prolonged healing is usual and neurosensory symptoms including local paresthesias may remain even after the lesion has healed. Experimental vinca lesions in mice have occurred, however, only after prolonged intradermal administration suggesting a local hypersensitivity etiology.[43] The use of intradermal steroids have not reduced or prevented the toxic effects of vinca extravasation.[44] Increasing the absorption and fluid resorption of the drug from the tissues with the use of hyaluronidase has been effective in vinca alkaloid extravasation. The dissolution of hyaluronic acid bonds responsible for the tightness of the apposition of tissue planes by

Table 3.2 Recommended chemotherapy extravasation antidotes[45]

Chemotherapy	Recommended antidotal maneuvers	Specific regimens
Alkylating agents Mechlorethamine	0.17 M sodium thiosulfate	Mix 4 ml of 10% sodium thiosulfate USP with 6 ml sterile water for injection of 2 ml into site for each mg of drug extravasated
Cisplatin,[a] mitomycin C	50% (v/v) dimethyl sulfoxide (Sol Rimso-50[R], Research Products Inc.)	Apply 1.5 ml topically to mitomycin site every 6 h for 7–14 days. Allow to air dry
DNA intercalating agents Doxorubicin, daunomycin, others	Cold application	Apply immediately without pressure, rotate on and off for 24 h
	50% (v/v) DMSO solution (optional)	Apply 1.5 ml topically on site every 6 h for 14 days; allow to air dry
Plant alkaloids Vinblastine, vincristine	150 units hyaluronidase (Wydase[R], Wyeth Laboratories)	Reconstitute 150 U in 1–3 ml of saline, inject into site using original needle if possible
	Warm pack	Apply to site without pressure after hyaluronidase
Epipodophyllotoxins[a]	150 units hyaluronidase	Use same schedule as vincas for VM-26 and VP-16

[a] Treatment not typically recommended since the drug is not ulcerogenic unless a large amount of highly concentrated solution is extravasated.

hyaluronidase may result in the enhanced systemic uptake of the extravasated drug. As a single agent, hyaluronidase is not toxic. Hyaluronidase is contra-indicated in the use of anthracycline type extravasation as well as injection into or near tumors. The usual recommended dose for hyaluronidase has been 150 units (turbidity reducing units of enzymatic activity).

Table 3.2 provides a synopsis of recommended treatments for the extravasa-tion of commonly used chemotherapeutic agents.

Alopecia

Certainly one of the most emotionally injurious toxicities of chemotherapy is the loss of hair. This toxicity contributes to the intolerance of those chemother-apeutic agents which cause alopecia. Hair grows in a tricyclic manner and approximately 85 per cent of the follicles are in an active growth cycle and thus sensitive to repeated doses of chemotherapeutic agents. Although the hair root usually begins to separate approximately 4 weeks after the initial doses of chemotherapy, regrowth may occur despite continued treatment, with new hair appearing in 3–6 months. Considerable effort has been expended to prevent chemotherapy induced hair loss, including the use of scalp tourniquets or cool-ing devices which reduce blood flow.

Those drugs which have a rapid uptake and a short half-life, such as Adria-mycin and vincristine, are the most amenable to local techniques of decreasing scalp blood flow. Utilizing a tourniquet technique has achieved some success in a non-randomized concurrent control study of 31 evaluable patients.[46] Multiple studies of hypothermia of the scalp during anthracycline use have shown reason-able protection of the hair as long as the dose does not exceed 50 mg per treatment. The prevention of hair loss from cyclophosphamide-containing regi-mens is not as successful because of the 6-hour half-life of the active drug. Although scalp hypothermia has been moderately successful, possible growth of scalp metastasis in the protected area has been a concern. Even though the incidence of scalp metastasis is well below 1 per cent,[47,48] the following guide-lines for selection of patients for the use of scalp hypothermia are recommended:[49]

- patients undergoing an Adriamycin-containing chemotherapy with palliative intent or patients with solid tumors rarely metastasizing to the scalp;
- patients not receiving other potent epilating agents and not undergoing cranial irradiation;
- patients with good performance status, normal hepatic function and willing to undergo the temporary discomfort of the scalp cooling.[50]

Pharmacologic therapy has been explored as a source of potential antidotes to the alopecia from chemotherapy. The Angora rabbit model demonstrated that the topical application of a 10 per cent α-tocopherol in DMSO solution did not provide any protection against doxorubicin-induced hair loss.[51] Rabbits fed an α-tocopherol-supplemented diet did seem to show evidence of protection against the doxorubicin-dependent inhibition of new hair growth. In a clinical study of 16 patients receiving Adriamycin plus 1600 IU orally of α-tocopherol per day, 11 did not have alopecia.[52] Unfortunately when confirmation was attempted[53,54] the oral administration of α-tocopherol did not change the natural course of alopecia.

Minoxidil, an antihypertensive agent which was found to induce hypertrichosis, has been evaluated for the treatment of alopecia secondary to chemotherapy. Minoxidil has been used to attempt to prevent alopecia during chemotherapy for gynecologic malignancies and it has been shown that the topical application has no benefit in the prevention of chemotherapy-induced alopecia.[55,56] It is conceivable that post-chemotherapy minoxidil could be used to accelerate the growth of patients' hair; however, as a preventive agent, 2 per cent minoxidil applied topically does not seem to alter the expected hair loss.

Other concepts have included the use of the amino acid L-cysteine and vitamin A (Gelacet) which was somewhat encouraging in a rabbit model.[57] ImuVert, a biologic response modifier derived from the bacterium *Serratia marcescens* seems to offer protection against alopecia in rats.[58] Interestingly, application of topical epidermal growth factor (EGF) on rats who are receiving high doses of cytosine arabinoside has prevented hair loss, although it did not prevent alopecia from other chemotherapeutic agents.[59] Developing new chemotherapeutic agents in which the analogs induce less alopecia have been accomplished in the cases of mitoxantrone and epiadriamycin.

In conclusion, although the alopecia of cancer chemotherapy is not currently preventable, there are still active compounds which require further investigation and meanwhile scalp hypothermia may provide reasonable reduction in alopecia in some situations.

MANAGEMENT OF NEUROTOXICITY

Direct toxic effects of chemotherapeutic agents on the central nervous system are manifest by seizures, encephalopathy, chemical meningitis, leukoencephalopathy, dementia, hemiparesis and coma. These effects are primarily dose-dependent or are associated with intrathecal adminstration. Alleviation of these CNS toxicities, once induced, necessitates immediate cessation of the chemotherapy and institution of supportive treatment. Prevention of peripheral nerve injury as well as damage to the VIIIth cranial nerve, however, has been addressed with protective agents and prophylactic therapy. Axons and the metabolic integrity of the myelin sheath are sensitive to chemotherapeutic agents. The agents most

Table 3.3 Drugs associated with peripheral neuropathy

Cisplatin
Carboplatin
Vindesine
Vinblastine
Vincristine
Vinorelbine
Etoposide
Altretamine
Paclitaxel
Docetaxel

directly associated with peripheral nerve demyelinization and interruption of function are listed in Table 3.3.

Variables that make evaluation of neurotoxicity difficult include pre-existing neurologic diseases as well as medical conditions which could induce primary neurologic deficits in and of themselves, such as diabetes, syphilis, neurologic complications of cancer, CNS disorders, vascular compromise, alcohol abuse and metabolic disorders which affect serum magnesium, calcium and potassium.

Cisplatin type

Peripheral neuropathy as an adverse effect of cisplatin was reported in 1978.[60] Scattered case reports appeared in the literature thereafter and, by 1983, peripheral neuropathy was a widely known adverse effect of cisplatin.[61-63] A recent review of English-language literature described this neurologic toxicity in 170 of 1444 patients who received cisplatin, showing a toxic effect in 11.8 per cent of patients. The important parameter which determines the onset of neuropathy is cumulative dose, with only 15 per cent of cases of neuropathy occurring below cumulative cisplatin doses of 300 mg/m^2.[64] The most consistent signs of early peripheral neuropathy are loss of vibratory sensation in toes and decreased ankle jerk reflex which, although detectable, are seldom patient complaints. Paresthesia is often the first symptom noted by the patient, at median cumulative doses of 400 mg/m^2 and above. Diminished vibratory sensation in the toes, ankles and legs, paresthesias in the feet and loss of ankle and knee jerk reflex are common symptoms. Cisplatin neuropathy is primarily sensory and predictably progressive beginning with the loss of vibratory sensation distally which becomes more proximal and may be accompanied by a loss of other deep tendon reflexes. Loss of touch and pain sensation is unusual although fine motor coordination difficulties can occur, usually with higher cumulative doses (600–750 mg/m^2).[65] Gait difficulties are probably a consequence of proprioceptive sensory loss since motor loss is rarely described, although there are reports of muscle weakness.[66]

Careful electrophysiological and pathologic studies have shown that the lesions are a combination of axonal degeneration and demyelination, especially of long sensory nerves. Concentrations of platinum have been shown in the sural and other peripheral nerves (including dorsal root ganglia) which are ten times greater than concentrations in the spinal cord and brain.[67] This may explain why central neurological effects of platinum are much rarer, although they can occur. The outcome of peripheral neuropathy after cessation of cisplatin therapy is variable. Many patients will experience improvement in their symptoms over a period of months but it is also possible to observe deterioration of neuropathy even several months after cisplatin therapy has stopped. Long-term survivors were studied and a 60 per cent incidence of persistent neuropathy was found.[68] Patients 49–106 months after a cumulative dose of 600 mg/m^2 (in combination with bleomycin and vinblastine) were examined and the incidence of symptomatic paresthesia was 37 per cent (although it had been 83 per cent immediately after therapy) and neurological signs could be detected in 73 per cent of patients.[69]

Attempts to diminish this dose-limiting toxicity of the platinum compounds have been vigorous and currently concentrate on the amino thiols amifostine and ACTH analog (ORG-2766). Using the threshold of vibration perception as measured by vibrometer, women treated for ovarian cancer with cisplatin and cyclophosphamide had neuropathy attenuated by ORG-2766.[70] ORG-2766 accelerates the functional recovery from sciatic nerve damage in the rat when locally applied at the site of injury utilizing a peptide-impregnated biodegradable gelatin foam matrix and biodegradable microspheres.[71]

In a prospective study of 69 patients receiving combination chemotherapy, including cisplatin, protection from neurotoxicity by amifostine was shown. The patients receiving amifostine had both a lower incidence of neuropathy as measured by an examination by a neurologist, and tolerated higher cumulative doses of cisplatin.[72] Another experience with high-dose cisplatin in the treatment of malignant melanoma confirmed the lower incidence of peripheral neuropathy when high-dose cisplatin was combined with amifostine.[73] In this currently ongoing study only two of twenty-two patients have experienced any neuropathy when utilizing doses of cisplatin >100 mg/m^2.

Cisplatin has been associated with toxicity to the VIIIth cranial nerve in 7–90 per cent of the patients receiving up to 120 mg/m^2.[74] Although the mechanism of ototoxicity is not well defined, it is known that cisplatin experimentally affects the first outer hair cells of basilar turn of the cochlea with progressive damage to the more apical hair cells. Subclinical changes are first shown by audiograms in the high-frequency range (from 4000 to 8000 Hz). Tinnitus may precede the hearing loss, usually as high-pitched sounds (4000 to 6000 Hz). Tinnitus is thought to result from damage to the cuticular plates and fused stereocilia of the basilar outer hair cells with degeneration of the spiral ganglion cells and cochlear neurons.[75–78] As the dose of cisplatin is increased or cumulative dose rises, the hearing loss involves lower frequencies (from 2000 to 4000 Hz). These frequencies are associated with the spoken word; there is some reversibility and it is usual that the hearing loss is bilateral. There are occasional cases of vestibular toxicity.[79] The degree of toxicity may be actually increased by rapid drug delivery, pre-existing hearing loss due to the use of diuretics, dehydration or pre-existing vestibular abnormalities.[80–82] Although careful pretreatment and post-treatment audiograms have not been accomplished in many clinical trials, one trial in ovarian cancer using 200 mg/m^2 of cisplatin carefully documented 80 per cent of patients with a greater than 30 dB decline in the 4000–8000 Hz range and 33 per cent of those had clinically relevant hearing loss.[83] Al Sarraf *et al.*, utilizing 100 mg/m^2 of cisplatin, demonstrated a significant hearing loss in 15 per cent of patients.[84] In two malignant melanoma trials utilizing high-dose cisplatin, significant ototoxicity was demonstrated in only 2 per cent and 6 per cent respectively by utilizing amifostine as a protector.

Although these studies are encouraging, the current standard approach is careful observation of the patient for the early onset of neurotoxic effects, and determination of the benefit of continued therapy.

Vinca alkaloid neurotoxicity

The dose-limiting toxicity of the vinca alkaloids begins with the loss of deep tendon reflexes and may progress to distal sensory loss as well as motor weakness and muscle atrophy. Co-administration of oral glutamic acid has been reported to alter the peripheral neuropathy; however, the mechanism of action is unknown.[85] Survival of a patient with inadvertent high-dose vincristine intrathecal adminstration was thought to be associated with immediate drainage of the cerebrospinal fluid, the administration of intravenous glutamic acid and perfusion of the ventricular lumbar space with 2.5 per cent fresh frozen plasma in lactated Ringer's solution.[86,87]

Like the vinca alkaloids, Paclitaxel induces aberrations in microtubule metabolism, specifically resulting in stable and non-functional polymerized microtubules. Microtubules are important in neuronal function and thus it is not surprising that in phase I Paclitaxel studies peripheral neurotoxicity occurred, consisting of numbness, stocking-glove paresthesia and hyperesthesia.[88]

Methotrexate neurotoxicity

Although systemic high-dose or intrathecal therapy with methotrexate may occasionally produce a myelopathy with paraplegia or cauda equina syndrome, accidental overdose of methotrexate requires rapid central spinal fluid drainage with ventricular lumbar profusion and high-dose leucovorin rescue both intrathecally and systemically with alkaline diuresis for the best possible chance for survival and recovery of neurologic function.[89,90]

MANAGEMENT OF NEPHROTOXICITY

The kidney and the liver are the primary sites for excretion of chemotherapeutic agents. Drugs may be metabolized by the kidney or simply concentrated and excreted as a metabolite or an unchanged compound. Anatomic abnormalities of the urinary system can alter drastically the toxicity of chemotherapeutic agents, but with a normal kidney, both filtration and active and passive transport carry drugs across the glomerulus and/or the renal tubules. The amount of drug actually removed depends on the glomerular filtration rate (a reflection of renal blood flow), the rate of non-renal metabolism and the normal operation of the urinary collection system.

Measurements of renal function have traditionally depended upon methods of measuring the filtration rate across the glomerulus and the efficiency of that system (e.g. serum creatinine). Inulin and creatinine clearances are the usual methods of estimating glomerular filtration rate (GFR). Creatinine is filtered and secreted by the kidney and the serum creatinine concentration is altered by the rate of production and excretion as well as the volume of creatinine distribution and the non-creatinine chromogen contribution. Both creatinine and inulin clearances have the potential for inaccuracy and new radioactive tracers such as chromium-51-labeled EDTA (ethylenediaminetetraacetic acid), and technetium-99-labeled DTPA (diethylenetriaminepentaacetic acid) and iodine-labeled ditrizoate and iothalamate are thought to be more accurate measurements; however, one cannot directly compare values from the more standard determinations of GFR[91] (i.e. creatinine clearance).

Specific chemotherapeutic agents associated with nephrotoxicity are the platinums, nitrosoureas, antibiotics, alkylating agents and biologics.

The drug *cis*-dichlorodiammineplatinum underwent trials in the early 1970s and nephrotoxicity was clearly established. Dentino and co-workers in 1978 described cases of renal toxicity in young men with testicular cancer who were treated with 100 mg/m^2 of cisplatin every 3 weeks.[92] These studies clearly established that regular and persistent decreases in glomerular filtration rate after the second course of treatment were present in at least 40 per cent of patients. Decreases in GFR were persistent for at least 2 years, as was magnesium wasting in at least a third of the patients, some still requiring magnesium supplementation at 2 years of follow-up. Platinum can be measured in the kidney months after treatment; however, this has not been shown to be clinically relevant in that further deterioration of renal function has not been noted after the completion of treatment. In most instances there is some improvement in GFR after treatment is completed; however, the younger the patient the more the improvement as a general rule. It has been demonstrated that nephrotoxicity is related to the peak platinum concentration in the plasma but there is controversy in the degree of additional importance of total dose over time.

Although the renal toxicity of cisplatin has been recognized for 20 years, its precise mechanism still remains the subject of research. Renal toxicity is most certainly dose-related and cumulative, although abrupt, irreversible renal failure has been associated with even a single dose (which was administered without hydration).[93] In both animal and human studies the predominant lesion is tubular, with light and electron microscopic evidence of hyaline droplets in proximal tubular cells, degeneration of the tubular basement membranes, and focal tubular necrosis.[94] The tubular injury is no surprise, in that renal tubules concentrate both toxic products and metabolites to locally higher concentrations than exist in the blood. Additionally, renal tubular cells are capable of oxidative and reductive activity of the administered chemotherapeutic agents. This includes the cytochrome p450 oxidases and hydroperoxidases, in addition to the reductive glutathione transferases. Thus the observation of magnesium wasting after cisplatin therapy is directly related to the additional damage of the renal tubule's ability to reabsorb solutes and maintain an electrolyte balance. Additional damage is evident when cisplatin is administered either with or after other renal toxins, such as aminoglycosides, indocin, amphotericin, cytoxan, methotrexate, ifosfamide, mitomycin C, and the nitrosoureas.

To estimate renal injury most trials have utilized either GFR or serum creatinine but it is clear that these can lead to underestimation of renal injuries, due to problems in collection or techniques using nomograms to calculate creatinine clearance. Additionally, cachexia and reduced creatinine production, which is a common condition in advanced cancer patients, can lead to lower estimates of renal injury. At the least, serum creatinine values are a less sensitive measure of renal damage because the levels only increase after destruction of a large number of nephrons. By contrast, protein excretion, when examined in terms of β_2-microglobulin, N-acetyl-β-D-glucosaminidase, alanine aminopeptidase, and adenosine deaminase binding protein, has been associated[95] with detection of subclinical nephrotoxicity.[96–98] This sensitive detection of toxicity is the result of tubular damage which prevents the reabsorption of filtered proteins and the excretion of necrotic tubular cells as well.

Hydration decreases the nephrotoxicity of cisplatin administration, as does saline loading. Cisplatin, in doses of between 100 and 200mg/m^2, has been given safely with 3 per cent saline diuresis, 24-hour hydration and furosemide being given 30 minutes before cisplatin.[99] This regimen results in less than 10 per cent clinically relevant renal toxicity, with the exception of hypomagnesia.

Agents which have been shown to demonstrate protection of the kidney from the toxic effects of cisplatin are sodium thiosulfate, DDTC (diethyldithiocarbamate), thiourea, acetazolamide, sodium-2-mercaptoethanesulfonate (mesna), ORG-2766 (an ACTH analog), phosphamycin, buthionine sulfoximine (BSO) and amifostine. Whether any of these agents offer any advantage over saline diuresis is under investigation. In depth discussions of protective agents are summarized in reviews by McCulloch *et al.*, Gandara *et al.*, Ozols, and Vogelzang.[100-103]

Nephrotoxicity may not be dose-limiting (up to 200 mg/m^2) when cisplatin is administered according to currently established practices of hydration, saline loading and diuresis. Even with these techniques there is subclinical renal damage with increasing doses of not only cisplatin but carboplatin as well. In melanoma and ovarian cancer the degree of renal injury is lessened with the use of amifostine. In an ovarian cancer trial using the criterion defined in the protocol for delaying cisplatin administration (i.e. serum creatinine less than 1.5 mg/dl by day 25), comparison of the two treatment groups showed that prolonged increased serum creatinine levels occurred more frequently in the arm not utilizing amifostine (14.6 per cent vs. 3.3 per cent). In a metastatic melanoma trial of high-dose cisplatin plus amifostine, there was a 10 per cent incidence of reversible nephrotoxicity, which compares favorably with the 16–25 per cent incidence of renal toxicity reported in other published studies of high-dose cisplatin with vigorous hydration.[104] DDTC has shown both dose- and time-dependent renal protection from cisplatin toxicity[105] but did not alter the bone marrow suppression, and additionally DDTC has been associated with a high incidence of a mixed autonomic hyperactivity with infusion. Further development of DDTC has been discontinued after adverse findings in a phase III controlled trial.[106]

It would seem then that some amelioration of nephrotoxicity is possible. If the current dose-limiting neurotoxicity of cisplatin is conquered and the dose can be further escalated beyond 200 mg/m^2, the combination of renal protectors and saline diuresis could allow for further escalation of the dose of cisplatin to provide a greater clinical response.

MANAGEMENT OF CARDIOTOXICITY

Cardiotoxicity of the anthracyclines as well as the other drugs discussed in this section are manifest by immediate dysrhythmia, coronary artery spasm resulting in angina, and/or latent or persistent arrhythmias as a result of congestive heart failure secondary to either direct or indirect effects on the cardiac muscle. The acute toxicities which are reversible and are unrelated to dosage are usually thought to be unrelated as well to subsequent heart failure. The more chronic changes that result from a cumulative dose effect are diagnosed by the signs of myocardial failure and can be documented by radionuclide angiocardiography, echocardiography and indium-111-antimyosin scintigraphy.[107] The latent effects, that is the persistent arrhythmias and/or gradual onset of congestive heart failure, may arise months to years after the administration of either anthracyclines or high-dose alkylating agents.

Anthracycline cardiotoxicity

With the demonstration of anthracycline cardiac toxicity, immediate attempts were made to reduce the dose-limiting side-effects. The cumulative probability of developing doxorubicin-induced congestive failure is less than 10 per cent, when total doses are below 600 mg/m^2.[108] Other contributing factors are pre-existing cardiac disease, mediastinal irradiation, age, nutritional status, hypertension, diabetes and the administration of other cardiotoxic drugs. Children seem to be especially susceptible to cardiac toxicity when radiation to the chest and anthracyclines are combined.[109]

Pathologic changes in the heart secondary to anthracycline administration are characterized by loss of myofibrils, swollen and altered mitrochondria, enlarged nuclei and nucleoli, increased numbers of lysosomes, cytoplasmic vacuolization and accumulation of lipid.[110,111] Anthracycline cardiotoxicity has been thought to be related to free radical formation with additional increased peroxidation, catalase activity, glutathione peroxidase levels and diaphorase activity. Additional changes are increased membrane permeability, altered calcium metabolism, alteration in mitochondrial respiratory activity, increased size and number of lysosomes and myofibrilar loss. Protection against these identified biochemical effects has concentrated on the free radical scavengers which are known to be able to limit free radical damage and lipid peroxidation induced by anthracyclines. Calcium channel blockers have also been studied in attempts to alter cardiac toxicity. Other drugs which have been studied are ICRF-159[112–114] and *N*-acetylcysteine.[115,116]

Perhaps the most successful clinical trials to date involve the use of the water-soluble ICRF-187 [+(1,2-bis-3,5-dioxopiperazinyl-1-yl propane)], an analog of EDTA which is thought to protect the heart by removing free iron necessary for the hydroxyl radical formation and liquid peroxidation induced by the anthracyclines. In a randomized trial of breast cancer patients treated with a combination of 5-fluorouracil, doxorubicin and cyclophosphamide, when treatment was preceded by ICRF-187 100 mg/m^2 IV, cardiac protection was demonstrated.[117] Clinical congestive heart failure developed in two patients in the treated group whereas twenty developed those signs in the control group. This study additionally has shown that the use of ICRF-187 permits significantly greater doses of doxorubicin to be administered to patients, thus hopefully translating into better response rates. Although the addition of ICRF-187 appears to add additional myelosuppression, it has not been clinically significant. The use of an iron chelator is thought to inhibit hydroxyl radical formation in heart tissue which is relatively low in catalase and superoxide dismutase (enzymes which are involved in detoxifying oxygen free-radicals). This results in subsequent peroxidation of membrane lipids. Iron complexed with anthracyclines enables transfer of electrons to molecular oxygen. ICRF-187 binds both free iron and copper, and in early studies it was suggested that the cardiotoxic agent may be the complexes of drug and metal.[118,119] Therefore, chelation of the metal ions should prevent or reduce the formation of metal–drug complexes, thus yielding the protective effect seen in the numerous clinical and preclinical studies. This protection did not block the antitumor effect of the drug in preclinical work.[120]

ICRF-197, a transcyclobutane analog, has shown cardiac protection in a rat model system with perhaps fewer side-effects.[121] Free radical scavengers such as α-tocopherol have been shown to offer protection in mouse models from the cardiotoxicity of anthracyclines;[122] however, in clinical trials by Legha et al.[123] Weitzman et al.[124] and Whittaker and Al-Ismail[125] no effect was seen with the use of α-tocopherol and doxorubicin. Ubiquinone (coenzyme Q_{10}), an important redox molecule which has a structure similar to that of an anthracycline, was used in twenty-two patients and suggested diminished cardiac toxicity.[126] Calcium channel blockers have been used to attempt to protect against anthracycline cardiotoxicity based on the hypothesis that an additional toxicity of anthracycline may be due to increased calcium concentration in myocardial cells, resulting in cell death. The protective effect of calcium channel blockers that was found in rabbits was not substantiated in a multicentered trial utilizing daunomycin in the treatment of acute myelogenous leukemia. Patients were randomized to 120 mg daily of verapamil administered orally and no significant difference was seen in cardiotoxidity between the verapamil and non-verapamil group.[127] Nifedipine was combined with α-tocopherol but was found not to offer protection.[128] Amifostine, an oxygen free radical scavenger is being evaluated in preclinical systems.

An additional attempt to reduce the cardiotoxicity of anthracyclines has involved the exploration of numerous analogs.[129] The most important of these currently is mitoxantrone, an anthroquinone structurally similar to the anthracyclines which has been shown to be less cardiotoxic than daunomycin. The risk of cardiotoxicity does not apparently begin to rise significantly until a dose of about 160 mg/m^2 is reached.[130] Of the other analogs, idarubicin, epirubicin and esorubicin all seem to be less cardiotoxic than doxorubicin in animal models.[131,132]

Alternative schedules have also been used to explore the concept of longer biologic half-life and either lower, more frequent doses or continuous infusion techniques that might produce less cardiotoxicity. With doxorubicin, weekly low-dose administration resulted in a lower incidence of doxorubicin-induced cardiomyopathy and maintained therapeutic efficacy.[133] Continuous infusion over 96 hours given every 3 weeks did seem to show some decrease in cardiotoxicity, but the slight increase in therapeutic activity of this schedule was not statistically significant.[134] Utilizing the technique of encapsulating anthracyclines within a lipsomal structure, cardiotoxicity of doxorubicin has been shown to be reduced, probably secondary to a decreased cardiac uptake of the drug without compromising the antitumor effect.[135]

5-Fluorouracil cardiotoxicity

Table 3.4 lists the manifestations of cardiotoxicity reported with 5-fluorouracil (5-FU) administration. The incidence of 5-FU cardiotoxicity appears to be less than 10 per cent: an incidence of 1.6 per cent was reported when 5-FU was given alone or in combination with other agents.[136] Although the mechanism of cardiotoxicity remains undefined, coronary artery spasm, arrhythmia and abnormalities in the coagulation system, specifically an increase in the fibrinopeptide A levels and a decrease in the level of function of tissue plasminogen activator have all been considered as possible etiologies. It is known that patients with underlying coronary artery disease and mediastinal irradiation are

Table 3.4 5-FU cardiac events

Supraventricular tachycardia
Angina
Ventricular tachycardia
Congestive heart failure
Reversible cardiomyopathy
Myocardial infarction
Sudden death

more likely to suffer cardiac manifestations. In an attempt to prevent coronary vessel spasm, when fifty-eight esophageal or advanced head and neck carcinoma patients were treated prophylactically with verapamil 120 mg three times daily, the signs of ischemia appeared in 12 per cent of the patients as compared to 13 per cent in the previously studied historical control group, thus showing no effect on the incidence of ischemic change or coronary artery spasm.[137] The incidence of 5-FU cardiotoxicity was more evident when patients were continuously monitored with a Holter monitor and 68 per cent demonstrated ST-segment depression during 5-FU infusion.[138]

Alkylating agents, specifically cylcophosphamide and ifosfamide, are known to cause cardiac toxicity in the form of supraventricular arrhythmias and ST–T wave changes, as well as fatal myocardial necrosis. Fatal cardiac complications occurred in 19 per cent of patients when high doses of cyclophosphamide (180 mg/kg) were given; at doses in the range of 240 mg/kg the incidence was thought to be at least 25 per cent.[139,140] Attempts to produce pro-drugs similar to nitrogen mustard resulted in the knowledge that activation was achieved by hepatic enzymes.[141] Phosphoramide mustard is recognized as the responsible active agent of cylcophosphamide and ifosfamide. The bladder toxicity of both drugs is thought to be more related to the acrolein entity of metabolism. Toxicity to the bladder can be eliminated with the use of a thiol primarily made available in the bladder mucosa (mesna). This spares the urethelium from the ifosfamide phosphorene bladder toxicity. Other thiols which have a more systemic effect, such as amifostine, may have an ameliorating effect on the cardiac toxicity when alkylating agents are used in high doses, as in bone marrow transplantation.

Newer biologic therapies have also been shown to be cardiotoxic; specifically interleukin-2 and lymphocyte-activated killer cells have been associated with arrhythmias, in addition to ischemic changes in several patients.[142] More recently, techniques of administering this therapy with lower fluid volumes and screening patients for prior ischemic heart disease have reduced the incidence of cardiac events. The cardiotoxicities of interferon are cardiac arrhythmias, dilated cardiomyopathy and ischemic symptoms which have included sudden death.[143] The etiology is unknown; however, perhaps coronary spasm and peripheral vascular effects resulting in cardiac stress may be the most likely etiology. Additional considerations could be stimulation of an autoimmune or inflammatory reaction; however, evidence for this has not been borne out by endomyocardial biopsies. In patients with pre-existing ischemic heart disease, interferon should be used with caution and routine electrocardiograms should precede the initiation of high-dose therapy. Cardiotoxic consequences are reversible after the cessation of drug therapy.

Bleomycin has been associated with occasional cardiotoxicity in the form of pericarditis and additionally has shown to perhaps initiate angina pectoris and Raynauds' phenomenon in a study by Stefenelli and Rosin.[144] Other drugs which have been associated with occasional cardiac toxicity are actinomycin D and mitomycin C.

MANAGEMENT OF PULMONARY TOXICITY

By 1980, pulmonary toxicity of antineoplastic therapy was associated with 13 different cytotoxic agents.[145] Those agents commonly associated with pulmonary toxicity are bleomycin, methotrexate, mitomycin, the nitrosoureas and interleukin-2. Although the incidence is somewhat dependent upon dose and route of administration of chemotherapy, the addition of prior radiotherapy and oxygen therapy can adversely affect the incidence and severity of pulmonary toxicity. Supplemental oxygen enhances the toxicity of both bleomycin and mitocycin as well as the nitrosoureas. The etiology of pulmonary damage is thought to be injury to the capillary epithelium mediated by oxygen free-radical induction, but later focal interstitial fibrosis is also a common injury.[146] Additionally, active fibrosis with proliferating smooth muscle cells, as well as dysplastic pneumocytes, eosinophilia, angitis and cellular edema may play a part. Because the mechanism of injury appears to be mediated by oxygen free-radicals, antioxidants may inhibit this injury and there may be a synergistic toxic effect of other free-radical generating chemotherapeutic agents and/or radiation. Oxygen administration probably enhances the potential for free-radical production, thus increasing the toxicity to the lung. Lung damage can also be acute and may precipitate acute respiratory distress syndrome and, with survival, can result in pulmonary fibrosis.

The clinical and physical findings of pulmonary compromise may be nonspecific; however, close attention to pulmonary examination including auscultation, blood gases and chest radiographs may be necessary early and often. Gallium scans may show diffuse uptake and may be helpful in evaluation of the severity of injury.[147] Often in the setting of acute respiratory distress in an immunocompromised host, an infectious etiology must be evaluated by bronchoscopy with transbronchial or open lung biopsy. In those who are not as acutely ill the diffusing capacity ($D_L CO$) has been the most useful pulmonary function test, to detect early interstitial changes.

Bleomycin is an active agent in the treatment of Hodgkin's disease, non-Hodgkin's lymphoma and germ-cell tumors, and it is in these patients that the identification of bleomycin toxicity has been clarified. Bleomycin alone is capable of inducing pulmonary fibrosis, but in combination with radiotherapy a 19 per cent incidence of pulmonary toxicity has been seen.[148] Blum *et al.* stated that once the cumulative dose of 450 units of bleomycin is reached, the incidence of pulmonary toxicity rises dramatically.[149] Thus therapies utilizing cumulative doses of 400–500 units have resulted in up to a 50 per cent incidence of pulmonary toxicity.[150] Most studies which employ lower doses report below 5 per cent toxicity.

The therapies for bleomycin lung toxicity have concentrated on attempts to prevent pulmonary fibrosis prophylactically since only supportive therapy for established fibrosis is possible. Corticosteroids were used in a study in germ-cell tumors by Jensen *et al.*[151] and the conclusion was that high-dose steroid administration did not reduce the frequency of pulmonary toxicity. Steroids did not alter bronchial lavage cell profiles and based on lung weights and extravascular albumen determinations animals showed no modulation of lung injury.[152]

Antioxidants may have some benefit in that activated bleomycin has been shown to release superoxide radicals. High levels of antioxidants might limit the activation of bleomycin in the lung and subsequently limit pulmonary injury, and one study, using liposome-encapsulated enzymes has shown some promise.[153]

N-Acetylcysteine is known to inhibit the lung collagen deposition following bleomycin administration.[154] Likewise the pulmonary injury secondary to bleomycin is exacerbated by higher concentrations of O_2,[155] and O_2 free-radical scavengers (e.g. amifostine) have been found to reduce bleomycin mutagenicity and toxicity.[156]

Iron chelators such as desferrioxamine have actually been shown to enhance the lung injury produced by bleomycin. Thus, the availability of iron within lung tissue does not appear to be an important factor in the development of pulmonary toxicity.[157,158] Bleomycin is eliminated by a renal mechanism through the kidneys and is commonly combined with cisplatin in therapeutic regimens. In a patient with renal insufficiency, a dose of only 60 units resulted in fatal pulmonary toxicity.[159] Bleomycin has a rapid plasma clearance with a terminal half-life of 90 minutes. A large renal excretion of the unchanged drug and a 70 per cent 24-hour excretion necessitates great caution in renal-insufficient patients when using bleomycin. Ambroxol is an agent which is apparently capable of increasing the secretory activity of the type 2 pneumocyte, the source of lung surfactant. Ambroxol has delayed the appearance of bleomycin lung toxicity in a rat model.[160] By utilizing the technique of continuous infusion of bleomycin, a decrease in bleomycin lung toxicity has also been shown.[161] Bleomycin analogs have also been developed in an attempt to minimize pulmonary toxicity, most prominently pepleomycin.[162]

Mitomycin pulmonary toxicity is variable and can range from 3 to 36 per cent.[163] This may not be a dose-related phenomenon and may result from interaction of concomitant cyclophosphamide, radiation therapy or even oxygen therapy. Mitomycin is one of the few drugs that can cause a capillary leak syndrome resulting in pleural effusion. Biopsy-proven pulmonary toxicity secondary to mitomycin was studied and although no specific pulmonary pathologic changes were found, dramatic improvement was seen with glucocorticoids given as prednisone 20 mg three times daily and in one case methyl prednisolone 60 mg every 6 hours, showing radiographic and clinical improvement.[164]

The nitrosoureas have also been shown to induce pulmonary fibrosis and in a study by Gaetani in which BCNU and CCNU were used in the treatment of malignant gliomas, a randomized trial utilizing ambroxol 120 mg per day for 40 days after the chemotherapy course compared with a control group of patients who received a placebo with the otherwise same dose and schedule of chemotherapy, showed a significant improvement in pulmonary functional parameters. Ambroxol is thought to enhance alveolar surfactant synthesis as well as modulate inflammatory cell efflux to the alveolar capillary structures.[165] Nitrosourea-induced fibrosis can be latent. In survivors among thirty-one children treated for brain tumors with carmustine, eight of whom were available for detailed study 13–17 years from treatment, all survivors studied had a restrictive spirometric defect. Interstitial fibrosis was seen by light and electron microscopy with damage to epithelial and endothelial cells as well. Latent lung fibrosis, in this study of nitrosoureas, does not seem to support a dose effect (above 1500 mg/m^2 has been associated with a higher risk of early onset lung fibrosis) in that only two of the long-term survivors had received greater than 1500 mg/m^2. It is probable, therefore, that all patients have some degree of acute subclinical injury leading to a varying degree of persistent lung fibrosis. It is known that pre-exisiting lung disease is an important variable in predicting the risk of lung toxicity with nitrosourea therapy.

Busulfan when used in the treatment of chronic myeloid leukemia (CML) was the first alkylator known to be associated with pulmonary toxicity. Pathologic changes have included hyperplasia and dysplasia of the type 2 pneumocytes and pulmonary ossification. This damage usually occurs after a long latent period averaging 3 years or longer, but may occur early after therapy.[166] Cyclophosphamide requires metabolic activation and it has been suggested that acrolein is the active metabolic agent which can result in pulmonary toxicity.[167] Exogenous thiol administration with amifostine before cyclophosphamide protected mice against this lung damage whereas sodium thiosulfate did not. Although mesna does protect the bladder epithelium from the acrolein toxicity, a systemic thiol is necessary to protect the pulmonary parenchyma. Ifosfamide, an analog of cyclophosphamide, is reported to cause interstitial pneumonitis.[168]

The antimetabolites methotrexate, ara-C, and fludarabine have all been uncommonly associated with pulmonary endothelial injury, capillary, diffuse alveolar damage and hypersensitivity. Corticosteroids have been used therapeutically and may hasten the resolution of the pneumonitis.[169] High-dose methotrexate and trimetrexate pulmonary toxicities have been ameliorated with use of leucovorin.

The biologic response modifiers have been reported to cause pulmonary edema, especially with the use of IL-2 lymphocyte-activated killer cells. High concentrations of IL-2 may have a direct effect on the pulmonary parenchyma resulting in a capillary leak syndrome.[170] Apparently tumor necrosis factor is the agent responsible for IL-2 toxicity and the cardiorespiratory effects. GM-CSF (granulocyte macrophage colony-stimulating factor) when given by continuous infusion has been associated with dyspnea 2–6 hours after starting the therapy. This may be related to aggregation of neutrophils pooling in the pulmonary vasculature and careful attention to proper hydration is necessary.[171]

MANAGEMENT OF GASTROINTESTINAL TOXICITY

The gastrointestinal mucosa cells, like the bone marrow and gonadal cells, are sensitive to chemotherapeutic agents due to their high growth fraction. Most of the gastrointestinal crypt cells are made up of undifferentiated cells which gradually migrate from the crypt to the villus and gradually undergo differentiation. It has been shown that most normal gastrointestinal tissue can renew itself after injury in less than a day.[172] Throughout the gastrointestinal mucosa as DNA synthesis takes place, rapidly dividing cells are much more susceptible to chemotherapeutic attack and the toxic effects of radiation therapy. The resultant toxic effects on the gastrointestinal system are nausea, vomiting, mucositis, malabsorption, diarrhea, constipation and resultant gastrointestinal infection secondary to fungal or bacterial overgrowth, and are discussed in detail in a review by Mitchell and Schein.[173] Mucosal injury is most commonly caused by methotrexate, the antibiotic tumor agents, 5-FU and the vinca alkaloids. Attempts to protect the gastrointestinal mucosa against the toxic effects of these chemotherapeutic agents have not resulted in many therapies available in the clinic as yet. When methotrexate is given in normal or high dose, monitoring the mucosal toxicity and the prophylactic use of leucovorin are able to ameliorate and blunt gastrointestinal toxicity.[174]

Animal studies of 5-FU gastrointestinal toxicity have shown that administration of the RNA base uridine blocked this toxicity in mice through an inhibition of RNA synthesis in the gastrointestinal epithelium. The combination of high-dose 5-FU utilizing uridine infusions decreased toxicity and did not influence the therapeutic index in a B16 melanoma cell line.[175,176]

The study of the effect of radiation on the gastrointestinal mucosa originates from whole-body irradiation and the study of lethal irradiation accidents in which a mechanism of death is severe damage to the intestinal epithelium. In 1973 it was shown that the jejunum could be protected with prior administration of amifostine at a dose-modifying factor (DMF) of 1.6–2.1 in mice and rats when exposed to ionizing radiation.[177] Liver protection was observed by measuring the active metabolic product of amifostine, WR-1065, in the Balb/c mouse liver after exposure to radiation. The DMF was 2.0–2.7. The limitation to the therapeutic radiation of metastatic lesions in the liver is the radiation-sensitive hepatocyte. Localized protection of the liver utilizing phosphorothioate radioprotectors attached to neoglycoalbumin, a synthetic ligand for the hepatocyte-specific receptor, hepatic-binding protein, has been attempted but the results have been inconclusive.[178]

A randomized trial of placebo vs. amifostine was given to dogs 30 minutes before a 10 Gy abdominal radiation. Observations of crypt cell necrosis, villus blunting, measurement of plasma diamineoxidase activity and observation for evidence of intestinal malabsorption all demonstrated a significant improvement in the amifostine-treated animals. This experiment secondarily demonstrated enhancement of hematopoietic cell survival, thus increasing the antimicrobial defenses.[179]

MANAGEMENT OF ENDOCRINOLOGIC TOXICITY

The common endocrinologic effect of cytotoxic chemotherapies is gonadal damage (ovary and testes) in addition to effects on thyroid, adrenal and pancreatic function. Therapeutic radiation treatment of brain tumors and head and neck cancer affect the pituitary, thyroid and parathyroid, but with radiation therapy treatments involving the abdomen and pelvis, the adrenal gland, ovary and pancreas may also be affected.

Recent years have seen curative therapy develop for Hodgkin's disease, germ cell tumors, choriocarcinoma and leukemia. Premature ovarian and testicular failure are common with these aggressive therapies. In a study of children treated for Hodgkin's disease with both radiation therapy and mechlorethamine, Oncovin (vincristine) procarbazine and prednisone (MOPP) chemotherapy, it was found that of males treated with radiation alone to the pelvis, only half were later able to father a child and the other half were oligospermic. Of those treated with MOPP therapy, 83 per cent demonstrated absolute azoospermia with no evidence of recovery after 11 years of follow-up. Eighty-seven per cent of the females had normal menses. Of those females who underwent pelvic irradiation without prior oophoropexy, none maintained ovarian function. After six cycles of MOPP therapy ovarian injury was directly related to the number of cycles of chemotherapy; however, most had the return of normal menstrual function.[180] A similar study[181] of ninety-two male patients treated for Hodgkin's disease showed some testicular atrophy in 97 per cent of patients. The testosterone levels did not differ from before and after treatment; however, the follicle-stimulating hormone (FSH) rose from pretreatment levels of 179 $\pm$ 22 ng/ml to 529 $\pm$ 102 ng/ml after treatment. Luteinizing hormone (LH) also rose post-chemotherapy. The irreversible azoospermia is thought to result from alkylating agents such as nitrogen mustard (mechlorethamine), chlorambucil and cyclophosphamide.[182] The regimen for Hodgkin's disease was modified to exclude the mechlorethamene and with a current regimen, ABVD (doxorubicin, bleomycin, vinblastine and dacarbazine), spermatogenesis recovery was observed in 67 per cent of patients treated with ABVD alone versus 25 per cent recovery with MOPP-treated patients.[183] In seventy-nine men with Hodgkin's disease, their pretreatment sperm concentration, motility progression, post-thaw motility and post-thaw progression were all significantly decreased when compared to normal controls prior to any therapy. Post-treatment semen analysis showed azoospermia in 80 per cent of those patients. However, despite these lower values, cryopreservation and artificial insemination do offer a partial solution for this toxic effect.[184]

Primary germ-cell tumors have been cured by platinum-based chemotherapeutic regimens. The long-term effects of such treatment showed abnormalities of thyroid-stimulating hormone (TSH), FSH and LH, but serum testosterone was normal.[185] Although the initial treatments for germ-cell cancers may not employ alkylating agents, the effect on spermatozoa and testicular volume was shown to be significantly reduced by cisplatin-based therapy. Cisplatin-based chemotherapy may lead to a persistent impairment in Leydig cell function as manifest by elevated LH levels.[186] Sertoli and Leydig cell function have been evaluated in men with cisplatin-induced testicular damage using serum immunoactive inhibin, FSH, LH and testosterone concentrations. Inhibin and testosterone levels were not significantly different from controls whereas median FSH and LH levels were significantly higher statistically than in controls.[187] Long-term follow-up of testicular cancer patients has demonstrated that gonadal toxicity is related to the patient's pretreatment gonadal function and age, in addition to the treatment of the malignancy.[188]

Attempts to protectively limit gonadal function during chemotherapy with the use of medroxyprogesterone acetate (500 mg daily beginning on day 1 of chemotherapy for testicular cancer) have demonstrated that although higher FSH levels were maintained and testosterone was significantly lower in the treated patients as opposed to the controls, there was no difference between the groups regarding the recovery of sperm cell production after chemotherapy. Although the medroxyprogesterone induced medical castration during intensive chemotherapy in testicular cancer, it was ineffective in protecting the testes against treatment-induced damage to spermatogenesis.[189] An attempt by Kreuser *et al.* to use LH-releasing hormone acetate (LHRHA) on spermatogenic stem cells in patients with germ-cell cancers was not successful. He effectively suppressed FSH, LH and testosterone levels during prechemotherapeutic administration of LHRHA and azoospermia was demonstrated. At the cessation of chemotherapy median FSH levels and sperm density normalized 24 months after chemotherapy and the control patients, who did not receive the LHRHA administration, also recovered within 24 months of therapy demonstrating no difference between the two groups.[190]

In summary, the effects of cancer treatment on the reproductive system are often profound and have lasting effects on both the testes and ovary. Germ-cell production is altered with the magnitude of the effect related to the pubertal status of the patient, the chemotherapeutic agents given, dosages or drug combinations administered and whether radiation therapy is employed with the treatment program. Primary testicular injury is related to the depletion of the germinal epithelial lining in the seminiferous tubules. Alkylating agents produce the most profound germinal aplasia and permanent infertility in the majority of patients. The ovarian injury following combination chemotherapy is related to the age of the patient at the time of treatment and overall 50 per cent of women treated with combination chemotherapy become amenorrheic, the frequency in women older than 35 may be as high as 90 per cent.[191] To date it has been shown that interventions to protect the gonads from cytotoxic agents have been unsuccessful. The use of buserelin (LHRH ethylamide) did not afford protection for the ovaries.[192] In animal studies, antioxidants and *N*-acetylcysteine have been used[193] and further attempts to protect normal tissue with aminothiols should be entertained. It is also known that adequate spermatogoneal supply can be regenerated even after greater than 99 per cent stem cell kill;[194] therefore, theoretically spermatogenesis may gradually recover in some cytotoxic-damaged human testes years later.[195]

Thyroid disease, especially hypothyroidism, is common in patients after treatment for Hodgkin's disease with mantle irradiation. In 1677 patients whose thyroid received some irradiation in the treatment of Hodgkin's disease at Stanford University, the actuarial risk of thyroid disease 20 years after treatment was 52 per cent. Graves' hyperthyroidism developed as well and the risk was 7–20 times that for normal subjects. Six patients developed papillary follicular cancers of the thyroid. An increased incidence of thyroid dysfunction has also been seen in pediatric patients undergoing bone marrow transplantation.[196] Compensated hypothyroidism occurred in one quarter of patients approximately a year after bone marrow transplantation. Spinal irradiation resulting from treatment of childhood leukemia or brain tumors has also resulted in primary thyroid dysfunction in approximately 23 per cent of the patients.[197] Attempts to suppress the normal thyroid function while undergoing radiation therapy have not been successful as a protective treatment to date. Treatment of radiation-induced hypothyroidism with thyroid hormone replacement is usually uncomplicated, once diagnosed; however, shielding techniques and careful treatment planning are currently the only mechanisms available to prophylactically minimize thyroid damage. Use of active thiols such as amifostine has been shown to protect salivary gland function in head and neck radiation, and conceivably experiments could be designed to determine whether the thyroid gland could also be protected.

MANAGEMENT OF MUTAGENICITY

The induction of altered DNA by radiation or chemotherapeutic agents is known to pose a significant risk of treatment-related malignancy. Secondary leukemia incidence is increased over the normal population in those treated for Hodgkin's disease, malignant lymphoma, multiple myeloma, small cell carcinoma of the lung, breast, ovarian and gastronintestinal cancer.[198] Although combination chemotherapy and irradiation can be curative, the carcinogenic potential of these modalities has been documented. The leukemogenic potential of the alkylating agents, nitrosoureas and procarbazine has been shown and is supported by the chromosomal abnormalities seen after the use of these agents.[199,200] Milas *et al.* in 1984 demonstrated that amifostine administered prior to irradiation significantly reduced the incidence of radiation-induced tumors in C3H mice.[201] Nagy and Grdina also demonstrated protection against nitrogen mustard and bleomycin-induced mutagenicity in V79 cells.[156] Clinical evidence of this protection against mutagenicity has not been shown to date; however, further study of amifostine, cystamine, diethyldithiocarbamate, sodium thiosulfate and *N*-acetylcysteine may lead to significant protection against mutagenesis, neoplastic transformation and carcinogenesis.[202]

REFERENCES

1. NIH Publication no. 87–2955, *Closing in on cancer, solving a 5000-year-old mystery*. National Cancer Institute, Bethesda, MD, USA, 1987.
2. Slevin ML, Stubbs L, Plant HJ *et al*. Attitudes to chemotherapy: comparing views of patients with cancer with those of doctors, nurses, and general public. *British Medical Journal* 1990; **300**: 1458–60.
3. Hryniuk W, Levine MN. Analysis of dose intensity for adjuvant chemotherapy trials in stage II breast cancer. *Journal of Clinical Oncology* 1986; **4**: 1162–70.
4. Rozencweig M, Von Hoff DD, Staquet MJ *et al*. Animal toxicology for early clinical trials with anticancer agents. *Cancer Clinical Trials* 1981; **4**: 21–8.
5. Hryniuk W, Levine MN. Analysis of dose intensity for adjuvant chemotherapy trials in stage II breast cancer. *Journal of Clinical Oncology* 1986; **4**: 1162–70.
6. Cavalli F, Sonntag RW, Jungi F *et al*. VP-16–213 monotherapy for remission induction of small cell lung cancer. A randomized trial using three dosage schedules. *Cancer Treatment Reports* 1978; **62**: 467–75.
7. Hrynuik WM, Figueredo A, Goodyear M. Application of dose intensity to problems in chemotherapy of breast and colorectal cancer. *Seminars in Oncology* 1987; **14** (Suppl. 4): 12–19.
8. Levin L, Hrynuik W. Dose intensity analysis of chemotherapy regimens in ovarian carcinoma. *Journal of Clinical Oncology* 1987; **5**: 756–67.
9. DeVita V, Hubbard S, Longo D: The chemotherapy of lymphomas. Looking back, moving forward. *Cancer Research* 1987; **47** 5810–324.
10. Torti FM, Bristow MR, Howes AE *et al*. Reduced cardiotoxicity of doxorubicin

delivered on a weekly schedule. Assessment by endomyocardial biopsy. *Annals of Internal Medicine* 1983; **99**: 745–9.

11. Lokich JJ, Ahlgren JD, Cantrell J *et al*. A prospective randomized comparison of protracted infusional 5-fluorouracil with or without weekly bolus cisplatin in metastatic colorectal carcinoma. *Cancer* 1991; **67**: 14–19.

12. Beck S. Impact of a systemic oral care protocol on stomatitis after chemotherapy. *Cancer and Nursing* 1979; **2**: 185–99.

13. Oliff A, Bleyer WA, Poplack DG. Methotrexate induced oral mucositis and salivary methotrexate concentrations. *Cancer Chemotherapy and Pharmacology* 1979; **2**: 225.

14. Bruckner HW, Bertino JR. Absorption of leucovorin (NSC-3590) from a 'mouthwash'. *Cancer Chemotherapy Reports* 1975; **59**: 575.

15. Sodicoff M, Conger AD, Pratt NE, Trepper P. Radioprotection by WR-2721 against long-term chronic damage to the rat parotid gland. *Radiation Research* 1976; **76**: 172–9.

16. Tanaka Y. Clinical experiences with a chemical radioprotector in tumor radiotherapy: WR-2721. In: *Modification of radiosensitivity in cancer treatment*. Tokyo: Academic Press, 1984: 61–81.

17. Niibe H, Takahashi I, Mitsuhashi N. An evaluation of the clinical usefulness of amifostine (YM-08310), radioprotective agent. *Journal of the Japanese Society of Cancer Therapy* 1985; **20**(5): 984–93.

18. Lampertia, Ziskin MC, Bergy E, Gorlowski J, Sodicoff M. *Journal of Radiation Research* 1990; **124**(2): 194–200.

19. Jung-Ah K, Baker DG, Hahn SS, Goodchild NT, Constable WC. Topical use of *N*-acetylcysteine forreduction of skin reaction to radiation therapy. *Seminars in Oncology* 1983; **10**(1) (Suppl. 1): 86–91.

20. Ensminger WD, Frei E. The prevention of methotrexate toxicity by thymidine infusions in humans. *Cancer Research* 1977; **37**: 1857–63.

21. Capizzi RL. Improvement in the therapeutic index of methotrexate (NSC 740) by asparaginase (NSC 109229). *Cancer Chemotherapy Reports* 1975; **6**: 37–41.

22. Blyer WA. The clinical pharmacology of methotrexate. *Cancer* 1978; **41**: 36–51.

23. Howell SB, Wung W, Taetle R *et al*. Modulation of 5-fluorouracil toxicity by allopurinol in man. *Cancer* 1981; **48**: 1281–9.

24. Peters GJ, Van Dijk K, Laurensse E *et al*. *In vitro* biochemical and *in vivo* biologic studies of the uridine 'rescue' of 5-fluorouracil. *British Journal of Cancer* 1988; **57**: 259–65.

25. Groeningen CJ, Petes GJ, Leyva A *et al*. Reversal of 5-fluorouracil induced myelosuppression by prolonged administration of high dose uridine. *Journal of National Cancer Institute* 1989; **81**: 157–62.

26. Hruban RH, Yardley JH, Donehower RC *et al*. Taxol toxicity. Epithelial necrosis in the gastrointestinal tract associated with polymerized microtubule accumulation and mitotic arrest. *Cancer* 1989; **63**: 1944–50.

27. Larson DL. Treatment of tissue extravasation by antitumor agents. *Cancer* 1982; **49**: 1796–9.

28. Lane P, Vichi P, Bain DL, Tritton TR. Temperature dependence studies of adriamycin uptake and cytotoxicity. *Cancer Research* 1987; **47**: 4038–42.

29. Dorr RT, Alberts DS. Vinca alkaloid skin toxicity: Antidote and drug disposition studies in the mouse. *Journal of the National Cancer Institute* 1985; **74**: 113–20.

30. Luedke D, Sun Woo Y, Luedle S, Godefroid R. Doxorubicin (D) induced soft tissue necrosis: Occurrence despite pH manipulation. *Proceedings of the American Association for Cancer Research and the American Society of Clinical Oncology* 1980; **21**: 330.

31. Barr RD, Sertic J. Soft-tissue necrosis induced by extravasated cancer chemother-

apeutic agents: A study of active intervention. *British Journal of Cancer* 1981; **44**: 267–9.

32. Ludwig CV, Stoll H, Obrist R. Prevention of cytotoxic drug-induced skin ulcers with dimethylsulfoxide (DMSO) and alpha-tocopherol. *European Journal of Clinical Oncology* 1987; **23**: 327–9.

33. Desai MH, Teres D. Prevention of doxorubicin-induced skin ulcers in the rat and pig with dimethyl sulfoxide (DMSO). *Cancer Treatment Reports* 1982; **66**: 1371–4.

34. Olver IN, Schwarz MA. Use of dimethyl sulfoxide in limiting tissue damage caused by extravasation of doxorubicin. *Cancer Treatment Reports* 1983; **67**: 407–8.

35. Olver IN, Aisner J, Hament A *et al.* A prospective study of topical dimethylsulfoxide for treating anthracycline extravasation. *Journal of Clinical Oncology* 1988; **6**: 1732–5.

36. Balazsovits JAE, Mayer LD, Bally MB *et al.* Analysis of the effect of liposome encapsulation on the vesicant properties, acute and cardiac toxicities, and antitumor efficacy of doxorubicin. *Cancer Chemotherapy and Pharmacology* 1989; **23**: 81–6.

37. Forssen EA, Tokes AZ. Attenuation of dermal toxicity of doxorubicin by liposome encapsulation. *Cancer Treatment Reports* 1983; **67**: 481–4.

38. Soble MJ, Dorr RT, Plezia P, Breckenridge S. Dose-dependent skin ulcers in mice treated with DNA binding antitumor antibiotics. *Cancer Chemotherapy and Pharmacology* 1987; **20**: 33–6.

39. Hatiboglu I, Mihich E, Moore GE, Nichol CA. Use of sodium thiosulfate as a neutralizing agent during regional administration of nitrogen mustard: An experimental study. *Annals of Surgery* 1962; **156**: 994–1001.

40. Bonadonna G, Karnofsky DA. Protection studies with sodium thiosulfate against methyl bis(B-chloroethylamine hydrochloride) and its ethyleinmonium derivative. *Clinical Pharmacology and Therapeutics* 1965; **6**: 50–4.

41. Dorr RT, Soble M, Liddil JD, Keller JH. Mitomycin C skin toxicity studies in mice: Reduced ulceration and altered pharmacokinetics with topical dimethyl sulfoxide. *Journal of Clinical Oncology* 1986; **4**: 1399–404.

42. Ludwig CV, Stoll H, Obrist R. Prevention of ocytotoxic drug-induced skin ulcers with dimethylsulfoxide (DMSO) and alpha-tocopherol. *European Journal of Clinical Oncology* 1987; **23**: 327–9.

43. Buchanan GR, Buchsbaum HJ, O'Banion K, Gojer B. Extravasation of dactinomycin, vincristine, and cisplatin: Studies in an animal model. *Medical and Pediatric Oncology* 1985; **13**: 375–80.

44. Harrison B, Godefroid R, Sun Woo Y, Luedke D, Luedke S. Histopathological evolution of vincristine (VCR) skin toxicity and treatment with local dexamethasone (DXM). *Proceedings of the American Society of Clinical Oncology* 1983; **2**: 86.

45. Dorr RT. Antidotes to vesicant chemotherapy extravasation. *Haematological Oncology: Blood Reviews* 1990; **4**: 56.

46. Pesce A, Cassuto JP, Joyner MV. Scalp tourniquet in the prevention of chemotherapy-induced alopecia. *New England Journal of Medicine* 1978; **298**: 1204–5.

47. Dean JC, Griffith KS, Cetas TC. Scalp hypothermia: a comparison of ice packs and the cold cap in the prevention of doxorubicin-induced alopecia. *Journal of Clinical Oncology* 1983; **1**: 33–7.

48. Kiser J, Weston S, Büsching G. Wann ist der Einstatz der Skalphypothermie wirklich sinnvoll? In: Glaus A, Senn HJ eds. *Unterstützende Pflege bei Krebspatienten.* Berlin: Springer-Verlag, 1987.

49. Joss RA, Kiser J, Weston S, Brunner KW. Fighting alopecia in cancer chemotherapy. *Recent Results in Cancer Research* 1988; **108**: 117–26.

50. Hillen HFP, Breed WPM, Botman CJ. Scalp cooling by cold air for the prevention of chemotherapy-induced alopecia. *Netherlands Journal of Medicine* 1990; **37**: 231–5.

51. Powis G, Kooistra KL. Doxorubicin-induced hair loss in the Angora rabbit: a study

of treatments to protect against the hair loss. *Cancer Chemotherapy and Pharmacology* 1987; **20**: 291–6.

52. Wood LA. Possible prevention of Adriamycin-induced alopecia by tocopherol. *New England Journal of Medicine* 1985; **312**: 1060.

53. Perez JE, Macchiavelli M, Leone Ba. High-dose alpha-tocopheral as a preventive of doxorubicin-induced alopecia. *Cancer Treatment Reports* 1986; **70**: 1213–14.

54. Martin-Jimenez M, Diaz-Rubio E, Gonzalez A, Larriba JE. Failure of high-dose tocopherol to prevent alopecia induced by doxorubicin. *New England Journal of Medicine* 1986; **315**: 894–895.

55. DeVillez RL. The therapeutic use of topical Minoxidil. *Dermatologic Clinics* 1990; **8**: 367–75.

56. Granai CO, Frederickson, H, Gajewski W, Goodman A, Goldstein A, Baden H. The use of minoxidil to attempt to prevent alopecia during chemotherapy for gynecologic malignancies. *European Journal of Gynaecologic Oncology* 1991; **12**: 129–32.

57. Zografos E. Medikamentöse Prophylaxemöglichkeiten der zytostatikabedingten Alopezie. *Tierexperimentelle Arbeit. Krankenhausarzt* 1984; **57**: 620–2.

58. Hussein AM, Jimenez JJ, McCall CA, Yunis AA. Protection from chemotherapy-induced alopecia in a rat model. *Science* 1990; **249**: 1564–6.

59. Walken E, Jimenez JJ. Preventing hair loss. *Cancer Research* 1992; **52**: 413–15.

60. Kedar A, Cohen ME, Freeman AI. Peripheral neuropathy as a complication of cis-dichlorodiammineplatinum II treatment: A case report. *Cancer Treatment Reports* 1978; **62**: 819–21.

61. Ashraf M, Scotchel PL, Krall JM *et al*. Cis-platinum-induced hypomagnesemia and peripheral neuropathy. *Gynecological Oncology* 1983; **16**: 309–18.

62. Thompson SW, Davis LE, Kornfeld M *et al*. Cisplatin neuropathy, clinical, electro-physiologic, morphologic and toxicologic studies. *Cancer* 1984; **54**: 1269–75.

63. Roelofs RI, Hrushesky W, Rogin J *et al*. Peripheral sensory neuropathy and cisplatin chemotherapy. *Neurology* 1984; **34**: 934–8.

64. Cersosimo RJ. Cisplatin neurotoxicity. *Cancer Treatment Reviews* 1989; **16**: 195–211.

65. Gershenson DM, Wharton JT, Herson J *et al*. Single agent cisplatinum therapy for advanced ovarian cancer. *Obstetrics and Gynecology* 1978; **58**: 487–96.

66. Lokich JJ. Phase I study of cis-diamminedichloroplatinum II administered as a constant 5-day infusion. *Cancer Treatment Reports* 1980; **64**: 905–8.

67. Thompson SW, Davis LE, Kornfield M *et al*. Cisplatin neuropathy, clinical, electro-physiologic, morphologic and toxicologic studies. *Cancer* 1984; **54**: 1269–75.

68. van der Hoop RG, van der Burg MEL, ten Bokkel Huinink WW *et al*. Incidence of neuropathy in 395 patients with ovarian cancer treated with or without cisplatin. *Cancer* 1990; **66**: 1697–1702.

69. Hansen SW, Helweg-Larsen S, Trojaborg W. Long term neurotoxicity in patients treated with cisplatin, vinblastine and bleomycin for metastatic germ cell cancer. *Journal of Clinical Oncology* 1989; **7**(10): 1457–61.

70. van der Hoop RG, Vecht CJ, van der Burg ME, Elderson A *et al*. Prevention of cisplatin neurotoxicity with an ACTH(4–9) analogue in patients with ovarian cancer. *New England Journal of Medicine* 1990; **322**(2): 89–94.

71. van der Zee CE, Brakkee JH, Gispen WH. Alpha-MSH and Org. 2766 in peripheral nerve regeneration: different routes of delivery. *European Journal of Pharmacology* 1988; **147**(3): 351–7.

72. Mollman JE, Glover DJ, Hogan M, Furman RE. Cisplatin neuropathy. Risk factors, prognosis and protection by WR-2721. *Cancer* 1988; **61**: 2192–5.

73. Avril MF, Ortoli JC, Fortier-Beaulieu M *et al*. High dose cisplatin (C) and WR-2721 in metastatic melanoma. *Proceedings of American Society of Clinical Oncology* 1992; **11**(1181): 334.

74. Ellerby R. Phase I clinical trial with 5 FU (NSC 19893) and cis-platinum (II) diaminechloride (NSC 119875). *Cancer* 1974; **34**: 1005–10.
75. Chapman P. Rapid onset hearing loss after cisplatin therapy. *Case Reports and Literature Review* 1982; **86**: 259.
76. Helson L. Cis-platinum ototoxicity. *Clinical Toxicology* 1978; **13**: 469.
77. Estrem S. Cis-diamminedichloroplatinum (II): Ototoxicity in the guinea pig. *Otolaryngology – Head and Neck Surgery* 1981; **89**: 638.
78. Fleishman R. Ototoxicity of cis-dichlorodiammine platinum (II) in the guinea pig. *Toxicology and Applied Pharmacology* 1975; **33**: 320.
79. Schaeffer SD, Wright CG, Post JD, Frenkel EP. Cis-platinum vestibular toxicity. *Cancer* 1981; **47**: 857–9.
80. Strauss M. Cis-platinum ototoxicity: Clinical experience and temporal bone histopathology. *Laryngoscope* 1983; **93**: 1554.
81. Vermorken JB. Ototoxicity of cis-diammine dichloroplatinum (II): influence of dose, schedule and mode of administration. *European Journal of Cancer and Clinical Oncology* 1983; **19**: 53.
82. Walker EM, Jr. Nephrotoxic and ototoxic agents. *Clinical Toxicology I. Clinics in Laboratory Medicine* 1990; **10**(2): 323–45.
83. Pollera C. Very high-dose cisplatin-induced ototoxicity: a preliminary report on early and long-term effects. *Cancer Chemotherapy and Pharmacology* 1988; **21**: 61–4.
84. Al-Sarraf M, Fletcher W, Oishi N *et al.* Cisplatin hydration with and without mannitol diuresis and refractory disseminated malignant melanoma: A Southwest Oncology Group study. *Cancer Treatment Reports* 1982; **66**(1): 31–5.
85. MacDonald DR. Neurotoxicity of chemotherapeutic agents. In: *The chemotherapeutic chemotherapy source book*. Perry Michael C ed. New York: Williams & Wilkins, 1992: 666–79.
86. Dyke RW. Treatment of inadvertent intrathecal injection of vincristine. *New England Journal of Medicine* 1989; **321**: 1270–1.
87. Jackson DV, Wells HB, Atkins JN *et al.* Amelioration of vincristine neurotoxicity by gluconic acid. *American Journal of Medicine* 1988; **84**: 1016–22.
88. Donehower RC, Rowinsky EK, Grochow LB *et al.* Phase I trial of taxol in patients with advanced cancer. *Cancer Treatment Reports* 1987; **71**: 1171–7.
89. Spiegel RJ, Cooper PR, Blum RH, Speyer JL, McBride D, Mangiar DIJ. Treatment of massive intrathecal methotrexate overdose by ventricular lumbar profusion. *New England Journal of Medicine* 1984; **311**: 386–8.
90. Addiego JE, Jr, Ridgway D, Blyer WA. The acute management of intrathecal methotrexate overdose: pharmacologic rationale and guidelines. *Journal of Pediatrics* 1981; **98**: 825–8.
91. Barbour GL, Crum CK, Boyd CM, Reeves RD, Rastogi SP, Patterson, RM. Comparison of inulin iothalamate and technetium 99 DTPA for measurement of glomerula filtration rate. *Journal of Nuclear Medicine* 1976; **17**: 316–20.
92. Dentino M, Luft FC, Yum MN, Williams SD, Einhorn LH. Long term effect of cis-diamminedichloride platinum (CdDP) on renal function and structure in man. *Cancer* 1978; **41**: 1274–81.
93. Vokes EE, Ackland SP, Vogelzang NJ. Cisplatin, carboplatin and gallium nitrate. In: Lokich JJ ed. *Cancer chemotherapy by infusion*. Chicago: Precept Press, 1990: 176–96.
94. Weiner MW, Jacobs C. Mechanism of cis-platin nephrotoxicity. *Federation Proceedings of Clinical Research* 1983; **42**: 2974.
95. Goren MP, Forastiere AA, Wright RW, Horowitz ME, Dodge RK, Kamen BA, Viar MF, Pratt CB. Carboplatin (CBDCA), iproplatin (CHIP) and high dose cisplatin in hypertonic saline evaluated for tubular nephrotoxicity. *Cancer Chemotherapy and Pharmacology* 1987; **19**: 57–60.

96. Goren MP, Wright RK, Horowitz ME, Meyer WH. Enhancement of methotrexate nephrotoxicity after cisplatin therapy. *Cancer* 1986; **58**: 2617–21.

97. Goren MP, Wright RK, Pratt CB *et al*. Potentiation of ifosfamide neurotoxicity, hematotoxicity, and tubular nephrotoxicity by prior cis-diamminedichloroplatinum (II) therapy. *Cancer Research* 1987; **47**: 1457–60.

98. Goren MP, Wright RK, Horowitz ME *et al*. Ifosfamide-induced subclinical tubular nephrotoxicity despite mesna. *Cancer Treatment Report* 1987; **71**: 127–30.

99. Ozols R. Cisplatin dose intensity. *Seminars in Oncology* 1989; **16**: 23.

100. McCulloch W, Scheffler BJ, Schein PS. New protective agents for bone marrow in cancer therapy. *Clinical Science Review* 1991; **9**: 279–87.

101. Gandara DR, Wiebe VJ, Perez EA, Makuch RW, De Gregorio MW. Cisplatin rescue therapy: experience with sodium thiosulfate, WR-2721, and diethyldithiocarbamate. *Critical Reviews in Oncology/Hematology* 1990; **10**: 353–63.

102. Ozols R. Cisplatin dose intensity. *Seminars in Oncology* 1989; **16**: 22–30.

103. Vogelzang NJ. Nephrotoxicity from chemotherapy: Prevention and management. *Oncology* 1991; **5**: 97–102.

104. Glover D, Glick JH, Weiler C, Yuhas J, Kligerman MM. Phase I trials of WR-2721 and cis-platinum. *Journal of Radiation Oncology Biology and Physics* 1984; **10**: 1781–4.

105. Berry JM. Sikie BI, Halsey J *et al*. A phase I trial of diethyldithiocarbamate as a modifier of cisplatin toxicity. *Proceedings of the American Society of Clinical Oncology* 1989; **8**: 69.

106. Estorch M, Ignasi C, Berna L *et al*. Indium-111-antimyosin cintigraphy after doxorubicin therapy in patients with advanced breast cancer. *Journal of Nuclear Medicine* 1990; **31**: 1965–9.

107. Rothenberg ML, Ostchega Y, Steinberg SM *et al*. High-dose cisplatin with diethyldithiocarbamate chemoprotection in treatment of women with relapsed ovarian cancer. *Journal of the National Cancer Institute* 1988; **80**(18): 1488–92.

108. Von Hoff DD, Layard MW, Basa P, Davis HL Jr, Von Hoff AL, Rozencweig M, Muggia FM. Risk factors for doxorubicin-induced congestive heart failure. *Annals of Internal Medicine* 1979; **91**: 710–17.

109. Steinherz L, Steinherz P. Delayed cardiac toxicity from anthyracycline therapy. *Pediatrician* 1991; **18**: 49–52.

110. Billingham ME, Mason JW, Bristow MR, Daniels JR. Anthracycline cardiomyopathy monitored by morphologic changes. *Cancer Treatment Reports* 1987; **62**: 865–72.

111. Powis G. Toxicity of free radical froming anticancer agents; In: Powis G, Hacker MP eds. *Toxicity of anticancer drugs*. New York: Pergamon Press, 1991: 113.

112. Herman EH, Ferrans VJ, Bhat HB, Witiak DT. Reduction of chronic doxorubicin cardiotoxicity in beagle dogs by bis-morpholinomethyl derivative of razoxane (ICRF-159). *Cancer Chemotherapy and Pharmacology* 1987; **19**: 277–81.

113. Speyer JL, Green MD. ICRF-187 permits longer treatment with doxorubicin in women with breast cancer. *Journal of Clinical Oncology* 1992; **10**(1): 117–27.

114. Whittaker JA, Al-Ismail SA. Effect of digoxin and vitamin E in preventing cardiac damage caused by doxorubicin in acute myeloid leukemia. *British Medical Journal* 1984; **288**: 283–4.

115. Unverferth DV, Jagadeesh JM, Unverferth MS, Magorien RD, Leier CV, Balcerzak SP. Attempts to prevent doxorubicin induced acute human myocardial morphologic damage with acetyl cysteine. *Journal of the National Cancer Institute* 1983; **71**: 917–20.

116. DeLeonardis V, Neri B *et al*. Reduction of cardiac toxicity of anthracyclines by L-carnitine – primary overview of clinical data. *International Journal of Clinical Pharmacology Research* 1985; **5**: 137–42.

117. Speyer JL, Green MD. ICRF-187 permits longer treatment with doxorubicin in women with breast cancer. *Journal of Clinical Oncology* 1992; **10**(1): 117–27.
118. Herman EH, Ferrans VJ, Bhat HB, Witiak DT. Reduction of chronic doxorubicin cardiotoxicity in beagle dogs by bis-morpholinomethyl derivative of razoxane (ICRF-159). *Cancer Chemotherapy and Pharmacology* 1987; **19**: 277–81.
119. Myers CE, Gianni L, Simone CB, Klecker R, Greene R. Oxidative destruction of erythrocyte ghost membranes catalyzed by the doxorubicin–iron complex. *Biochemistry* 1982; **21**: 1707.
120. Wadler S, Green MD, Muggia FM. Synergistic activity of doxorubicin and the bisdioxopiperazine (ICRF-187) against the murine sarcoma S-180 cell line. *Cancer Research* 1986; **46**: 1176–81.
121. Yeung TK, Jeffery WA, Long J, Wilding D, Hopewell JW, Creighton AM. ICRF 197: a new agent for protecting against drug-induced cardiotoxicity. *Annals of Oncology* 1992; **3**(Suppl. 1): abstract no. 222.
122. Myers CE, McGuire WP, Yeung R. Adriamycin amelioration of toxicity by alpha tocopherol. *Cancer Treatment Reports* 1976; **60**: 961–2.
123. Legha SS, Wang YM, Mackay B, Ewer M, Hortobagy GN, Benjamin RS, Ali MK. Clinical and pharmacologic investigation of the effects of α-tocopherol on Adriamycin cardiotoxicity. *Annals of the New York Academy of Sciences* 1982; **393**: 411.
124. Weitzman SA, Lorell B, Carey RW, Kaufman S, Stossel TP. Prospective study of tocopherol prophylaxis for anthracycline cardiac toxicity. *Current Therapeutic Research*.
125. Whittaker JA, Al-Ismail SA. Effect of digoxin and vitamin E in preventing cardiac damage caused by doxorubicin in acute myeloid leukemia. *British Medical Journal* 1984; **288**: 283–4.
126. Folkers K, Wolaniuk A. Research on coenzyme Q10 in clinical medicine an in immunomodulation. *Drugs Under Experimental and Clinical Research* 1985; **11**: 539–45.
127. Kraft J, Grille W, Appelt M *et al*. Effects of verapamil on anthracycline induced cardiomyopathy: preliminary results of a prospective multicenter trial. *Haematology and Blood Transfusion* 1990; **33**: 566–70.
128. Lenzhofer R, Ganzinger U, Rameis H, Moser K. Acute cardiac toxicity in patients after doxorubicin treatment and the effect of combined tocopherol and nifedipine pretreatment. *Journal of Cancer Research and Clinical Oncology* 1983; **106**: 143–7.
129. Weiss RB, Sarosy G, Clagett-Carr K, Russo M, Leyland-Jones B. Anthracycline analogs: the past, present and future. *Cancer Chemotherapy and Pharmacology* 1986; **18**: 185–97.
130. Posner LE, Dukart G, Goldberg J, Bernstein T, Cartwright K. Mitoxantrone: an overview of safety and toxicity. *Investigational New Drugs* 1985; **3**: 123–32.
131. Jain KK, Casper ES, Geller NL *et al*. A prospective randomized comparison of epirubicin and doxorubicin in patients with advanced breast cancer. *Journal of Clinical Oncology* 1985; **3**: 818–26.
132. Cassaza AM. Effects of modifications in position 4 of the chromaphore or in position 4 prime of the amino sugar on the anti-tumor activity and toxicity of daunarubicin and doxorubicin. In: Crook ST, Reich SD eds. *Anthracyclines: current status and new developments*. New York: Academic Press, 1980: 403–30.
133. Anders RJ, Shanes JG, Zeller FP. Lower incidence of doxorubicin-induced cardiomyopathy by once-a-week low-dose administration. *American Heart Journal* 1986; **111**: 755–9.
134. Hortobagyi GN, Frye D, Buzdar AU *et al*. Decreased cardiac toxicity of doxorubicin administered by continuous intravenous infusion in combination chemotherapy for metastatic breast carcinoma. *Cancer* 1989; **63**: 37–45.
135. Herman EH, Romman A *et al*. Prevention of chronic doxorubicin cardiotoxicity in beagles by liposomal encapsulation. *Cancer Research* 1983; **43**: 5427–32.

136. LaBianca R, Beretta G, Clerici M, Fraschini P, Luporini G. Cardiac toxicity of 5-fluorouracil: A study of 1,083 patients. *Tumori* 1982; **68**: 505–10.
137. Eskilsson J, Albertsson M. Failure of preventing 5-fluorouracil cardiotoxicity by prophylactic treatment with verapamil. *Acta Oncologica* 1990; **29**(8): 1001–3.
138. Rezkala S, Kloner RA, Ensley J, Al-Sarraf M, Revels S, Olivenstein A. *et al.* Continuous ambulatory ECG monitoring during fluorouracil therapy: A prospective study. *Journal of Clinical Oncology* 1989; **7**: 509–14.
139. Gottdiener JS, Appelbaum FR, Ferrans VJ, Deisseroth A, Ziegler J. Cardiotoxicity with high dose cyclophosphamide therapy. *Archives of Internal Medicine* 1981; **141**: 758–63.
140. Santos GW, Sensenbrenner LL, Burke PJ *et al.* Marrow transplantation in man following cyclophosphamide. *Transplantation Proceedings* 1971; **3**: 400–4.
141. Foley GE, Freedman OM, Drolet BP. Studies in the mechanism of activation of cytoxan – evidence of activation *in vivo* and *in vitro*. *Cancer Research* 1961; **21**: 57–63.
142. Margolin KA, Rayner AA, Hawkins MJ *et al.* Interleukin 2 in lymphokine activated killer cell therapy of solid tumors: Analysis of toxicity and management guidelines. *Journal of Clinical Oncology* 1989; **7**: 486–98.
143. Sonnenblick M, Rosin A. Cardiotoxicity of interferon: review of 44 cases. *Chest* **99**(3): 557–61.
144. Stefenelli T, Kuzmits R. Acute vascular toxicity after combination chemotherapy with cisplatin, vinblastin and bleomycin for vesticular cancer. *European Heart Journal* 1988; **9**: 552–6.
145. Weiss RB, Muggia FM. Cytotoxic drug induced pulmonary disease update. *American Journal of Medicine* 1980; **68**: 259–66.
146. Kayser K, Gabius HJ, Carl S *et al.* Alterations in human lung parenchyma after cytostatic therapy. *APMIS* 1991; **99**: 121–8.
147. Wells JD, Huskison WT, Davenport OL. Gallium citrate Ga 67 accumulation in pulmonary lesions after chemotherapy (MOPP). *Southern Medical Journal* 1986; **79**(10): 1293–5.
148. Catane R, Swade JG, Turrisi AT *et al.* Pulmonary toxicity after radiation and bleomycin: a review. *Radiation Oncology, Biology and Physics* 1979; **5**: 1513–18.
149. Blum RH, Carter SK, Agre K. A clinical review of bleomycin – a new anti-neoplastic agent. *Cancer* 1973; **31**: 903.
150. Cooper AD, White DA, Matthay RA. State of the art of drug-induced pulmonary disease. *American Review of Respiratory Diseases* 1986; **133**: 321–40.
151. Jensen JL, Goel R, Venner PM. The effect of corticosteroid administration on bleomycin lung toxicity. *Cancer* 1990; **65**(6): 1291–7.
152. Hay J, Haslam PL, Staple LH, Laurent GJ. Role of iron and oxygen in bleomycin induced pulmonary edema. In: Altura ABM, Davis E eds. *Advances in microcirculation*, Basel, Switzerland: Karger, vol. 13. 1987: 239–55.
153. Padmanabahn RV, Gudapaty R, Liener IE, Schwartz BA, Hoidal JR. Protection against pulmonary oxygen toxicity in rats by the intratracheal administration of liposome encapsulated super oxide dismutase or catalase. *American Review of Respiratory Diseases* 1985; **132**: 164–7.
154. Hay J, Shahzeidi S, Laurent G. Mechanisms of bleomycin-induced lung damage. *Archives of Toxicology* 1991; **65**: 89.
155. Toledo CH, Ross WE, Hood CI, Block ER. Potentiation of bleomycin toxicity to oxygen. *Cancer Treatment Reports* 1982; **66**(2): 359–62.
156. Nagy B, Grdina DJ. Protective effects of 2[(aminopropyl)amino] ethanethiol against bleomycin and nitrogen mustard-induced mutagenicity in V79 cells. *International Journal of Radiation Oncology, Biology Physics* 1986; **12**: 1475–8.
157. Ward HE, Nicholson A. Desferrioxamine infusion does not inhibit bleomycin-induced lung damage in the rat. *American Review of Respiratory Diseases* 1986; **133**: 317.

158. Hay J, Shahzeidi S, Laurent G. Mechanisms of bleomycin-induced lung damage. *Archives of Toxicology* 1991; **65**: 81–94.
159. McLeod BV, Lawrence J, Smith DW *et al.* Fatal bleomycin toxicity from a low cumulative dose in a patient with renal insufficiency. *Cancer* 1987; **60**: 2617–20.
160. Luisetti M, Pozzi E *et al.* Ambroxol and bleomycin-induced pulmonary toxicity: experimental and clinical aspects. Paper presented at the *First International Symposium on Organ Directed Toxicities of Anticancer Drugs*, 1987: 57.
161. Sikich BI. Bleomycin chemotherapy. In: Sikic BI, Rozencweig M, Carter SK eds. *Bleomycin Chemotherapy.* New York: Academic Press, 1985: 247–54.
162. Villani F, Pizzini L, Rossi D. Evaluation of pulmonary toxicity induced by pepleomycin. *Tumori* 1988; **74**: 429–32.
163. Doll DC, Weiss RB, Issel BF. Mitomycin: 10 years after approval. *Marketing Journal of Clinical Oncology* 1985; **3**: 276–86.
164. Chang A, Kuebler J, Phillip, Pandya KJ *et al.* Pulmonary toxicity induced by mitomycin C is highly responsive to glucocorticoids. *Cancer* 1986; **57**: 2285–90.
165. Gaetani P, Silvani V, Butti G, Spanu G, Rossi A, Knerich R. Nitrosourea derivatives – induced pulmonary toxicity in patients treated for malignant brain tumors. Early subclinical detection and its prevention. *European Journal of Cancer Clinical Oncology* 1987; **23**: 267–71.
166. Hankins DG, Sanders S, MacDonald FM *et al.* Pulmonary toxicity recurring after a six week course of busulfan therapy and after subsequent therapy with uracil mustard. *Chest* 1978; **73**: 415–16.
167. Patell JM, Block ER, Hood CR. Biochemical indices of cyclophosphamide-induced lung toxicity. *Toxicology and Applied Pharmacology* 1984; **76**: 128–38.
168. Baker WJ, Fistell SJ, Jones RV *et al.* Interstitial pneumonitis associated with hyphosphamide therapy. *Cancer* 1990; **65**: 2217–21.
169. Sostman HD, Matthay RA, Putman CE, Smith GJW. Methotrexate-induced pneumonitis. *Medicine* 1976; **55**: 371–88.
170. Glauser FL, DeBlois G, Bechard D, Flower AA, Merchant R, Fairman P. Review of cardiopulmonary toxicity of adoptive immunotherapy. *American Journal of Medical Science* 1988; **296**: 406–12.
171. Herrmann F, Schulz G. Hematopoetic responses in patients with advanced malignancy treated with recombinant human GMCSF. *Journal of Clinical Oncology* 1989; **7**: 159–67.
172. Deschner C, Lipkim D. Proliferation and differentiation of gastrointestinal cells in relation to therapy. *Medical Clinics of North America* 1975; **55**: 601–12.
173. Mitchell EP, Schein PS. Gastrointestinal toxicity of chemotherapeutic agents. In: Perry Michael C ed. *The chemotherapy source book.* New York: Williams & Wilkins 1992: 620–34.
174. Jacobs WA. Methotrexate: clinical pharmacology; current status and therapeutic guidelines. *Cancer Treatment Reviews* 1977; **4**: 87–101.
175. Houghton JA, Houghton PJ, Wooten RS. Mechanism of induction of gastrointestinal toxicity in the mouse by 5-fluorouracil, 5-fluorouradine and 5-fluoro-2'-deoxyuradine. *Cancer Research* 1979; **39**: 2406.
176. Klubes P, Cerna I. Use of uridine rescue to enhance the antitumor selectivity of 5-fluorouracil. *Cancer Research* 1983; **43**: 3183–6.
177. Phillips TL, Kane L, Utley JF. Radioprotection of tumor in normal tissues by thiophosphate compounds. *Cancer* 1973; **32**: 528–35.
178. Wu GY, Wu CH, Stockert RJ *et al.* Model for specific rescue of normal hepatocytes during methotrexate treatment of hepatic malignancy. *Proceedings of the National Academy of Sciences, USA* 1983; **80**: 3078–80.
179. Dubois A. Aspects of radiation induced gastrointestinal injury. *Radioprotection, Pharmacology and Therapeutics* 1988; **39**: 67–72.
180. Ortin TT, Shostak CA, Donaldson SS. Gonadal status and reproductive function following treatment for Hodgkin's disease in childhood. The Stanford experience. *International Journal of Radiation Oncology, Biology, Physics* 1990; **19**(4): 1099.

181. Charak BS, Gupta R, Mandrekar P *et al.* Testicular dysfunction after cyclophosphamide, vincristine, procarbazine and prednisone chemotherapy for advanced Hodgkin's Disease. *Cancer* 1990; **65**(9): 1903–6.
182. Fairley KF, Barrie JU, Johnson W. Sterility and testicular atrophy related to cyclophosphamide therapy. *Lancet* 1972; **1**: 568–9.
183. Anselmo AP, Cartoni C, Bellantuono P, Maurizi-Envich R, Aboulkair N, Ermini M. Risk of infertility in patients with Hodgkin's disease treated with ABVD versus ABVD/MOPP. *Haematologica* 1990; **75**(2): 155–8.
184. Redman JR, Bajorunas DR, Goldstein MC *et al.* Semen preservation and artificial insemination for Hodgkin's disease. *Journal of Clinical Oncology* 1987; **2**: 233–8.
185. Stewart NS, Woodroffe CM, Grundy R, Cullen MH. Long-term toxicity of chemotherapy for testicular cancer: The cost of cure. *British Journal of Cancer* 1990; **3**: 479–84.
186. Hansen SW, Berthelsen JG, von-der-Maase H. Long-term fertility in Leydig cell function in patients treated for germ cell cancer with cisplatin, vinblastine and bleomycin versus surveillance. *Journal of Clinical Oncology* 1990: **10**: 1695–8.
187. Tsatsoulis A, Shalet SM, Morris ID, de Kretser DM. Immunoactive inhabin as a marker of Sertoli cell function following cytotoxic damage to the human testes. *Hormone Research* 1990; **34**: 254–9.
188. Aass N, Fossa SD, Theodorsen L, Norman N. Prediction of long-term gonadal toxicity after standard treatment for testicular cancer. *European Journal of Cancer* 1991; **9**: 1087–91.
189. Fossa SD, Klepp O. Lack of gonadal protection by medroxy progesterone acetate induced transient medical castration during chemotherapy for testicular cancer. *British Journal of Urology* 1988; **5**: 449–53.
190. Kreuser ED, Hetzel WD, Hautmann R, Pfeiffer EF. Reproductive toxicity with and without LHRHA administration during adjuvant chemotherapy in patients with germ cell tumors. *Hormone, Metabolic Research* 1990; **22**(9): 494–8.
191. Gradishar WJ, Schilsky RL. Effects of cancer treatment on the reproductive system. *Critical Reviews in Oncology and Hematology* 1988; **8**(2): 153–71.
192. Waxman JH, Ahmed R, Smith D *et al.* Failure to preserve fertility in patients with Hodgkin's Disease. *Cancer Chemotherapy Pharmacology* 1987; **19**: 159–62.
193. Horstman MG, Meadows GG, Yost GS. Separate mechanisms for procarbazenes spermatotoxicity in anticancer activity. *Cancer Research* 1987; **47**: 1547–50.
194. Clifton DK, Bremner WJ. The effect of testicular radiation on spermatogenesis in man. *Journal of Andrology* 1983; **4**: 387–92.
195. Chapman R. Gonadal toxicity and teratogenicity. In: Perry Michael C ed. *The chemotherapy source book*. Baltimore: Williams & Wilkins, 1992, 710–53.
196. Gatsanis E, Shapiro RS. Thyroid dysfunction following bone marrow transplantation long term follow-up of eighty pediatric patients. *Journal of Bone Marrow Transplantation* 1990; **5**: 335–40.
197. Livesey EA, Hindmarsh PC. Endocrine disorders following treatment of childhood brain tumors. *British Journal of Cancer* 1990; **4**: 622–5.
198. Kantarjian HM, Keating MJ. Therapy related leukemia and myelodisplastic syndrome, *Seminars in Oncology* 1987; **14**(4): 435–43.
199. Rieche K. Carcinogenicity of antineoplastic agents in man. *Cancer Treatment Reviews* 1984; **11**: 39–67.
200. Kyle, R. Seond malignancies associated with chemotherapeutic agents. *Seminars in Oncology* 1982; **9**: 131–42.
201. Milas L, Hunter N, Stephens LC, Peters L. Inhibition of radiation carcinogenesis in mice by S-2-(3-aminopropylamino)-ethylphosphorothioic acid. *Cancer Research* 1984; **44**: 5567–69.
202. Grdina DJ, Nagy B, Sigdestad CP. Radioprotectors in the treatment therapy to reduce risk in seconday tumor induction. *Pharmacology and Therapeutics* 1988; **39**: 21–5.

CHAPTER 4

Chronopharmacology and avoidance of anticancer drug toxicity

ROTISLAV VYZULA, GEORG A BJARNASON AND WILLIAM JM HRUSHESKY

INTRODUCTION

The primary goal of clinical pharmacology is to develop a rational basis for the treatment of disease. In oncology, highly toxic agents are used that possess narrow therapeutic indices and so the effective use of chemotherapeutic agents requires a higher level of pharmacologic understanding than in any other sub-speciality of internal medicine.

The objective of this chapter is to provide fundamental information on drug toxicity in humans which is dependent upon the optimal circadian timing of the administration of many important anticancer drugs. Safe drug use requires a few initial steps: (1) determination of safe dosage range; (2) choice of an appropriate route of administration; (3) awareness of the incidence and course of potentially life-threatening toxicities; (4) awareness of routes of drug elimination and adjustment of dose to accommodate organ dysfunction; and (5) knowledge of drug–host interactions as influenced by their circadian timing to maximize favorable efficacy and minimize toxicity. Each of these points should be considered in developing a new anticancer therapy or in using any unfamiliar protocol for the first time. This brief article focuses solely upon the circadian scheduling of cytotoxic therapy.

CHRONOBIOLOGY

Quantitative study of biodynamics clearly demonstrates that all biophysical and biochemical processes vary with respect to time in a regular and predictable periodic manner across several rhythmic frequencies.[1,2] In 1647, the Italian scientist Sanctorius constructed a huge balance, where he could sit each day as he took his meals. For roughly 30 years he weighed himself several times each day, and noted regular changes in his physical condition. He found that his weight fluctuated with daily rhythms that paralleled the rise and set of the sun and his weight also fluctuated on a 30-day cycle and this was accompanied by a similar reflection in the turbidity of his urine.

Biological rhythms have since been established for a wide range of species. Recently additional hard evidence for the existence of endogenous biological rhythms and for precise molecular time-keeping mechanisms, 'clock genes', first documented for *Drosophila melanogaster* by Konopka and Benzer,[3] has been produced.

CIRCADIAN CHRONOPHARMACOLOGY OF ANTINEOPLASTIC AGENTS

A better understanding of temporal changes in drug effects as a function of the agents' circadian timing is achievable by considering two important concepts: first, the reproducible temporal changes in the biological handling of drugs, their chronopharmacokinetics, and second, the temporal variation in the sensitivity of target tissues to these drugs, their chronopharmacodynamics. From a practical point of view, the expression of a drug effect will depend on what stage of a programmed function is featured when the agent reaches the cell. Thus chrono-pharmacologists are confronted with new facts that need to be explained to and understood by traditionally schooled physiologists and pharmacologists. Chronopharmacokinetics and chronopharmacodynamics redefine the dynamics of pharmacology and adjust them to present knowledge as it applies to circadian change in drug handling and drug action.

Chronopharmacokinetics

Chronopharmacokinetics is the study of the reproducible and predictable temporal variation in absorption, distribution, metabolism and elimination of drugs. The chronopharmacokinetic behavior of over 100 drugs has been described in animals and humans.[4] Non-trivial temporal variations have been documented in drug absorption and distribution,[5] metabolism,[6] and excretion.[7,8] This has been well-documented *in vivo* for many drugs metabolized through the P-450 system, probably due to reproducible within-day temporal variation in the microsomal concentration of the various P-450 isoenzymes. Reproducible circadian variation has also been documented in the activity of at least thirteen major hepatic drug-metabolizing enzyme systems, including those responsible for hepatic glucuronidation and sulfatation, as well as glutathione conjugation.[9,10]

Chronopharmacodynamics

Rhythmic changes in the susceptibility of a biosystem are well documented for many cytoxic agents, both *in vivo* and *in vitro*, for cells removed at specific circadian phases. Sometimes the susceptibility can be explained and quantified in terms of bioperiodic changes in the concentration of receptors of a given system for a given drug,[11–13] or the cellular defense mechanisms such as oxygen free-radical defense mechanisms, such as glutathione and the concentration of other non-protein-bound sulfhydryl compounds.[14–17]

Chronotoxicology is the best-documented domain of chronopharmacology.[18–25] How to increase the tolerance of an anticancer agent is a critical question for oncologists. Chronotherapeutic approaches have already been adapted for agents such as corticoids, non-steroid anti-inflammatory drugs, antihistamines and theophyllines.

Modern chronopharmacology investigates drugs' effects (a) as a function of biological timing and (b) upon parameters characterizing the endogenous bioperiodicities. Chronopharmacologists now face a new challenge in the search for reliable markers of rhythms: to find the circadian rhythm parameters (e.g. acrophase) of variables to guide chronotherapy, and to estimate the chronophysiological status of each patient.

The clinical investigations of circadian optimization of chemotherapy have to date been based upon prior findings in murine models. Murine data demonstrating 'best administration times' that diminish side-effects are currently available for twenty antineoplastic agents. Some data are also available for time dependent tumor control in mouse and rat models.

FLUOROPYRIMIDINES

Floxuridine and 5-fluorouridine preclinical studies

Animal studies have shown floxuridine (FUDR) bolus[26] and continuous infusion[27] to be highly circadian-stage dependent both with regard to toxicity and antitumor activity. Single boluses of FUDR in doses from 1000 mg/kg to 2000 mg/kg were given at one of six equally distributed circadian stages to more than 300 CD2F1 mice. The best tolerance was found in the daily late activity span [18–20 hours after daily light onset (HALO)].

Roemeling and Hrushesky performed a preclinical study with seven equal doses of intravenous continuous-infusion FUDR infused either at a variable rate or at a constant rate in female F344 rats.[28] For the variable-rate infusion, peaking at six different times, the daily dose of FUDR was divided into four 6-hour portions of 68 per cent, 15 per cent, 2 per cent and 15 per cent to achieve a quasisinusoidal pattern. Rats receiving FUDR either by variable-rate infusion with the peak between late activity and early daily sleep at (22–04 HALO) or by constant-rate infusion lived significantly longer than rats receiving FUDR by variable-rate infusion with peaks at other circadian stages. Autopsies revealed toxic affects to the intestines and bone marrow as causes of death. The circadian infusion pattern peaking late in the daily activity phase was better tolerated and had superior antitumor activity than a constant infusion against a transplanted tumor.

Gonzales et al.[29] concurrently tested the lethal toxicity of a single intraperitoneal 5-fluorouridine (5-FU) and FUDR bolus injection at one of six different time points in Balb-c mice. 5-FU was least toxic in late rest (10 HALO), whereas FUDR was least toxic in early rest (2 HALO).

Gardner and Plumb[30] found that the impairment of water absorption by small intestine *in vitro* and the incidence of diarrhea *in vivo* differed as a function of treatment time when 5-FU was given to rats. The intestinal toxicity was minimal after treatment in late activity (19 HALO) when the maximum number of small intestine mucosa cells were in the postmitotic resting phase (G_1) and less susceptible to the effects from 5-FU.

FUDR and 5-FU clinical studies

Roemeling and Hrushesky compared a circadian patterned variable-rate infusion of 5-fluoro-2'-deoxyuridine (floxuridine, FUDR) with a maximal flow rate in the late afternoon/early evening and minimum flow rate during the early morning hours to a constant rate infusion in fifty-four patients with widespread cancer.[31] The daily drug dose was divided into four portions: 15 per cent (from 9.00 to 15.00), 68 per cent (15.00–21.00), 15 per cent (21.00–3.00), 2 per cent (3.00–9.00). Results were: 50 per cent of patients on constant-rate infusion had nausea or vomiting versus 19 per cent on time-modified infusion. Ninety-three per cent of those on constant-rate infusion had diarrhea of mild to severe grade versus 6 per cent of the patients on variable-rate infusion, whose toxicity was only mild. Even at high dose intensity, cumulative drug toxicity was absent for bone marrow, heart, kidney, lungs and liver. Patients receiving time-modified FUDR infusion tolerated an average of > 1.45-fold more drug per unit time while evincing minimal toxicity. FUDR infusion was found to have activity against progressive metastatic renal cell cancer (RCC).

In another study Hrushesky *et al.* treated sixty-eight unselected patients with progressive metastatic RCC with continuous circadian infusion FUDR.[32] Thirty-seven per cent of these patients had previously received and failed systemic treatment. Using implantable pumps for autonomic drug delivery, FUDR was continously infused for 14 days at monthly intervals. Complete responses (CR; 7.1 per cent); and partial responses (PR; 12.5 per cent) were observed (objective response rate, CR + PR = 19.6 per cent). In a subgroup of seven assessable patients receiving hepatic arterial FUDR, they observed one CR and three PRs (CR + PR = 57.2 per cent).

The clinical data available indicate that the combination of 5-FU and leucovorin (LV) is more effective in shrinking tumors than 5-FU alone in patients with metastatic colorectal cancer. In a phase II trial in patients with metastatic colorectal cancer, 5-FU, LV and oxaliplatin were infused continuously for 5 days every 3 weeks. Oxaliplatin was infused for 12 hours with peak delivery at 4 pm, and 5-FU and LV were infused concurrently for 12 hours with peak delivery at 4 pm. Objective response was seen in 58 per cent.

This circadian regimen has now been compared to a flat delivery of the same drugs in a prospective phase III clinical trial in 186 patients with metastatic colorectal cancer.[33] Patients on the circadian arm had less toxicity with regard to both stomatitis (Grade 3–4 in 15 per cent vs. 75 per cent, $P < 0.0001$), hand–foot syndrome ($P < 0.03$), neutropenia ($p < 0.03$) and neuropathy (15 per cent vs. 29 per cent, $P < 0.05$). In spite of less toxicity, the median dose intensity (mg/m^2 per week) for 5-FU over six planned cycles was significantly higher on the circadian arm (1013 vs. 815, $P = 0.00001$). The objective response rate was also significantly better on the circadian arm (49.5 per cent vs. 30 per cent, $P = 0.007$).

Bjarnason *et al.* determined the maximum tolerated dose (MTD: ≥ 50 per cent of patients with ≥ grade 2 toxicity) for 5-FU and LV, given as a continuous circadian infusion over 14 days, with 64 per cent of the daily dose given over 7 hours around 3–4 a.m.[34] LV was first escalated by 5 mg/m^2 per day to 20 mg/m^2 per day, followed by escalation of 5-FU by 50mg/m^2 per day. Patients who developed ≥ grade 2 toxicity had the peak of the infusion shifted from 3–4 a.m. to 9–10 p.m., to determine if this reduced toxicity. In six patients developing ≥ grade 2 toxicity the peak of the infusion was shifted to 9–10 p.m. Toxicity was reduced in all six and further dose escalation was possible in three patients. This study demonstrates the potential fallacy of relying solely on experimental data to determine the optimal time of drug delivery in clinical trials.

Mechanism responsible for fluoropyrimidine circadian pharmacodynamics

Serial biopsies of rectal mucosa every 3 hours for 24 hours from twenty-four human volunteers in both the fed and fasted states, reveal that there is a much greater *in vitro* uptake of [^{3}H]thymidine (presumably reflecting DNA synthesis) in colonic epithelial cells removed during the early morning hours (4 hours prior to usual awakening) than later in the day and evening.[35] This circadian stage coincidence of minimal [^{3}H]thymidine uptake and minimal FUDR toxicity in colon epithelial cells is intriguing and warrants further study.

Both 5-FU and FUDR are most active against cells undergoing DNA synthesis. DNA synthesis in all tissues studied throughout the circadian cycle is not randomly distributed throughout the day.[36] Depending on dose and duration of infusion, the gut, skin, and bone marrow are the primary targets of fluoropyrimidine toxicity. Human skin, bone marrow, and human colorectal mucosa have each been found to exhibit marked circadian rhythms in DNA synthesis.[37]

The activites of the enzymes important in the activation of FUDR to FdUMP (i.e. dehydrouracil dehydrogenase, uridine phosphorylase and thymidine phosphorylase) have been shown to be subject to circadian rhythms in mouse liver;[38] however, assessment of the exact contribution of these enzymes to the crisp, high-amplitude circadian rhythm in FUDR toxicity and efficacy requires further work in murine and human systems.

The activity of dihydropyrimidine dehydrogenase (DPD), the rate-limiting enzyme for fluoropyrimidine catabolism, is highly circadian stage-dependent ($P < 0.0001$) in liver,[39] with a peak in late rest (10 HALO). Harris has subsequently shown that this leads to a circadian variation of 5-FU catabolism in the isolated perfused rat liver with the peak and trough elimination rates of 5-FU in late activity (19 HALO) and mid-rest (7 HALO) respectively. There was a reciprocal relationship between the elimination rates of 5-FU and 5-FU catabolites.[40]

ANTHRACYCLINES (ALONE OR IN COMBINATION WITH OTHER AGENTS)

Doxorubicin preclinical study

Early chronotoxicity studies of intraperitoneal doxorubicin in hybrid mice and F344 rats[41] demonstrated its profound circadian pharmacodynamics. When doxorubicin was given in early activity (14 HALO), it was much better tolerated than when given in early rest (2 HALO).

Hrushesky *et al.*[42] described two studies using lower doses of doxorubicin and cisplatin. Drug effects on the host and tumor were tested at six different circadian stages. Study 1 was designed primarily to test the effect of doxorubicin as a single agent at each of six different circadian stages. Study 2 was designed to test the effect of doxorubicin adminstered only at the best circadian stages. Study 2 was designed to test the effect of doxorubicin administered only at the best circadian time in combination with cisplatin at one of six different circadian stages. In study 1 least weight loss, e.g. toxicity, occurred following treatment at 10 HALO (late night), while most weight loss was observed after treatment at 22 HALO (late dark). In study 2, different timing of cisplatin resulted in the least weight loss at 14 and 18 HALO, while most weight loss occurred following treatment at 2 and 6 HALO. More rats survived longer if they were treated with doxorubicin at 10 HALO (just before daily awakening) in combination with cisplatin at 18 HALO (late afternoon for humans). Several studies by other investigators have confirmed these findings.

Clinical study

Hrushesky *et al.* have also carried out a clinical study of these agents.[42] The patients had advanced malignancy (ovarian cancer and transitional cell cancer of the bladder). The first clinical study was performed to test two different circadian time schedules of the same combination of doxorubicin and cisplatin with equal doses and drug sequence. This first clinical protocol randomized intial doxorubicin treatment time between 06.00 and 18.00. Cisplatin followed each doxorubicin infusion by 12 hours. Cisplatin-induced nephrotocixity was statistically greater following morning cisplatin administration compared to evening administration. Bone marrow toxicity (neutropenia and thrombocytopenia) was less when doxorubicin was given at 06.00 and cisplatin 18.00 than when the doxorubicin was given at 18.00 followed by cisplatin at 06.00. The morning doxorubicin schedule resulted in statistically significantly less depressed nadir counts and in full recovery of all counts to pretreatment levels. Those patients who received cisplatin at 06.00 had more vomiting episodes, which tended to begin sooner and last longer.

In another non-crossover study in patients with ovarian cancer, circadian schedule A was morning doxorubicin followed by evening cisplatin; schedule B was evening doxorubicin followed by morning cisplatin. Because of leukopenia, most patients treated on schedule B had to have greater than 33 per cent doxorubicin dose reduction and many of them had to have treatment delays of greater than 2 weeks as opposed to those on schedule A. Less nephrotoxicity was seen when cisplatin was given at 18.00 as compared to 06.00. Neurotoxicity, chronic anemia, and transfusion requirement were each statistically signifcantly different in favor of morning doxorubicin and evening cisplatin.[43]

Mechanism

The explanation for the mechanism of circadian toxicity differences for doxorubicin may be secondary to its activation into a free-radical intermediate. The availability of the main free-radical scavenger, reduced glutathione, is circadian-stage dependent, with peak levels at the time of lowest drug toxicity.[44,45] Some of the bone marrow toxicity and all of the cardiac toxicity of doxorubicin may be related to the NADPH-dependent, doxorubicin semiquinone-mediated generation of free-radicals, such as hydroxyl and superoxide anions,[46] that can be detoxified by a number of pathways, primarily the glutathione cycle. A circadian rhythm of several-fold in amplitude in the level of total glutathione and GSH in cardiac tissue has been documented in mice[16] and rats,[47] with highest levels in the early activity span, corresponding to the time of lowest lethal toxicity of IV doxorubicin in these animals.

For cisplatin, the mechanism of circadian toxicity is thought to be related to the kidney. Both normal kidney function and cisplatin pharmacokinetics are circadian-stage dependent.[48,49] It has been shown in rats that mortality results from nephrotoxicity. This was proven by monitoring blood urea and by microscopic section of the severely damaged kidneys. Kidney damage was most extensive in the proximal convoluted tubules. A brush border lysosomal enzyme, β-N-acetylglucosaminidase (NAG), was found to be released into the urine proportionately to the degree of renal dysfunction induced by cisplatin. This enzyme was present in urine in normal animals, and its baseline concentration was found to display a high-amplitude circadian rhythm. If cisplatin was given at a favorable circadian stage, these rats did not demonstrate much NAG rise and had little renal damage with only a small rise in blood urea nitrogen (BUN).[42]

Cytosine arabinoside

A single fixed dose of cytosine arabinoside (ara-C) administered daily for 6 days to mice, was found to be least toxic when given in the rest span (2.5–7 HALO). The same dose of ara-C killed 15 per cent of the animals if given in the rest span compared to 75 per cent if given in the activity span.[50,51] Haus et al.[65] applied this finding to the treatment of leukemic mice. In one group of animals the doses at the various injection times varied in amount according to a sinusoidal pattern, and another group of animals received the same total doses. A doubling of survival was observed in the sinusoidally treated group (23 per cent) as compared to the group given constant doses (11 per cent). Hromas et al.[52] used flow cytometry to look at the effect of ara-C on the chronobiology of the bone marrow DNA synthesis in mice. At all times, ara-C flattened the rhythm of bone marrow DNA synthesis; however, it had its greatest effect if given when there were relatively more cells moving into S-phase (18 HALO) or in S-phase (0 HALO) as compared to when few cells were in S-phase (12 HALO) or when cells were leaving S-phase (6 HALO).

When vincristine was added to the best schedule of ara-C and cyclophosphamide described above, best results (52 per cent cure rate) were achieved when vincristine was given in late activity (23 HALO). When methylprednisolone was added to this three-drug scheme, best results where obtained when prednisolone was given in early activity (11 HALO or 14 HALO).[53] No clinical studies have followed up these exciting results.

Methotrexate

Intravenous methotrexate was found to be most toxic in rats in late activity (23.5 HALO), with least toxicity in terms of marrow, renal and liver toxicity in mid-activity (17.5 HALO).[54] The time of day of maximum toxicity coincided with the nadir for plasma corticosterone concentration. In subsequent studies by the same authors high plasma levels of exogenously administered corticosterone protected against methotrexate toxicity, whereas suppressed levels markedly increased toxicity unrelated to time.[55] Additionally, giving oral melatonin daily for 6 weeks, prior to methotrexate treatment, increased its toxicity at all time points.[56]

6-Mercaptopurine and methotrexate

The course of 118 children with acute lymphoblastic leukemia (ALL), who had achieved complete remission with a standard induction protocol and had also received meningeal prophylaxis with intrathecal methotrexate and cranial irradiation, was reviewed.[57] Maintenance therapy consisted of daily 6-mercaptopurine (6-MP), weekly methotrexate (MTX), and monthly vincristine and prednisone. For compliance reasons, eighty-two children took their 6-MP and MTX in the morning and thirty-six children took these medications in the evening. Regression analysis showed that, for those children surviving free of disease for longer than 78 weeks, the risk of relapsing was 4.6 times greater for the morning schedule than for the evening schedule ($P = 0.006$).

The antileukemic effect of 6-MP is related to the incorporation of 6-MP-derived nucleotides (6-TGN) into DNA. The red blood cell concentration of 6-TGN achieved after a standard dose of 6-MP was very variable, not correlated with the dose of 6-MP, but predictive of outcome in children on maintenance therapy (6-MP given in the morning after overnight fasting) for ALL.[58] Thus giving a constant dose of MTX and 6-MP, without modification with regard to achieved serum concentrations or induced toxicity, may expose these children to very different amounts of drugs over time, and can impact on their ultimate prognosis.

Plant alkaloids

The time for least toxicity in mice varies considerably for agents in this class. Vincristine[59] is least toxic in early activity (13 HALO); vinblastine[60] is least toxic in mid-activity (18 HALO). Etoposide[61] is best tolerated in late rest (7–11 HALO). It should be noted, however, that the solvent for VP-16 was more toxic to rodents than the combination of solvent and VP-16,[62] and therefore these data may not truly reflect the circadian pharmacodynamics of VP-16. The toxic responses to both the VP-16 + solvent and solvent alone were time-dependent and the lethality patterns were about 180° out of phase with one another. Focan et al.,[63] have demonstrated a circadian variation in vindesine serum concentration in nine patients receiving this drug as a 48-hour continuous constant-rate infusion, with peak at about mid-day. In a study of thirty-four patients receiving cisplatin (given at 6 p.m. daily for 3 days) and etoposide (given at either 7 a.m. or 7 p.m. daily for 3 days), less hematological toxicity was found in the group receiving etoposide at 7 a.m.[64]

PRACTICAL IMPLICATIONS

Preclinical and clinical trials carried out to date have confirmed that optimal timing of chemotherapy can lead to decreased toxicity. This is certainly a very important finding in this era of heightened interest in the quality of life of cancer patients. Several clinical studies have clearly demonstrated that maximal safe dose intensity is also dependent upon the time of drug therapy. There are compelling experimental data suggesting that the therapeutic index of commonly applied anticancer agents can be improved by the optimal circadian timing of treatment. Additional prospective randomized studies are required to demonstrate if a better response rate and/or survival can be achieved in patients given chemotherapy based on these principles.

Toxicity is an important end-point in itself in patients receiving chemotherapy. Chemotherapy-induced toxicity impacts on the quality of life for these patients and increases costs for the health-care system. Even if we observe similar response rates but less toxicity, by using chronochemotherapy, something important has been gained. Toxicity becomes a very important issue with regard to adjuvant treatment. A large proportion of patients receiving adjuvant treatment are not destined to have recurrence of their cancer, but receive adjuvant chemotherapy as an insurance policy against future relapse. It is therefore very important to be able to offer patients in this situation both a safe and effective chemotherapy.

Evidence from studies with chronochemotherapy, both in animals and humans, confirms that this scheduling method reduces bone marrow toxicity and also other types of toxicity such as gastrointestinal and renal toxicity. This scheduling method therefore offers the possibility of giving more dose-intensive chemotherapy without more toxicity, and could work well in conjunction with other strategies for high-dose chemotherapy. It should be noted that dose intensity is in itself a time-dependent variable, since both the pharmacokinetics and pharmacodynamics of the major anticancer agents are dependent on the time of delivery. This fact complicates even further the practice of dose-intensity calculations.

We are still at an early stage with regard to understanding the mechanisms responsible for circadian dependency of toxicity and efficacy. Interindividual variation in the best timing for certain drugs is a potential problem. Ideally the best treatment time should be determined for each individual according to measurable internal marker rhythms. More work is needed in this area to optimize the benefits of chronochemotherapy for each patient.

In summary, the circadian timing of anticancer drugs markedly affects their pharmacology, toxicology and efficacy. In giving cytotoxic cancer therapy without regard to its circadian timing, as in the case of continuous infusions, the timing of the peak drug infusion rate will result in apparently variable and poorly reproducible therapeutic results and unnecessary drug toxicity. This simple strategy can with little or no delay improve the quality of life of every cancer patient currently receiving cytotoxic therapy with the agents that have to date been studied.

REFERENCES

1. Aschoff J. Comparative physiology; diurnal rhythms. *Annual Review of Physiology* 1963; **25** 581.
2. Bünning E. *Die physiologische Uhr.* Berlin: Springer-Verlag, 1963.
3. Konopka RJ, Benzer S. Clock mutants of *Drosophila melanogaster. Proceedings of the National Academy of Sciences, USA* 1971; **68**(9): 2112–16.
4. Reinberg A, Smolensky MH. Circadian changes of drug disposition in man. *Clinical Pharmacokinetics* 1982; **7**: 401–20.
5. Bruguerolle B. Temporal aspects of drug absorption and drug distribution. In: Lemmer B ed. *Chronopharmacology: cellular and biochemical interactions.* New York: Marcel Dekker, 1989: 3–13.
6. Belanger MP, Labreque G. Temporal aspects of drug metabolism. In: Lemmer B ed. *Chronopharmacology: cellular and biochemical interactions.* New York Marcel Dekker, 1989: 15–34.
7. Waterhouse JM, Minors DS. Temporal aspects of renal drug elimination. In: Lemmer B ed. *Chronopharmacology: cellular and biochemical interactions.* New York: Marcel Dekker, 1989: 35–50.
8. Koopman MG, Krediet RT, Arisz L. Circadian rhythms and the kidney. *Netherlands Journal of Medicine* 1985; **28**: 416–23.
9. North C, Feuers RJ, Scheving LE, Pauli JE, Tsai TH, Casciano DA. Circadian organization of thirteen liver and six brain enzymes of the mouse. *American Journal of Anatomy* 1981; **162**: 184–99.
10. Radzialowski FM, Bousquet WF. Daily rhythmic variation in hepatic drug metabolism in rat and mouse. *Journal of Pharmacology and Experimental Therapeutics* 1968; **163** (1): 229–38.
11. Hughes A, Jacabon HI, Wagner RK, Jungblut PW. Ovarian independent fluctuations of estradiol receptor levels in mammalian tissues. *Molecular and Cellular Endocrinology* 1976; **5**: 379–88.
12. Wirz-Justice A. Neurophsychopharmacology and biological rhythms. In: Mendlewics J ed. *Biological rhythms and behavior.* Basel: Karger, 1982.
13. Wirz-Justice A, Wehr TA, Goodwin FK *et al.* Antidepressant drugs slow circadian rhythm in behaviour and brain neurotransmitter receptors. *Psychopharmacology Bulletin* 1980; **16**: 45.
14. Adams J, Carmichael J, Wolf CR. Altered mouse bone marrow glutathione transferase levels in response to cytotoxins. *Cancer Research* 1985; **45**: 1669–73.
15. Beollamy WT, Alberts DS, Dorr RT. Daily variation in non-protein sulfhydryl levels of human bone marrow. *European Journal of Cancer and Clinical Oncology* 1988; **24**(11): 1759–62.
16. Hrushesky WJM, Dell I, Eaton J, Halberg F. Circadian-stage-dependent effect of doxorubicin upon reduced glutathione in the murine heart. *Proceedings of the Annual Meeting of the American Association for Cancer Research* 1982; **23**: 12 (abstract).
17. Smaaland R, Svardal AM, Lote K, Ueland PM, Laerum OD. Glutathione content in human bone marrow and circadian stage relation to DNA synthesis. *Journal of the National Cancer Institute* 1991; **83**: 1092–8.
18. Reinberg A, Smolensky M, Labreque G. New aspects in chronopharmacology. *Annual Review of Chronopharmacology* 1986; **2**: 3–26.
19. Cal JC, Dorian C, Catroux P, Cambar J. Nephrotoxicity of heavy metals and antibiotics. In: Lemmer B ed. *Chronopharmacology.* New York: Marcel Dekker, 1989.
20. Levi F, Bailleul F, Metzger G *et al.* Adriamycin chronotherapy of advanced breast

cancer with a progammable implantable drug administration device (DAD). *Annual Review of Chronopharmacology* 1986; **3**: 237–40.

21. Reinberg A, Smolensky MH. *Biological rhythms and medicine* New York: Springer-Verlag, 1983.
22. Wirz-Justice A. Circadian rhythms in mammalian neurotransmitter receptors. *Progress in Neurobiology* 1987; **29**: 219–59.
23. Hrushesky WJM. Chemotherapy timing: an important variable in toxicity and response. In: Perry M, Yarbo J eds. *Toxicity of chemotherapy*. New York: Grune & Stratton, 1984: 449–77.
24. Reinberg A, Halberg F. Circadian chronopharmacology. *Annual Review of Pharmacology* 1971; **11**: 455–92.
25. Lévi F. Chronobiologie et cancer. *Pathologie Biologie* 1987; **35**: 960–8.
26. von Roemeling R, Hrushesky WJM. Circadian pattern of continuous FUDR infusion reduces toxicity. In: Pauli JE, Scheving LE eds. *Advances in chronobiology*, part B. New York: Allen R Liss 1987: 357–73.
27. von Roemeling R, Mormont MC, Walker K, Olshefski R. Cancer control depends upon the circadian shape of continuous FUDR infusion. *Proceedings of the Annual Meeting of the American Association for Cancer Research* 1987; **28**: A1293 (abstract).
28. von Roemeling R, Hrushesky WJM. Determination of the therapeutic index of floxuridine by its circadian infusion pattern. *Journal of the National Cancer Institute* 1990; **82**: 386–93.
29. Gonzalez RB, Sothern RB, Thatcher G, Nguyen N, Hrushesky WJM. Substantial difference in timing of murine circadian susceptibility to 5-fluorouracil and FUDR. *Proceedings of the Annual Meeting of the American Association for Cancer Research* 1989; **30** A2452 (abstract).
30. Gardner MLG, Plumb JA. Diurnal variation in the intestinal toxicity of 5-fluorouracil in the rat. *Clinical Science* 1981; **61**: 717–22.
31. von Roemeling R, Hrushesky WJM. Circadian patterning of continuous floxuridine infusion reduces toxicity and allows higher dose intensity in patients with widespread cancer. *Journal of Clinical Oncology* 1989; **7**: 1710–19.
32. Hrushesky WJM, von Roemeling R, Lanning RM, Rabatin JT. Circadian-shaped infusion of floxuridine for progressive metastatic renal cell carcinoma. *Journal of Clinical Oncology* 1990; **8**: 1504–13.
33. Lévi F, Zidani R, Di Palma M *et al.* Improved therapeutic index through ambulatory circadian rhythm delivery of high dose 3-drug chemotherapy in a randomized Phase III multicenter trial. *Proceedings of the Annual Meeting of the American Society of Clinical Oncology*. 1994; **13**: A574. (abstract.)
34. Bjarnason GA, Kerr I, Doyle N, Macdonald M, Sone M. Phase I study of 5-fluorouracil and leucovorin by a 14 day circadian infusion in patients with metastatic adenocarcinoma. *Cancer Chemotherapy and Pharmacology* 1993; **33**(3): 221–8.
35. Buchi KN, Moore JG, Hrushesky WJM, Sothern RB, Rubin NH. Circadian rhythm of cellular proliferation in the human rectal mucosa. *Gastroenterology* 1991; **101**(2): 410–15.
36. Scheving LE, Tsai TH, Feuers RJ, Scheving LA. Cellular mechanism involved in the action of anticancer drugs. In: Lemmer B ed. *Chronopharmacology: cellular and biochemical interactions*. New York: Marcel Dekker, 1989: 317–69.
37. Hrushesky WJM. More evidence for circadian rhythm effects in cancer chemotherapy: the fluoropyrimidine story. *Cancer Cells* 1990; **2**: 65–8.
38. el Kouni MH, Naguib FMN, Cha S. Circadian rhythm of dihydrouracil dehydrogenase (DHUDase), uridine phosphorylase (UrdPase), and thymidine phosphorylase (dThdPase) in mouse liver. *FASEB Journal* 1989; **3**: A397.
39. Harris BE, Song R, HE Y, Diasio RB. Circadian rhythm of rat liver dihydropyrimidine dehydrogenase. *Biochemistry and Pharmacology* 1988; **37**(24): 4759–62.

40. Harris BE, Song R, Soong S, Diasio RB. Circadian variation of 5-fluorouracil catabolism in isolated perfused rat liver. *Cancer Research* 1989; **49**: 6610–14.
41. Kuhl JFW, Grage F, Halberg F, Rosene G, Scheving LE, Haus E. Ellen-effect: tolerance of adriamycin by mice and rats depend on circadian timing of injection. *International Journal of Chronobiology* 1973; **1**: 335–6.
42. Hrushesky WJM, von Roemeling R, Sothern RB. Circadian chronotherpay: From animal experiments to human cancer chemotherapy. In: Lemmer B, (ed.) *Chronopharmacology: cellular and biochemical interactions*. New York and Basel: Marcel Dekker 1989; 439–73.
43. Hrushesky WJM. Circadian timing of cancer chemotherapy. *Science* 1985; **228**: 73–5.
44. Hrushesky WJM, Dell I, Eaton J, Hallberg F. Circadian-stage-dependent effect of doxorubicin upon reduced glutathione in murine heart. *Proceedings of the American Association for Cancer Research* 1982; **23**: 12.
45. Lévi F. Chronopharmacology of anticancer agents and cancer chronotherapy. In: Kummerle H, (ed.) *International handbook of clinical pharmacology*, vol II-2.15.3.3. Landsberg am Lech: Ecomed 1987; 1–17.
46. Bachur NR, Gordon SL, Gee MW. A general mechanism for microsomal activation of quinone anticancer agents to free radicals. *Cancer Research* 1978; **38**: 1745–50.
47. Boor PJ. Cardiac glutathione: diurnal rhythm and variation in drug-induced cardiomyopathy. *Research Communications in Chemical Pathology and Pharmacology* **24**: 1979; 27–36.
48. Wesson LG. Electrolyte excretion in relation to diurnal cycles of renal function. *Medicine* 1964; **43**: 547–92.
49. Hecquet B. Meynadier J, Bonneterre J, Adenis L, Demaille A. Time dependency in plasmatic protein binding of cisplatin. *Cancer Treatment Reports* 1985; **69**: 79–82.
50. Cardoso SS, Scheving LE, Halberg F. Mortality of mice as influenced by the hour of the day of drug (ara-C) administration. *Pharmacologist* 1970; **12**: 302.
51. Scheving Le, Cardoso SS, Pauly JE, Halberg F, Haus E. Variation susceptibility of mice to the carcinostatic agent arabinosylcytosine. In: Scheving LE, Pauly JE eds. *Chronobiology*. Tokyo: Igaku-Shoin, 1974: 213–17.
52. Hromas RA, Hutchison JT, Markel DE, Scholes VE. Flow cytometric analysis of the effect of ara-C on the chronobiology of bone marrow DNA synthesis. *Chronobiologia* 1981; **8**: 369–73.
53. Burns ER, Scheving LE. Circadian optimization of the treatment of L1210 leukemia with 1-β-D-arabinofuranasylcytosine, cyclophosphamide, vincristine and methylprednisolone. *Chronobiologia* 1980; **7**: 41–51.
54. English J, Aherne GW, Marks V. The effect of timing of a single injection on the toxicity of methotrexate in the rat. *Cancer Chemotherpay and Pharmacology* 1982; **9**: 114–17.
55. English J, Aherne GW, Marks V. The effect of abolition of the endogenous corticosteroid rhythm on the circadian variation in methotrexate toxicity in the rat. *Cancer Chemotherapy and Pharmacology* 1987; **19**: 287–90.
56. English J, Aherne GW, Arend J. Effect of corticosteroids and melatonin on the circadian rhythm of methotrexate toxicity in the rat. In: Reinberg A, Smolensky M, Labrecque G eds. *Annual review of chronopharmacology, vol. 1*. Oxford: Pergamon Press, 1984: 145–8.
57. Rivard GE, Infante-Rivard C, Hoyoux C, Champagne J. Maintenance chemotherapy for childhood acute lymphoblastic leukemia: Better in the evening. *Lancet* 1985; **ii** (8467): 1264–6.
58. Lennard L, Lilleyman JS. Variable mercaptopurine metabolism and treatment outcome in childhood lymphoblastic leukemia. *Journal of Clinical Oncology* 1989; **7**(12): 1816–23.
59. Halberg F, Gupta B, Haus E *et al*. Steps toward a chronopolychemotherapy. In:

Proceedings of the 14th International Congress of Therapeutics Paris: L'Expansion Scientifique Francaise, 1977: 151–96.

60. Mormont MC, Berestka J, Mushiya T *et al.* Circadian dependence of vinblastine toxicity. In: Reinberg A, Smolensky M, Labrecque G eds. *Annual review of chronopharmacology*, vol. 3. Oxford: Pergamon Press, 1986: 187–90.

61. Lévi F, Mechkouri M, Roulon A *et al.* Circadian rhythm in tolerance of mice for etoposide. *Cancer Treatment Reports* 1985; **69**: 1443–5.

62. Tsai TH, Scheving LE. Murine circadian variation in susceptibility to epipodophillotoxin (VP16) as well as to the solvent alone in which it was suspended. In: Reinberg A, Smolensky M, Labrecque G eds. *Annual review of chronopharmacology*, vol. 3 Oxford: Pergamon Press, 1984: 389–92.

63. Focan C, Mazy JM, Zhou J, Rahmani R, Cano JP. Circadian variation of vindesine serum concentrations during continuous infusion. In: Reinberg A, Smolensky M, Labreque G eds. *Annual review of chronopharmacology*, vol. 5. Oxford: Pergamon Press, 1988: 411–14.

64. Krakowski I, Levi F, Mechkouri M *et al.* Dose intensity of etoposide (vp16)-cisplatin (cddp) depends upon dosing time. *Proceedings of the Annual Meeting of the American Association for Cancer Research* 1988; **29**: A776 (abstract).

65. Haus E, Halberg F, Scheving L *et al.* Increased tolerance of mice to arabinosylcytosine given on schedule adjusted to circadian system. *Science* 1972; **177**: 80–2.

PART 2

Therapy and biological agents

CHAPTER 5

The role of cytokines in the supportive care of the cancer patient

JOHN W SWEETENHAM

INTRODUCTION

In recent years, several recombinant human cytokines have become available for clinical use. There has been intense research activity at the preclinical and clinical level into the potential applications of these agents in patients with malignant disease.

To date, the haemopoietic cytokines have probably been the most widely tested agents. Their potential role in the supportive care of patients receiving myelosuppressive chemotherapy has been investigated in a number of clinical studies, including some recent randomized, placebo-controlled trials. However, the design of some of these trials has led to difficulties in their interpretation, and the value of these agents in the supportive care of patients receiving chemotherapy remains unclear. This chapter summarizes some of the recent studies using these agents as a supportive measure in cancer patients. The use of cytokines as 'mobilizing' agents for peripheral blood progenitor cells is covered in Chapter 1 and will not be covered here.

ERYTHROPOIETIN (EPO)

Anaemia is a common clinical problem in patients with cancer. In most published series, around 20 per cent of patients with cancer will develop symptomatic anaemia requiring red cell transfusion.[1,2] Although sometimes attributable to blood loss, or nutritional causes, its causes are multifactorial, although it is often classified as anaemia of chronic disease (ACD).[3,4] The degree of anaemia can be worsened by a number of treatment-related factors. Chemotherapy with myelotoxic drugs can worsen anaemia, as can radiotherapy. In addition, the use of nephrotoxic chemotherapy or antibiotics can contribute further to the anaemia.

Laboratory features

ACD is characterized by a slight reduction in red cell survival, erythroid hypoplasia in the bone marrow, reduced utilization of iron in the bone marrow and serum Epo levels which are inappropriately low to the haemoglobin.[5,6]

Although the precise causes of ACD in cancer patients are unclear, it is thought to be at least partly due to the secretion of tumour-related cytokines which have a negative effect on Epo production in the kidney.

Anaemia-related symptoms

Anaemia is thought to contribute substantially to the lethargy and malaise associated with cancer, and with patients receiving chemotherapy or radio-therapy. The contribution of mild anaemia to the decline in quality of life experienced by cancer patients is highlighted by the effects of Epo in the clinical studies reported to date (see below).

Treatment of anaemia has, until recently, relied on red blood cell transfusions. However, minor complications of red cell transfusions such as fever, rash and chills are common, occurring in about 20 per cent of patients.[7] Major complications such as allergic reactions, alloreactivity or hepatitis are also occasionally seen. In addition, red cell transfusions are disruptive for patients and their carers, requiring hospital attendance, and frequently requiring admission.

As a result of this, and of the observation that serum Epo levels are inappropriately low in this group of patients, plus the clinical experience in patients with chronic renal impairment[8,9] and HIV infection,[10] the use of recombinant Epo has been the subject of a number of studies in cancer patients.

Studies in untreated patients

Recombinant Epo has been assessed in several relatively small studies in cancer patients who are not receiving active therapy at the time of Epo treatment. In a study from Vienna, sixty-seven patients with a range of malignancies were treated in a phase II study of recombinant Epo at an initial subcutaneous dose of 150 U/kg, three times weekly.[11]

Patients were assessed at 3-weekly intervals over the first 9 weeks of treatment. Response was defined as an increase in the haemoglobin level of 2 g/l or greater compared with the baseline level. Patients who failed to respond were given increased doses in 50 IU increments to a maximum dose of 300 U/kg three times weekly.

These authors reported a 43 per cent response rate to Epo, with a median time to response of 4.9 weeks (range 1–20.3 weeks). Of the twenty-six responding patients, twenty-four responded within the first 12 weeks of therapy. Responding patients were followed on therapy for 1 year, and the response was maintained for the total 1-year period in most of these patients.

Although the number of patients was relatively small, differences in response rate were observed according to the underlying disease. For example, 78 per cent of patients with myeloma were classified as responders, compared with 45 per cent of those with breast cancer, and 33 per cent of those with colon cancer or lymphoid malignancy.

Only 11 per cent of the responders required blood transfusions during the study period, compared with 62 per cent of the non-responders. A survival difference was also observed between responders and non-responders, although it is likely that this reflects the nature of the underlying malignant diseases, rather than an effect of Epo therapy.

Although no formal quality of life assessment was performed, the WHO performance status of the responding patients increased significantly after 2 months of therapy. A second study from the same group produced similar observations, with a high response rate in patients with myeloma, and lower response rates in selected solid tumours including breast and colon cancer.

This same group have also conducted formal quality of life studies in patients receiving Epo.[12] A total of fifty-four patients with various solid and haematological malignancies were treated with recombinant Epo according to a similar regimen to that described above. A quality of life questionnaire was applied before the start of Epo, and at weeks 8 and 12 after treatment.

A close correlation was observed between response to Epo as determined by increase in haemoglobin levels, and mood (Fig. 5.1). In patients with a response of haemoglobin to Epo, there was a significant improvement in mood, feeling of well-being, social activities and appetite by week 8. After 12 weeks of therapy, all of the ten items assessed in the questionnaire had improved in responding patients. Increases in WHO performance status were also observed to correlate closely with response to Epo.

As in previous studies, there was superior survival in responding patients. Median survival for the non-responders was 4.1 months, compared with 12.0 months for the responders.

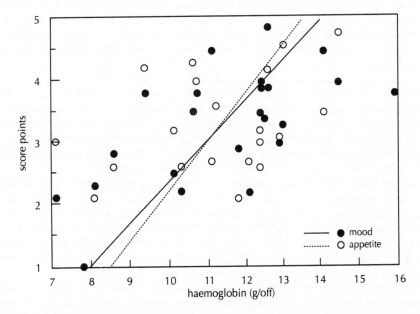

Fig. 5.1 Correlation between haemoglobin levels and mood and appetite for patients receiving recombinant erythropoietin. (With permission from ref. 12.)

Studies in patients receiving chemotherapy

The incidence of significant anaemia requiring blood transfusion in patients receiving combination chemotherapy for anaemia is fairly poorly documented, although rates as high as 40 per cent have been reported for patients receiving cisplatin-based therapy.[13,14] Several reports suggest a higher incidence of anaemia in patients receiving cisplatin, which may relate either to the underlying disease, or may be a consequence of the effect of cisplatin on erythropoietin production in the kidney.

Early reports of the use of recombinant Epo for patients having cisplatin-based treatment for a variety of solid tumours showed improvements in haemoglobin levels and reduction in transfusion requirements.[15–17] Abels has reported the results of a series of randomized placebo-controlled trials of Epo in cancer patients receiving no treatment, combination chemotherapy without cisplatin, or cisplatin-based therapy.[18] All patients were randomized to receive subcutaneous Epo or placebo according to various dosage regimens. Patients with haematological and solid malignancies were included, receiving a range of chemotherapy regimens.

The initial endogenous erythropoietin levels were measured in all patients and were lowest in the cisplatin group, possibly due to the nephrotoxic nature of cisplatin. Over the 12-week period of the study, the mean haematocrit increased significantly over control in all three groups (Fig. 5.2). The increase was greater in the chemotherapy-treated groups than in the untreated patients. This difference was reflected in a significantly lower transfusion requirement in the patients receiving Epo.

A relationship between response and tumour type was observed. Significant responses were seen in patients with lymphoma, breast and lung cancer, gastrointestinal and gynaecological malignancy. The increases for patients with CLL and myeloma did not achieve statistical significance. Improvements in quality of life were also reported, according to several criteria including daily activity and energy levels.

Overall, most trials have demonstrated that approximately 50 per cent of patients on chemotherapy receiving Epo will respond. In order to reduce the financial and emotional burden imposed by the use of Epo, the possibility of early prediction of response has been addressed by several groups. Ludwig *et al.* have investigated a number of potential predictive factors including serum levels of Epo, iron, ferritin, transferrin and transferrin receptor, WHO performance status, stem cell factor, C-reactive protein, and α_1-antitrypsin.[19]

None of these factors was predictive of response at the start of treatment. However, a predictive algorithm was constructed as follows: In patients in whom the serum Epo level was $\geq$ 100 mU/ml and the Hb had not increased by at least 5 g/l, response was highly unlikely, with a predictive power of 93 per cent. By contrast, if Epo levels had fallen below 100 mU/ml and Hb levels had increased by > 5 g/l, response was very likely, with a predictive power of 95 per cent. Serum ferritin levels could also be used to predict response.

Other studies have confirmed these observations, and it is now generally recommended that these or similar criteria be applied after 2 weeks of Epo therapy, to identify those patients in whom longer term treatment is likely to be beneficial.

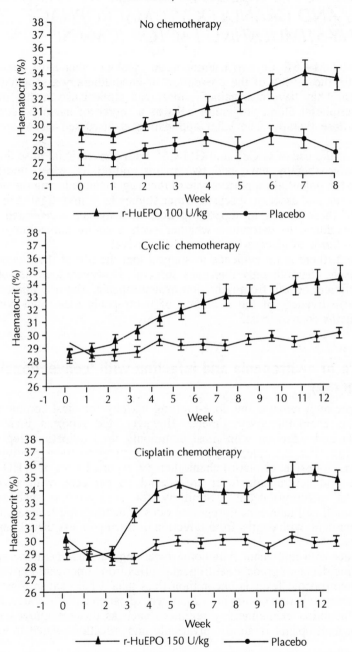

Fig. 5.2. Increases in haematocrit according to treatment arm in cancer patients receiving no chemotherapy, non-cisplatin-based chemotherapy, and cisplatin-based chemotherapy. (With permission from ref. 18.)

GRANULOCYTE COLONY-STIMULATING FACTOR (G-CSF) AND GRANULOCYTE/MACROPHAGE COLONY-STIMULATING FACTOR (GM-CSF)

G-CSF and GM-CSF are two haemopoietic cytokines that have been widely evaluated in the setting of the prevention of chemotherapy-associated myelo-suppression. They have also gained widespread clinical use in the 'mobiliza-tion' of peripheral blood progenitor cells as a source of haemopoietic rescue after high-dose therapy. The latter application is discussed elsewhere in this book.

Studies of the use of G-CSF and GM-CSF with conventional dose therapy or dose-intensive therapy have had two major end-points. Most studies have focused on the potential supportive role of these agents in reducing the incidence of neutropenia and associated sepsis. Other studies have investigated the poten-tial role of these agents in supporting dose-intensive or accelerated chemo-therapy schedules, to determine whether such dose-intensification improves outcome in terms of disease-free or overall survival.

At present, there is no evidence to suggest that the use of these agents with dose-intensive chemotherapy improves survival. However, there is some evi-dence of clinical benefit from reduction of neutropenia. The true clinical value, and cost-effectiveness of the reduction of neutropenia associated with these agents remains controversial.

Incidence of neutropenia and infection with 'conventional dose' chemotherapy

Myelosuppression remains the dose-limiting toxicity for most commonly used combination chemotherapy regimens. However, the reported incidence of neutropenia and infection with most commonly used outpatient regimens is relatively low. For example, in patients with testicular cancer receiving BEP (bleomycin, etoposide, cisplatin) chemotherapy, reported rates of WHO grade 4 leukopenia and neutropenic fever are around 16 per cent, with a very low incidence of infectious death.[20] Similarly, for solid tumours such as breast cancer or small cell lung cancer, reported rates of neutropenic fever are between 3 and 16 per cent, with deaths from infection occurring in less than 3 per cent in most series.[21–23]

In patients with malignant lymphoma receiving various chemotherapy regi-mens, the incidence of grade 4 neutropenia varies from 3 per cent to over 20 per cent, but neutropenic fever is uncommon (less than 5 per cent in most series), and death from infection occurs in 1–2 per cent of patients.[24,25] Clearly, for more intensive induction chemotherapy regimens such as those employed in acute leukaemia, neutropenia is almost invariable and infection-related mortality is high.[26]

Although neutropenic fever is rarely fatal, it remains a significant cause of extended hospital admission. Most patients developing neutropenic fever spend approximately 1 week in hospital.[27,28] This has obvious implications in terms of quality of life and the need for other supportive measures including blood products and antibiotics. Thus, although reductions in neutropenic fever may not impact significantly on mortality associated with conventional dose chemotherapy, they may result in other benefits. In addition, the prevention of neutropenic fever might, in theory, reduce the requirement for dose reductions of subsequent chemotherapy courses (although this has not been shown to have an adverse effect on survival when tested prospectively).

A number of randomized trials have assessed the effect of G- and GM-CSF on neutropenic fever in patients receiving chemotherapy. Two early studies were conducted in patients with small cell lung cancer (SCLC), receiving CAE chemotherapy (cyclophosphamide, doxorubicin, etoposide).[22,29] The results of both studies were broadly similar. In the trial reported by Crawford *et al.* the overall incidence of neutropenic fever in the control group was 40 per cent.[22] This was reduced to approximately 20 per cent in the group receiving G-CSF. There was an associated reduction in duration of antibiotic use and hospital stay.

However, there was no significant improvement in infectious mortality. Furthermore, no differences were observed in response or survival rates. The doses of chemotherapy used in these two trials were substantially higher than most standard chemotherapy regimens for small cell lung cancer. This is reflected in the relatively high incidence of neutropenic fever in the control arm. For example, Nichols *et al.* reviewed the use of several chemotherapy regimens for SCLC and reported only an 18 per cent incidence of neutropenic fever.[30] Median survival in these studies was comparable with that reported in the two G-CSF supported chemotherapy trials.

In summary, these trials demonstrate that the use of G-CSF with intensive chemotherapy for SCLC reduces the incidence of neutropenic fever, but with no effect on mortality, and no benefit from the use of more intensive, severely myelotoxic therapy.

Similar findings have been reported for patients with non-Hodgkin's lymphoma (NHL) receiving chemotherapy supported with G- or GM-CSF. In a study from Manchester, UK, patients with intermediate/high-grade NHL receiving weekly alternating chemotherapy with VAPEC-B (vincristine, doxorubicin, prednisone, etoposide, cyclophosphamide, bleomycin) were randomly allocated to G-CSF placebo (Fig 5.3).[31] The incidence of neutropenia was significantly lower among the treated group (37 per cent vs. 81 per cent), as was the incidence of neutropenic fever (22 per cent vs. 44 per cent). Gerhartz *et al.* reported the use of GM-CSF in a placebo-controlled trial in patients receiving COP-BLAM (cyclophosphamide, vincristine, prednisone, bleomycin, doxorubicin, methotrexate) chemotherapy for aggressive NHL.[32] The GM-CSF-treated group had a reduced incidence of neutropenic fever and duration of hospitalization (Fig. 5.4), but these improvements were only seen when the analysis was restricted to the 72 per cent of patients who tolerated GM-CSF therapy. No intention-to-treat analysis was performed, and the interpretation of the results is therefore problematic.

Other randomized studies using GM-CSF have been largely negative, including studies in testicular cancer and SCLC, where no reductions in neutrophil recovery or neutropenic fever were observed.[33–35]

The results of these and other trials have led to the publication of guidelines for the use of haemopoietic growth factors by the American Society of Clinical Oncology (ASCO).[36] The recommendations of this group are that primary

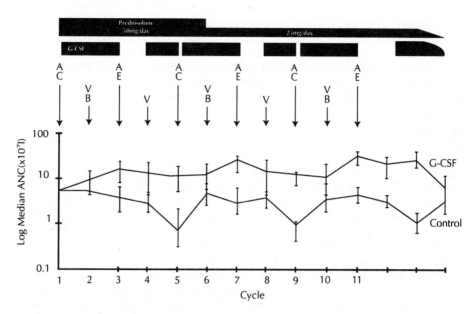

Fig. 5.3. Treatment schema and median neutrophil counts for patients receiving VAPEC-B +/− G-CSF for non-Hodgkin's lymphoma. (With permission from ref. 31.)

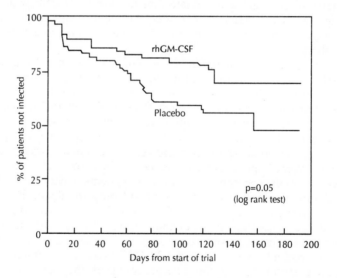

Fig. 5.4. Percentage of NHL patients treated with COP-BLAM +/− GM-CSF remaining free from infection. (With permission from ref. 32.)

administration of growth factors for supportive purposes should be restricted to those chemotherapy regimens in which the reported incidence of neutropenic fever is 40 per cent or greater. This conclusion is based primarily on the data reported in SCLC. Since the reported incidence of neutropenic fever for most commonly used outpatient regimens is much lower than this, the widespread use of these agents is not recommended. Furthermore, the recommendation is based on studies which used very intensive chemotherapy compared with accepted standard regimens, and their clinical benefit was doubtful. Whether the use of haemopoietic growth factors in these circumstances has real advantages over the conventional approach of chemotherapy dose reduction, in terms of cost-effectiveness, quality of life, etc., has not been formally evaluated.

The secondary use of these agents, in patients who have suffered an episode of neutropenic fever in a previous chemotherapy cycle has also been addressed. No randomized trials have been reported, but evidence from the study by Crawford *et al.* in which patients on the control arm were allowed to cross over to G-CSF treatment if they suffered an episode of febrile neutropenia, demonstrated a shorter period of neutropenia and reduced rate of neutropenic fever (100 per cent for cycle 1 vs. 23 per cent for cycle 2).[22] No improvement in survival can be demonstrated with this approach and it is recommended that chemotherapy dose reduction be used, rather than secondary growth factor administration, unless the period of neutropenia is excessively prolonged.

The use of G- or GM-CSF in established neutropenia

Several trials have investigated the use of these factors in patients with established neutropenic fever.[27,37–39] In the largest of these studies, patients with established neutropenia were treated with standard antibiotics and randomized to G-CSF or placebo until recovery of their neutrophil counts to $> 0.5 \times 10^9/l$.[37] The median duration of neutropenia was 1 day less in the treated group, but no difference was observed in the duration of fever or antibiotic therapy. Some positive benefits of G-CSF therapy were seen – there was a reduction in the number of patients requiring hospitalization for more than 11 days, and a reduction in antifungal therapy. Similar negative findings have been reported in studies using GM-CSF.

Again, no formal assessment of quality of life has been performed in these patients, but current recommendations are that growth factors should not be used in this situation. Similarly, for patients with established neutropenia who are afebrile, randomized studies of G- or GM-CSF have failed to show any benefit in terms of duration of neutropenia, or incidence of subsequent neutropenic fever.

CYTOKINES FOR THE TREATMENT AND PREVENTION OF THROMBOCYTOPENIA

The use of myeloid growth factors has reduced the incidence of neutropenia as a dose-limiting toxicity in the chemotherapy of cancer. As a result, and partly because of the increased dose intensity achieved with these agents, thrombocytopenia is assuming more importance in dose-intensive chemotherapy regimens.

Despite the use of modern methods of blood product support, including platelet transfusion, the reported incidence of mortality from haemorrhage in patients receiving intensive induction therapy for acute leukaemia has been over 20 per cent in some series.[40,41]

Prophylactic platelet transfusion for thrombocytopenia is standard practice, although some controversy has persisted regarding the appropriate level at which transfusion should be recommended.[42-45] However, there are complications arising from repeated platelet transfusion, including the risk of alloimmunization, and the disruption caused to patients by the necessity for platelet transfusion to be undertaken in hospital.[46,47]

There is therefore considerable potential to reduce transfusion requirements, provide safer, cost-effective therapy, and improve quality of life for patients if effective cytokine therapy for thrombocytopenia can be developed.

Current evidence suggests that many cytokines have some thrombopoietic activity, some of which have been shown to have clinical benefit. The potential for some newly developed agents, particularly thrombopoietin, is considerable. Some of the cytokines under investigation for thrombocytopenia are as follows.

Interleukin 3 (IL-3)

Interleukin 3 acts primarily on a relatively non-committed haemopoietic progenitor cell, and can stimulate all cell lines in human and murine systems, including megakaryocytes. In an early phase II clinical trial Ganser *et al.* demonstrated that platelet requirements of patients with bone marrow failure secondary to malignant infiltration could be reduced using IL-3.[48] Similar findings have been reported in small studies of chemotherapy-induced thrombocytopenia, although no large-scale randomized studies have been performed.[49,50]

PIXY 321 (GM-CSF/IL-3 fusion protein)

PIXY 321 is a synthetic cytokine produced by the end-to-end combination of GM-CSF and IL-3.[51] In an early report from a clinical study in women receiving cyclophosphamide, etoposide and cisplatin for breast cancer, significant reductions in platelet transfusions were reported for patients receiving PIXY 321 compared with other haemopoietic growth factors.[52]

Stem cell factor

Stem cell factor is thought to act on a very early multipotential haemopoietic progenitor cell. As a result, it is possible that it will produce reductions in chemotherapy-associated thrombocytopenia, although results of clinical trials are awaited.[53]

Thrombopoietin

Thrombopoietin was cloned in 1994 and has been shown to be a powerful stimulator of megakaryopoiesis *in vitro* and *in vivo*. In normal mice it has been shown to produce four-fold increases in platelet counts.[54] Preclinical studies are now underway, and this agent is likely to prove a major advance in the treatment of thrombobocytopenia in cancer patients with malignant marrow infiltration, or due to chemotherapy.

SUMMARY

The use of haemopoietic cytokines to support patients with cancer, particularly those receiving chemotherapy, has increased dramatically in the last 5 years. Despite the widespread use of the myeloid growth factors, their optimal use remains controversial, but few clear benefits, either in terms of survival parameters, cost-effectiveness measures, or beneficial effects on quality of life, have been demonstrated.

The use of erythropoietin has been reported from several centres. It appears to have beneficial effects in terms of reduced blood transfusions, and formal quality of life studies suggest benefits also. The advent of thrombopoietin for the treatment of thrombocytopenia has yet to be evaluated, but offers the promise of effective treatment, which may improve quality of life parameters.

Aspects of quality of life must, of course, include assessments of the toxicities of these agents. Most of these cytokines have similar toxicities such as mild chills, fevers, local reactions at the injection sites, and bone pain. The incidence of these toxicities has been between 15 per cent and 30 per cent with most agents, although they are rarely severe or dose-limiting. However, subsequent prospective studies of these agents will undoubtedly include quality of life endpoints which will enable accurate assessment of the tolerability and overall benefits of these cytokines.

REFERENCES

1. Mayer K. Transfusion support for leukemia and oncology patients. *Clinical Haematology* 1984; **13**: 93–8.
2. Skillings JR, Sridhar FG, Wong C *et al.* The frequency of red cell transfusions for anaemia in patients receiving chemotherapy. *American Journal of Clinical Oncology* 1993; **16**: 22–5.
3. Bunn HF. Anaemia associated with chronic disorders. In: *Harrison's Principles of Internal Medicine*, 11th edn. New York, McGraw-Hill, 1987: 1504–5.
4. Johnson RA, Roodman GD Hematologic manifestations of malignancy. *Disease-a-Month* 1989; **35**: 716–68.
5. Miller CB, Jones RJ, Piantadosis *et al.* Deceased erythropoietin response in patients with the anaemia of cancer, *New England Journal of Medicine* 1990; **332**: 1689–92.
6. Smith DH, Goldwasser E, Vokes EE. Serum immunoerythropoietin levels in patients with cancer receiving cisplatin-based chemotherapy. *Cancer* 1991; **68**: 1101–15.
7. Walker RH. Special report: transfusion risks. *American Journal of Clinical Pathology* 1987; **88**: 374–8.
8. Winearis CG, Oliver DO, Pippard MJ *et al.* effect of human erythropoietin derived from recombinant DNA on the anaemia of patients maintained by chronic dialysis. *Lancet* 1986; **2**: 1175–8.
9. Eschbach JW, Egrie JC, Downing MR *et al.* Correction of the anaemia of end stage renal disease with recombinant human erythropoietin. Results of a combined phase I and II clinical trial. *New England Journal of Medicine* 1987; **316**: 73–80.
10. Fischl M, Galpin JE, Levine JD *et al.* Recombinant human erythropoietin for patients with AIDS treated with zidovudine. *New England Journal of Medicine* 1990; **322**: 1488–93.
11. Ludwig H, Leitgeb C, Fritz E *et al.* Erythropoietin treatment of chronic anaemia of cancer. *European Journal of Cancer* 1993; **29A** (Suppl. 2): S8–12.

12. Leitgeb C, Pecherstorfer M, Fritz E *et al.* Quality of life in chronic anaemia of cancer during treatment with recombinant human erythropoietin. *Cancer* 1994; **73**: 2535–42.

13. Rossof AH, Slayton RE, Perlia CP. Preliminary clinical experience with cis-diamminedichloroplatinum (II) (NSC 119875, CACP). *Cancer* 1972; **30**: 1451–6.

14. von Hoff DD, Schilsky R, Reichert CM *et al.* Toxic effects of cisdichlorodiammineplatinum (II) in man. *Cancer Treatment Reports* 1979; **63**: 1527–31.

15. Cascinu S, Fedeli A, Fedeli FS *et al.* Cisplatin-associated anaemia treated with subcutaneous erythropoietin. A pilot study. *British Journal of Cancer* 1993; **67**: 156–8.

16. Gamucci T, Thorel MF, Frasca AM *et al.* Erythropoietin for the prevention of anaemia in neoplastic patients treated with cisplatin. *European Journal of Cancer* 1993; **29A** (Suppl. 2) S13–14.

17. James RD, Wilkinson PM, Belli F *et al.* Recombinant human erythropoietin in patients with ovarian carcinoma and anaemia secondary to cisplatin and carboplatin chemotherapy: preliminary results. *Acta Haematologica* 1992; **87** (Suppl. 1): 12–15.

18. Abels R. Erythropoietin for anaemia in cancer patients. *European Journal of Cancer* 1993; **29A** (Suppl. 2): S2–8.

19. Ludwig H, Fritz E, Leitgeb C *et al.* Prediction of response to erythropoietin treatment in chronic anemia of cancer. *Blood* 1994; **84**: 1056–63.

20. Nicholas CR, Williams SD, Loehrer PJ *et al.* Randomized study of cisplatin dose-intensity in poor-risk germ cell tumors: A Southeastern Cancer Study Group and Southwest Oncology Group protocol. *Journal of Clinical Oncology* 1991; **9**: 1163–72.

21. Budman DR, Korzun AH, Ainer J *et al.* A feasibility study of intensive CAF as outpatient adjuvant therapy for stage II breast cancer in a cooperative group: CALGB 8443. *Cancer Investigation* 1990; **8**: 571–5.

22. Crawford, J, Ozer H, Stoller R *et al.* Reduction by granulocyte colony stimulating factor of fever and neutropenia induced by chemotherapy in patients with small cell lung cancer (r-metHuG-CSF). *New England Journal of Medicine* 1991; **325**: 164–70.

23. Roth BJ, Johnson DH, Einhorn LH *et al.* Randomized study of cyclophosphamide, doxorubicin and vincristine versus etoposide and cisplatin versus alternation of these two regimens in extensive small-cell lung cancer. A phase III trial of the Southeastern Cancer Study Group. *Journal of Clincal Oncology* 1992; **10**: 282–91.

24. Fisher RI, Gaynor ER, Dahlberg S *et al.* Comparison of a standard regimen (CHOP) with three intensive chemotherpay regimens for advanced non-Hodgkin's lymphoma. *New England Journal of Medicine* 1993; **328**: 1002–6.

25. Canellos GP, Anderson JR, Propert KJ. *et al.* Chemotherapy of advanced Hodgkin's disease with MOPP, ABVD. or MOPP alternating with ABVD. *New England Journal of Medicine* 1992; **327**: 1478–84.

26. Dillman RO, Davis RB, Green MR *et al.* A comparative study of two different doses of cytarabine for acute myeloid leukemia: A phase III trial of the Cancer and Leukemia Group B. *Blood* 1991; **78**: 2520–6.

27. Riikonen P, Saarinen UM, Makipernaa A *et al.* rhGM-CSF in the treatment of fever and neutropenia: A double-blind placebo-controlled study in children with malignancy. *Proceedings of the American Society of Clinical Oncology* 1993; **12**: 442 (abstract).

28. Talcott JA, Finberg R, Mayer RJ *et al.* The medical course of cancer patients with fever and neutropenia. *Archives of Internal Medicine* 1988; **148**: 2561–8.

29. Trillet-Lenoir V, Green J, Manegold C *et al.* Recombinant granulocyte colony-stimulating factor reduces the infectious complications of cytotoxic chemotherapy. *European Journal of Cancer* 1993; **29**A: 319–24.

30. Nichols CR, Fox EP, Roth BJ *et al.* Incidence of neutropenic fever in patients treated with standard-dose combination chemotherpay for small cell lung cancer and the

cost impact of treatment with granulocyte colony-stimulating factor. *Journal of Clinical Oncology* 1994; **12**: 1245–9.

31. Pettengell R, Gurney H, Radford JA. *et al.* Granulocyte colony-stimulating factor to prevent dose-limiting neutropenia in non-Hodgkin's lymphoma: a randomized controlled trial. *Blood* 1992; **80**: 1430–6.

32. Gerhartz HH, Engelhard M, Meusers P *et al.* Randomized, double-blind, placebo-controlled, phase III study of recombinant human granulocyte-macrophage colony stimulating factor as adjunct to induction treatment of high grade malignant non-Hodgkin's lymphomas. *Blood* 1993; **82**: 2329–39.

33. Hamm JT, Schiller JH, Oken MM *et al.* Granulocyte-macrophage colony-stimulating factor (GM-CSF) in small cell carcinoma of the lung (SCCL). Preliminary analysis of a randomized controlled trial. *Proceedings of the American Society of Clinical Oncology* 1991; **10**: 255 (abstract).

34. Nichols C, Bajorin D, Schmoll HJ *et al.* VIP chemotherapy with/without GM-CSF for poor risk, relapsed or refractory germ cell tumors (GCT): Preliminary analysis of a randomized controlled trial. *Proceedings of the American society of Clinical Oncology* 1991; **10**: 167 (abstract).

35. Bunn PA, Crowley J, Hazuka M *et al.* The role of GM-CSF in limited stage SCLC: A randomized phase III study of the Southwest Oncology Group (SWOG). *Proceedings of the American Society of Clinical Oncology* 1992; **11**: 292 (abstract).

36. Americn Society of Clinical Oncology recommendations for the use of hematopoietic colony-stimulating factors: Evidence-based, clinical practice guidelines. *Journal of Clinical Oncology* 1994; **12**: 2471–508.

37. Maher D, Green M, Bishop J *et al.* Randomized, placebo-controlled trial of filgrastim (r-metHuG-CSF) in patients with febrile neutropenia (FN) following chemotherapy (CT). *Proceedings of the Americn Society of Clinical Oncology* 1993; **12**: 434 (abstract).

38. Biesma B, De Vries EG, Willemse PH *et al.* Efficacy and tolerability of recombinant human granulocyte-macrophage colony-stimulating factor in patients with chemotherapy-related leukopenia and fever. *European Journal of Cancer* 1990; **26**: 932–6.

39. Mayordomo JI, Rivera F, Diaz-Puente MT *et al.* decreasing morbidity and cost of treating febrile neutropenia by adding G-CSF and GM-CSF to standard antibiotic therapy: results of a randomized trial. *Proceedings of the American Society of Clinical Oncology* 1993; **12**: 437 (abstract).

40. Rees JKH, Gray RG, Swirsky D *et al.* Principal results in the MRC 8th Acute Myeloid Leukaemia Trial. *Lancet* 1986; **29**: 1236–42.

41. Tornebohm E, Lockner D, Paul C. A retrospective analysis of bleeding complications in 438 patients with acute leukemia during the years 1972–1991. *European Journal of Haematology* 1993; **50**: 160–7.

42. Han T, Stutzman L, Cohen E *et al.* Effect of platelet transfusion on haemorrhage in patients with acute leukemia. *Cancer* 1966; **19**: 1937–42.

43. Higby DJ, Cohen E, Holland JF *et al.* The prophylactic treatment of thrombocytopenic leukaemic patients in a double blind study. *Transfusion* 1974; **14**: 440–6.

44. Bodensteiner DC, Tilzer LL, Adams ME *et al.* Use of blood components in cancer patients with bleeding. *Hematology Oncology Clinics of North America* 1992; **6**: 1375–92.

45. National Institutes of Health. Consensus development conference on platelet transfusion therapy. *Journal of the American Medical Association* 1987; **257**: 1777–80.

46. Gmur J, von Felten A, Osterwalder B *et al.* Delayed alloimunisation using random single donor platelet transfusions: a prospective study in thrombocytopenic patients with acute leukemia. *Blood* 1983; **61**: 473–9.

47. Gmur J, Burger J, Sauter Chr *et al.* Allo-immunisation by leukocyte-rich or

leukocyte-poor random single donor platelet transfusion. *Progress in Clinical and Biology Research* 1990; **337**: 45–8.

48. Ganser A, Lindemann A, Seipelt G *et al*. Effects of recombinant human interleukin 3 in patients with normal hematopoiesis and in patients with bone marrow failure. Phase I/II study. *Blood* 1990; **76**: 666–9.

49. Hoelzer D, Seipelt G, Ganser A *et al*. Interleukin 3 alone and in combination with GM-CSF in the treatment of patients with neoplastic disease. *Seminars in Hematology* 1991; **28**: 17–24.

50. Biesma B, Willemse HB, Muilder NH *et al*. Effects of interleukin 3 after chemotherapy for advanced ovarian cancer. *Blood* 1992; **80**: 1141–8.

51. Vadhan-Raj S. PIXY 321 (GM-CSF/IL3 fusion protein): biology and early clinical development. *Stem Cells* 1994; **12**: 253–41.

52. Collins C, Livingston RB, Ellis G *et al*. Effect of PIXY 321 on hematological recovery after high dose cyclophosphamide, etoposide and cisplatin in women with breast cancer. *Blood* 1993; **82** 366a (abstract).

53. Piacibello W, Sanavio F, Bresso P *et al*. Stem cell factor improvement of proliferation and maintenance of haemopoietic progenitors in myelodysplastic syndromes. *Leukemia* 1994; **8**: 250–7.

54. Kaushansky K, Lok S, Holly RD *et al*. Promotion of megakaryocyte progenitor expansion and differentiation by the c-Mpl ligand thrombopoietin. *Nature* 1994; **369**: 571–4.

CHAPTER 6

Sepsis: the role of cytokines and possible strategies to interfere with their action

TOM VAN DER POLL AND SANDER JH VAN DEVENTER———

INTRODUCTION

Sepsis is an increasingly common cause of morbidity and mortality, especially in elderly and/or immunocompromized patients. Cancer patients are at considerable risk of developing sepsis, not only as a consequence of their debilitating disease, but more importantly as a result of the use of immunosuppressive and cytoreductive chemotherapy. Indeed, the increasing incidence of sepsis in recent decades can at least in part be explained by the introduction of cytotoxic agents in the treatment of malignancies. In the United States the annual number of discharge diagnoses of sepsis increased from 164 000 in 1979 to 425 000 in 1987.[1]

Sepsis can be defined as a clinical syndrome arising from a systemic inflammatory response to infection. Evidence has accumulated that the eventual clinical and laboratory features of sepsis result from a cascade of reactions that can be initiated by different microorganisms or parts of them. Sepsis is most frequently caused by Gram-negative bacteria, but can also occur as a consequence of Gram-positive bacteraemia, or infection with fungi, parasites and viruses. Classically, in patients with neutropenia Gram-negative bacilli have been the most commonly isolated pathogens, but in the past few years the incidence of Gram-positive infection has increased markedly, conceivably in part due to the widespread use of semipermanent indwelling venous catheters and decontamination regimens. It has become increasingly clear that the toxic sequelae of all these infectious agents result from the stimulation of a common 'sepsis cascade'. A large family of endogenous inflammatory mediators, collectively designated cytokines, plays an early and very important role in this sepsis cascade. In this chapter we will discuss the part of several cytokines in the pathogenesis of sepsis, as well as possible ways to interfere with their action as treatment modalities in septic patients.

Table 6.1 Cellular sources of cytokines

Cytokine	Main source
TNF	Monocytes
IL-1	Monocytes, endothelial cells, smooth muscle cells, keratinocytes
IL-6, IL-8	Monocytes, lymphocytes, fibroblasts, endothelial cells, smooth muscle cells, keratinocytes
IFN-γ	T lymphocytes

CYTOKINES

Cytokines are small proteins with molecular weights below 80 kDa that are produced and secreted by various cell types in response to various infectious stimuli (Table 6.1). Cytokines are extremely potent, exerting an amazing variety of biological effects at picomolar concentrations. Although most cytokines are structurally unrelated, they have multiple overlapping cell regulatory actions. They closely interact in a highly complex network, in which they reciprocally influence their synthesis rates and biological activities. Cytokines can induce other cytokines, can modulate the expression of specific cell surface receptors of other cytokines, can stimulate the production of natural inhibitors of other cytokines, and can synergistically, additively or antagonistically contribute to the actions of other cytokines.

Cytokines are involved in immunity and inflammation, and are essential for the orchestration of the host response to local infection. In sepsis, however, the invasive generalized infection leads to excessive systemic production of cytokines, which results in tissue toxicity and injury. Indeed, ample evidence exists indicating that this 'overproduction' of cytokines is the main event that initiates the sepsis cascade. Cytokines that have gained most attention as possible mediators of sepsis are tumour necrosis factor α, interleukin 1, interleukin 6, interleukin 8, and interferon γ.

Tumour necrosis factor α (TNF)

TNF has also been termed cachectin.[2] The protein was purified to homogeneity and sequenced by two different groups of investigators. Aggarwal *et al.*[2] isolated the factor that induced necrosis of tumours in cancer-bearing animals after administration of endotoxin, and named it 'tumour necrosis factor'. Beutler *et al.*[2] identified cachectin, a protein that they held responsible for cachexia in chronic infections. Shortly after their characterization, tumour necrosis factor and cachectin turned out to be one and the same protein. The human TNF gene is located on the short arm of chromosome 6, closely linked to the major histocompatability complex. TNF is translated as a 26 kDa prohormone, which is processed to a mature secreted form, consisting of 157 amino acids. TNF circulates as a compact trimer composed of three non-covalently bound 17 kDa polypeptides.

Interleukin 1 (IL-1)

IL-1 is the designation for two polypeptides, IL-1α and IL-1β, each encoded by a separate gene on chromosome 2.[3] Although the two proteins share only 26 per cent amino acid homology, they recognize the same cellular receptors and have highly similar biological activities. Both IL-1s are translated as 31 kDa precursor proteins, which are processed to mature peptides with molecular weights of 17 kDa. Several studies indicate that IL-1α is predominantly membrane-associated, whereas IL-1β is the major form that is secreted into the extracellular fluid. The recently cloned naturally occurring IL-1 receptor antagonist (see below) can also be viewed as a member of the IL-1 family.

Interleukin 6 (IL-6)

IL-6 was originally identified as a T-cell-derived protein that induced antibody production in B cells.[4] It is a glycoprotein of 23–30 kDa encoded on chromosome 7; the heterogeneity in size is related to the differential extent of glycosylation. Major actions of IL-6 include induction of B-cell differentiation and of hepatic acute phase protein synthesis.

Interleukin 8 (IL-8)

IL-8 can be distinguished from the earlier mentioned cytokines by its low molecular weight: natural IL-8 occurs as a 6–8 kDa doublet.[5] The IL-8 gene is located on chromosome 4, at a locus that also contains the genes for structurally and functionally related low molecular weight inflammatory proteins, such as platelet factor 4, β-thromboglobulin, and macrophage inflammatory proteins 1 and 2. Therefore, IL-8 is a member of a supergene family of small cytokines. Sequence analysis of mature IL-8 reveals that it exists in multiple forms that differ in truncation at the amino-terminus. The composition of IL-8 depends on the cells used to produce it. Interestingly, the conditions required to induce IL-8 in several *in vitro* systems show a large similarity with those necessary for IL-6 induction. Among the most important biological functions of IL-8 is the stimulation of various neutrophil functions.

Interferon γ (IFN-γ)

IFN-γ is part of a multigene family whose products can be divided into three main proteins: IFN-α, IFN-β and IFN-γ.[6] IFN-γ is encoded on chromosome 12 and synthesized mainly by activated T cells and by natural killer cells. IFN-γ has pronounced immunoregulatory effects, involving both cellular and humoral immunity. It sensitizes the host to the effects of TNF.

CYTOKINES AND THE PATHOGENESIS OF SEPSIS

Under physiological conditions cytokines are either not detected or detected at extremely low concentrations in the circulation by the currently available assays. In sepsis, however, the massive and systemic induction of cytokine synthesis leads to elevated serum levels of these proteins. TNF has been detected in 25–100 per cent of patients with sepsis.[7–9] In most studies TNF serum levels positively correlated with mortality rates. Increased serum concentrations of IL-6 and IL-8 can be found in 65–90 per cent of septic patients, in whom the levels of both cytokines appear to be strongly correlated.[10–12] As is the case for TNF, high IL-6 values are related to a poor clinical outcome. Variable circulating levels of IL-1 and IFN-γ have been reported in clinical sepsis.

In experimental models of sepsis TNF is the first cytokine to appear in the circulation (Fig. 6.1). Infusion of either a relatively low dose of endotoxin into healthy humans, or a lethal dose of live *Escherichia coli* into baboons results in detectable levels of TNF in the circulation after approximately 45 minutes, with peak levels occurring after 90 minutes.[13–15] In both models TNF release is transient. In lethal experimental sepsis TNF is no longer detectable in the circulation 6 hours after the bacterial infusion, which is several hours before the animals die from fulminant septic shock.[13] There is a close correlation between the magnitude of the bacterial challenge and the amount of TNF released, i.e. the levels of TNF detected in the lethal baboon studies are much higher than in the mild human volunteer studies. Interestingly, the clinical signs and symptoms associated with injection of endotoxin into normal humans, consisting of myalgia, headache and fever, start at the time TNF becomes detectable in the circulation. In addition, the extent of endotoxin-induced

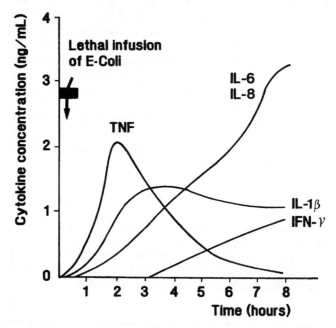

Fig. 6.1 The systemic appearance of cytokines after a lethal IV infusion of live *Escherichia coli* into baboons. TNF is the first cytokine that becomes detectable, followed by IL-1β. The kinetics of IL-6 and IL-8 secretion are remarkably similar; both cytokines appear after TNF and IL-1β. The absolute concentrations of these cytokines in the circulation vary from study to study; the levels given here should be considered as an indication.

clinical, haematological and metabolic responses are related to peak TNF concentrations, suggesting that TNF serves as an intermediate factor in endotoxin-provoked toxicity. Other cytokines appear shortly after TNF in experimental sepsis and endotoxaemia. The release of IL-6 closely parallels that of IL-8: administration of low-dose endotoxin to humans causes transient secretion of both mediators, whereas a lethal infusion of *E. coli* results in a continuous rise in their serum concentrations.[15-17] IL-1β and IFN-γ also follow TNF release; significant levels are only observed after severe bacterial challenges.[13,17]

The detection of elevated levels of cytokines in the circulation in experimental and clinical sepsis does not necessarily indicate a causal role in the pathogenesis of this syndrome. Much of our present knowledge of the part of cytokines in the sepsis cascade is derived from the development of, and subsequent studies with, recombinant forms of these mediators. Injection of high doses of either recombinant TNF or IL-1 into laboratory animals reproduces many of the clinical and metabolic features of sepsis.[18,19] Interestingly, the combined administration of both cytokines results in a synergistic systemic toxic effect, substantiating the tight interactions between the various members of the cytokine network.[19] Like TNF and IL-1, IL-6 and IL-8 are pyrogenic when administered to animals.[20,21] However, no significant toxicity has been reported following injection of IL-6 or IL-8. Conceivably, these latter cytokines are more 'downstream' components of the sepsis cascade, mediating more specific changes, and probably interfering with the actions of earlier induced cytokines. This is particular true for IL-6, which has been found to inhibit endotoxin-induced TNF and IL-1 production by mononuclear cells *in vitro*, and TNF release in mice *in vivo*.[22,23]

Relatively little is known about the biological effects of cytokines in humans. Most human studies involve trials in patients with widespread malignancies, in whom both TNF and IL-1 appear to be highly toxic. IL-6, recently given to patients with renal cell carcinoma, does not seem to elicit significant side-effects besides fever.[24] In a saline-controlled investigation in healthy volunteers a bolus intravenous injection of TNF induced a variety of changes in several organ systems, including activation of the coagulation and fibrinolytic systems,[25,26] activation of leukocytes,[27] as well as alterations in substrate turnovers and the endocrine environment that mimicked those found in sepsis.[28] Hence, both experimental and clinical evidence is available indicating that cytokines play an important role in the development of tissue injury in systemic infection.

MODULATION OF CYTOKINE ACTIVITY IN SEPSIS

The ultimate proof that cytokines are indeed critical for the initiation of the sepsis cascade is derived from investigations that addressed the efficacy of inhibiting cytokine production or activity in sepsis and endotoxaemia. In 1985 Beutler and colleagues were the first to report that passive immunization against TNF by pretreatment with a specific polyclonal antiserum to TNF protects mice against the lethal effect of intravenously administered endotoxin.[29] Since then the protective effect of immunoneutralization of TNF has been confirmed in a series of sepsis models. In addition, several other strategies to interfere with excessive cytokine activity have been developed (Fig. 6.2). Some of these

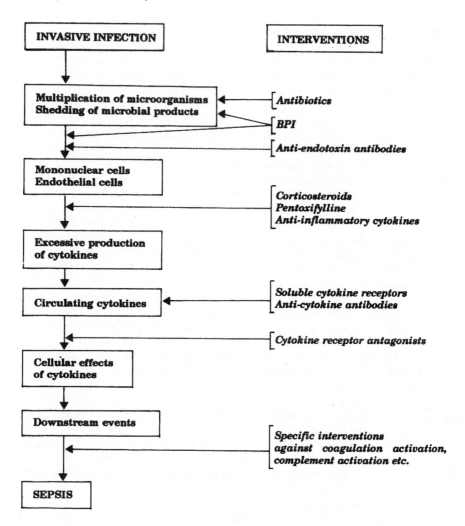

Fig. 6.2   Diagrammatic representation of the sepsis cascade and possible strategies to inhibit the action of cytokines in sepsis. See text for further explanation.

treatment modalities have now been evaluated in clinical trials with patients suffering from sepsis, whereas others are currently undergoing extensive investigations in large multicentre studies. Very little is known about the usefulness of these treatments in patients with acquired immunodeficiencies, such as subjects treated for malignancies with chemotherapy.

Inhibition of production of cytokines

Anti-endotoxin treatment

An approach to the inhibition of cytokine production that has gained attention is the neutralization of the agent responsible for the induction of excessive synthesis of these inflammatory proteins. In the case of Gram-negative sepsis the major inducer of cytokines is endotoxin, the lipopolysaccharide component of the outer membrane of Gram-negative bacteria. Endotoxin is composed of a lipid moiety, called lipid A, and a polysaccharide chain, the O-chain, that protrudes from the membrane into the environment. In an attempt to block endotoxin activity in Gram-negative sepsis, antibodies have been manufactured against several parts of endotoxin. The outer O-specific oligosaccharide side-chains are very immunogenic. Although anti-O antibodies are effective at inhibiting the effects of endotoxin, their clinical application is limited, because many O-serotypes exist, even within one bacterial species, and a particular antibody only binds one particular serotype. The inner part of the polysaccharide chain, the so-called endotoxin 'core', is more conserved. Antibodies directed against the core glycolipid, or against lipid A, which is the biologically active part of endotoxin, may be cross-reactive and may offer protection against most clinically relevant Gram-negative bacteria.

The first randomized trial that investigated the efficacy of anti-endotoxin antibodies was published in 1982.[30] In this study human antiserum was administered to 103 patients with Gram-negative bacteriaemia or focal Gram-negative infection. The antiserum was obtained by immunization of healthy volunteers with *Escherichia coli* 0111: B4 J5, a mutant bacterium that lacks the polysaccharide chain. The control group consisted of 109 patients with similar infections, and was treated with non-immune serum. Originally, 304 patients were enrolled in this trial; 92 patients were excluded from the analysis because they did not have culture proven Gram-negative infection. Although the outcome of the entire population was not reported, in the patients with documented Gram-negative infection treatment with polyclonal anti-J5-antiserum reduced mortality from 39 to 22 per cent.

These results could not be confirmed in a recent trial involving seventy-three children with severe infectious purpura.[31] In this study anti-J5 plasma did not change the course or mortality of these children. In another investigation anti-J5 was administered prophylactically to patients at risk of developing sepsis, e.g. after complicated abdominal surgery, after multiple trauma, and after massive aspiration.[32] Anti-J5 did not prevent the occurrence of Gram-negative infections, but the clinical course of these episodes was less severe when compared to control patients, and the risk of developing septic shock was significantly reduced. Subsequently the efficacy of purified IgG from a pool of plasma samples from volunteers immunized with *E. coli* J5 vaccine was tested in patients with a high likelihood of Gram-negative sepsis in the double-blind placebo-controlled 'Swiss–Dutch' study.[33] Of the eighty-nine evaluable patients, seventy-one turned out to have Gram-negative septic shock, thirty of whom were treated with the J5 IgG fraction, whereas forty-one were treated with a control IgG preparation prepared from a pool of blood donations. Disappointingly, no differences were found between the two treatment groups in any of the pre-defined study end-points.

Hyperimmunoglobulin has also been used in a prophylactic trial in patients at high risk of abdominal sepsis while in surgical intensive care units.[34] Hyper-immunoglobulin (IgG) made from the plasma of donors selected for their high levels of naturally occurring antibodies to *Salmonella minnesota* R595 lipo-polysaccharide, given weekly for up to 4 weeks, did not affect the incidence of mortality, systemic infections, septic shock, or focal infections, as compared with placebo. Remarkably, in this study, that included 329 patients in three treatment arms, a preparation of standard immunoglobulin did reduce the inci-dence of focal infections, as compared with placebo and hyperimmunoglobulin, whereas the rates of systemic infection, septic shock, and mortality were not affected. This apparent discrepancy remained unexplained.[35]

In the past few years several studies have been published that investigated the efficacy of monoclonal antibodies to endotoxin in patients with suspected Gram-negative sepsis. In the first study HA-1A, a human antilipid A IgM antibody derived from immunization with the J5 vaccine of a patient who was scheduled for a staging laparotomy that included splenectomy, was evaluated in a total of 543 patients with a presumptive diagnosis of Gram-negative sepsis.[36] HA-1A was administered to 262 patients as a single 100 mg intravenous dose dissolved in human serum albumin; 281 patients received placebo (human serum albumin alone). In the 200 patients with documented Gram-negative sepsis HA-1A significantly improved survival (reduction in 28-day mortality from 49 to 30 per cent). HA-1A was especially effective in patients with Gram-negative septic shock (reduction in 28-day mortality from 57 to 33 per cent). However, on an intention-to-treat basis HA-1A did not significantly affect clinical outcome (28-day mortality 39 per cent in HA-1A-treated patients vs. 43 per cent in control patients). Further, major concerns about this study appeared shortly after its publication in the literature,[37] and a second placebo-controlled phase III trial of HA-1A, requested by the Food and Drug Administration, was terminated after an interim-analysis of 1500 patients had revealed excess mortality in patients with-out Gram-negative bacteriaemia who received HA-1A.[38]

In another study E5 was used, a murine IgM antilipid A monoclonal anti-body developed from splenocytes immunized with J5 mutant *E. coli* cells.[39] In this study 486 patients received either two intravenous doses 24 hours apart of 2 mg/kg E5, or placebo. Among the 137 patients with documented Gram-negative infection who were not in shock on admission, E5 reduced mortality from 43 to 30 per cent. Mortality rates of the 179 patients with Gram-negative septic shock, as well as of the 152 patients who turned out not to have Gram-negative infection, were not different between the two treatment groups. As for HA-1A, E5 was not efficacious on an intention-to-treat basis.

It is beyond the scope of this chapter to fully discuss the criticism on the clinical anti-endotoxin trials. At present it is clear, however, that anti-endotoxin antibodies are not generally accepted as an essential treatment of patients with a presumptive diagnosis of Gram-negative sepsis. Additionally, there is no evidence that anti-endotoxin treatment should be given to patients at risk of developing sepsis. Further research is necessary to resolve these controversial issues.

Bactericidal/permeability increasing protein

Bactericidal/permeability increasing protein (BPI) is a natural product present in the azurophilic granules of neutrophils, which is cytotoxic for Gram-negative bacteria. BPI has a high affinity for lipopolysaccharide in the outer membrane of Gram-negative microorganisms, and is able to inhibit biological effects of purified endotoxin *in vitro*, as well as in animal experiments.[40,41] In whole blood exogenous administration of BPI or its bioactive fragments has been found to both inhibit the release of TNF elicited by live *E. coli*, and to increase killing of *E. coli*.[40] In human volunteers, recombinant BPI inhibited endotoxin-induced inflammatory responses.[42] These promising results suggest that BPI may be an important addition to currently available agents serving in the treatment of Gram-negative sepsis. BPI has two major advantages over other agents: firstly, it is a natural component of the antimicrobial system of the host, and secondly, it is the only factor known to date that has both bactericidal and endotoxin-neutralizing properties.

Corticosteroids

Corticosteroids are anti-inflammatory and antipyrogenic. They potently inhibit the production of both TNF and IL-1 at the transcriptional level.[2,3] Of importance, corticosteroids only reduce the synthesis of these cytokines when administered before the triggering agent. This may explain why none of the three large clinical trials that addressed the usefulness of corticosteroids in the treatment of sepsis found any evidence of benefit from steroids; steroid recipients even had significantly more secondary bacterial infections.[43-45] Hence, there is no support for the routine use of high-dose steroids in septic shock.

Pentoxifylline

Pentoxifylline is a xanthine derivative that blocks endotoxin-induced TNF synthesis by mononuclear cells *in vitro*,[46] as well as in healthy human volunteers *in vivo*.[14] It has been reported to have a high protective potential in septic shock in experimental animals.[47] Recently, we demonstrated that pentoxifylline inhibits endotoxin-induced coagulation activation, fibrinolytic activation and neutrophil degranulation in a chimpanzee model of sepsis.[48] Investigations with pentoxifylline in patients with sepsis have not been published. Therefore, it remains to be established whether this compound is of use in clinical practice.

Other cytokines

It has become evident that some members of the cytokine family are capable of downregulating the production of other members of this network. The inflammatory cytokine IL-10 has been found to reduce endotoxin-induced lethality in mice, which was associated with a reduction in TNF release.[49]

Binding of cytokines

Soluble cytokine receptors

Soluble receptors for several cytokines have been identified in biological fluids of humans and other species, including IL-2, IL-4, IL-6, IFN-γ, and TNF.[50] They represent truncated forms of the respective membrane receptors that lack trans-membrane and intracytoplasmic domains, but retain the ligand-binding extra-cellular part. The affinities of soluble receptors are commonly comparable to those of the membrane-associated receptors, and they therefore compete with the cellular receptors for binding of the free cytokine. This competition does not always result in inhibition of the activity of the particular cytokine; for example, the soluble receptor for IL-6 is capable of augmenting IL-6 bioactivity. Cur-rently available data indicate that soluble receptors for TNF may be of use in the management of sepsis. Two types of soluble TNF receptors have been isolated, corresponding with the types I and II transmembrane receptors, and each with the capacity to inhibit TNF activity.[51] Both soluble receptors circulate in increased amounts in patients with sepsis, which may be considered a host-defense mechanism.[51,52] Apparently, this inhibitory system is often insufficient to prevent the lethal consequences of high concentrations of TNF. Exogenous administration of these proteins may prove to be beneficial for the outcome of sepsis. Indeed, infusion of recombinant type I soluble TNF receptor into baboons with lethal *E. coli* sepsis attenuated haemodynamic collapse and cytokine release.[51] In addition, chimeric forms of soluble TNF receptors have been constructed, composed of two soluble receptors coupled to an IgG heavy chain, that have a high affinity for TNF and potently antagonized TNF activity *in vitro* and prevented endotoxin-induced death in rodents.[53] However, a recent study reported enhanced mortality in patients with sepsis treated with such a chimeric TNF receptor protein.[54] Explanations for this alarming finding could be an adverse effect of the compound (i.e. delayed release of bioactive TNF from the drug) or the fact that it is harmful to neutralize all TNF during sepsis.

Antibodies directed against cytokines

Much research has been carried out to evaluate the effects of neutralizing cytokines with specific antibodies. A series of studies have shown that anti-TNF treatment, consisting of either purified antiserum or monoclonal antibodies, is highly protective against lethality when given before, simultaneously or very shortly (30 minutes) after intravenous infusion of an LD_{100} dose of endotoxin or live bacteria.[55–57] Furthermore, passive immunization against TNF also strongly reduced the appearances of IL-1β and IL-6 in lethal bacteriaemia in baboons, indicating that TNF is an intermediate factor in the secretion of these other cytokines in sepsis.[58] Importantly, blocking TNF activity appears not to be beneficial in all forms of sepsis: in experimental models in which the bacterial challenge was administered intraperitoneally anti-TNF treatment did not improve clinical outcomes.[59] Recently, a number of studies addressing the efficacy of anti-TNF treatment in patients with sepsis have been published. In one study, anti-TNF therapy was associated with a trend toward higher mortality at 28 days, in the subgroup of patients without shock.[60] In a second trial of the same antibody, high dose treatment resulted in a trend toward increased overall mortality.[61] Hence, if these studies indicate that the neutralization of TNF activity exacerbates infection in patients with sepsis, the safety of anti-TNF treatment in the treatment of sepsis needs serious reconsideration.

Other anticytokine antibodies that have been more or less successful in experimental sepsis in animals include antibodies directed against IL-6 and IFN-γ. Anti-IL-6 monoclonal antibodies protected mice from lethality after LD_{100} doses of either lipopolysaccharide or TNF; however, this protection was no longer observed when the doses of endotoxin or TNF were slightly increased.[62] Anti-IFN-γ monoclonal antibodies also were capable of markedly reducing lethality induced by endotoxin in mice.[6,63]

Blocking of cytokine receptors

Cytokine receptors can be specifically bound by proteins that lack biological activity. To date, the only naturally occurring receptor antagonist identified is the IL-1 receptor antagonist (IL-1ra).[3] IL-1ra was first described as an IL-1 inhibitory activity in the supernatants of human monocytes cultured on adherent IgG, and in the urine of patients with fever and myelomonocytic leukaemia. IL-1ra is structurally related to IL-1α and IL-1β and binds to both known IL-1 receptors without eliciting any discernable biological responses. Several studies indicate that the production of IL-1ra is enhanced in infectious diseases, especially during sepsis. Endogenously produced IL-1ra may serve to limit the severity of disease by impairing the binding of IL-1 to its cellular receptors. Theoretically, administration of IL-1ra may therefore be beneficial in severe infections.

Indeed, exogenous IL-1ra has been reported to improve the outcomes of several disease states. IL-1ra strongly diminished lethality in septic shock models in various species.[3,64,65] In baboons challenged with a lethal dose of live *E. coli*, IL-1ra significantly attenuated haemodynamic collapse and improved survival.[65] In addition, the IL-6 response was reduced by IL-1ra treatment, indicating that apart from TNF (see above), IL-1 also acts as an intermediate factor in the appearance of IL-6 in sepsis. IL-1ra did not affect TNF levels. Importantly, IL-1ra was protective in some animal models when given up to 2 hours after lipopolysaccharide. Moreover, the protective effects of IL-1ra are not limited to infections caused by Gram-negative bacteria: IL-1ra also attenuated shock in staphylococcal bacteriaemia in rabbits.[3]

However, treatment of patients with sepsis with recombinant IL-1ra did not result in an increased survival.[66] Thus, as for anti-TNF strategies, the clinical use of IL-1ra has not proven efficacious.

Strategies to block 'downstream' events

As outlined above, the sepsis cascade is probably initiated by excessive stimulation of the cytokine network by bacteria or their products. Cytokines, and probably bacteria themselves, can subsequently activate other mediator systems, such as the coagulation system, the fibrinolytic system, the complement system and leukocytes. In the past few years several therapeutic strategies have been developed that aim to specifically interfere with these 'downstream' events. The coagulative response to endotoxin or live *E. coli* can be inhibited by either monoclonal antibodies directed against tissue factor (the essential cofactor for activation of the extrinsic pathway of the coagulation system) or factor VIIa, as well as by activated protein C. The administration of C1-esterase inhibitor may be useful to impair activation of both the complement system and the contact system. It is beyond the scope of this chapter to discuss these new treatment modalities in detail.

CONCLUSION

Cytokines play a pivotal role in the pathogenesis of sepsis. Excessive production of TNF, followed by the appearance of other cytokines, initiates a cascade of events that ultimately results in the classical clinical syndrome of sepsis characterized by multiple organ failure, shock and death. Although animal studies in which the excessive activity of proinflammatory cytokines was inhibited have been promising, clinical trials with anti-TNF or IL-1ra did not reveal any benefit (and sometimes even harm) for treated patients. Cancer patients might benefit from a better sepsis treatment in two ways: firstly, the outcome of sepsis, a disease that particularly threatens the ones with a weakened immunodefence, may improve, and secondly, some of these agents may be employed prophylactically in order to reduce the incidence of sepsis. It is without doubt that in the years to come the insights into the pathophysiology of sepsis will continue to grow rapidly. It is hoped that this increased knowledge will lead to a better treatment of this catastrophic illness in the near future.

Acknowledgement

We thank Mrs Gerdie Wentink for preparing the illustrations. Tom van der Poll is a fellow of the Royal Netherlands Academy of Arts and Sciences.

REFERENCES

1. Centers for Disease Control. Increase in National Hospital Discharge Survey rates for septicemia–United States 1979–1987. *MMWR. Morbidity and Mortality Weekly Report* 1990; **39**: 31–4.
2. Vassalli P. The pathophysiology of tumor necrosis factors. *Annual Reviews in Immunology* 1992; **10**: 411–52.
3. Dinarello CA. Interleukin-1 and interleukin-1 antagonism. *Blood* 1991; **77**: 1627–52.
4. Le J, Vilcek J. Biology of disease. Interleukin 6: a multifunctional cytokine regulating immune reactions and the acute phase protein response. *Laboratory Investigation* 1989; **61**: 588–602.
5. Van Damme J. Interleukin-8 and related molecules. In: Thomson AW ed. *The Cytokine Handbook*. London: Harcourt Brace Jovanich, 1991: 201–14.
6. Heremans H, Billiau A. The role of interferon-γ in inflammation. In: van Furth R ed. *Mononuclear Phagocytes*. Amsterdam: Kluwer Academic, 1992: 511–16.
7. Waage A, Halstensen A, Espevik T. Association between tumour necrosis factor in serum and fatal outcome in patients with meningococcal disease. *Lancet* 1987; **i**: 355–7.

8. Girardin E, Grau GE, Dayer J-M, Roux-Lombard P, the J5 study group, Lambert P-H. Tumor necrosis factor and interleukin 1 in the serum of children with severe infectious purpura. *New England Journal of Medicine* 1988; **319**: 397–400.

9. Calandra T, Baumgartner J-D, Grau GE *et al.*, the Swiss-Dutch J5 Immunoglobulin Study Group. Prognostic values of tumor necrosis factor, interleukin-1, interferon-α, and interferon-γ in the serum of patients with septic shock. *Journal of Infectious Diseases* 1990; **161**: 982–7.

10. Hack CE, de Groot ER, Felt-Bersma RJF *et al.* Increased plasma levels of interleukin-6 in sepsis. *Blood* 1989; **74**: 1704–10.

11. Calandra T, Gerain J, Heumann D, Baumgartner J-D, Glauser MP, the Swiss-Dutch J5 Immunoglobulin Study Group. High circulating levels of interleukin-6 in patients with septic shock: evolution during sepsis, prognostic value, and interplay with other cytokines. *American Journal of Medicine* 1991; **91**: 23–9.

12. Hack CE, Hart M, Strack van Schijndel RJM *et al.* Interleukin-8 in sepsis: relation to shock and inflammatory mediators. *Infection and Immunity* 1992; **60**: 2835–42.

13. Hesse DG, Tracey KJ, Fong Y *et al.* Cytokine appearance in human endotoxemia and primate bacteremia. *Surgery Gynecology and Obstetrics* 1988; **166**: 147–53.

14. Zabel P, Wolter DT, Schönharting MM, Schade UF. Oxpentifylline in endotoxemia. *Lancet* 1989; **ii**: 1474–7.

15. Van Deventer SJH, Büller HR, ten Cate JW, Aarden LA, Hack CE, Sturk A. Experimental endotoxemia in humans: analysis of cytokine release and coagulation, fibrinolytic and complement pathways. *Blood* 1990; **76**: 2520–6.

16. Van Deventer SJH, Hart M, van der Poll T, Hack CE, Aarden LA. Endotoxin and TNF-induced IL-8 release in humans. *Journal of Infectious Diseases* 1993; **167**: 461–4.

17. Van Zee KJ, DeForge LE, Fischer E *et al.* IL-8 in septic shock, endotoxemia, and after IL-1 administration. *Journal of Immunology* 1991; **146**: 3478–82.

18. Tracey KJ, Beutler B, Lowry SF *et al.* Shock and tissue injury induced by recombinant human cachectin. *Science* 1986; **234** 470–4.

19. Okusawa S, Gelfland JA, Ikejima T, Connolly RJ, Dinarello CA. Interleukin 1 induces a shock-like state in rabbits. Synergism with tumor necrosis factor and the effect of cyclooxygenase inhibition. *Journal of Clinical Investigation* 1988; **81**: 1162–72.

20. Helle M, Brakenhoff JPJ, de Groot ER, Aarden LA. Interleukin 6 is involved in interleukin 1-induced activities. *European Journal of Immunology* 1988; **18**: 957–9.

21. Van Zee KJ, Fischer E, Hawes AS *et al.* Effects of intravenous IL-8 administration in nonhuman primates. *Journal of Immunology* 1992; **148**: 1746–52.

22. Aderka D, Le J, Vilcek J. IL-6 inhibits lipopolysaccharide-induced tumor necrosis factor production in cultured human monocytes, U937 cells and in mice. *Journal of Immunology* 1989; **143**: 3517–23.

23. Schindler R, Mancilla J, Endres S, Ghorbani R, Clark SC, Dinarello CA. Correlations and interactions in the production of interleukin 6 (IL-6), IL-1 and tumor necrosis factor (TNF) in human blood mononuclear cells: IL-6 suppresses IL-1 and TNF. *Blood* 1990; **75**: 40–7.

24. Stouthard JML, Rorriyn JA, Van der Poll T *et al.* Endocrine and metabolic effects of interleukin-6 in humans. *American Journal of Physiology* 1995; **268**: E813–E819.

25. Van der Poll T, Büller HR, ten Cate H *et al.* Activation of coagulation after administration of tumor necrosis factor to normal subjects. *New England Journal of Medicine* 1990; **322**: 1622–7.

26. Van der Poll T, Levi M, Büller HR *et al.* Fibrinolytic response to tumor necrosis factor in healthy subjects. *Journal of Experimental Medicine* 1991; **174**: 729–32.

27. Van der Poll T, van Deventer SJH, Hack CE *et al.* Effects on leukocytes following injection of tumor necrosis factor into healthy humans. *Blood* 1992; **79**: 693–8.

28. Van der Poll T, Romijn JA, Endert E, Borm JJJ, Büller HR, Sauerwein HP. Tumor

necrosis factor mimics the metabolic response to acute infection in healthy humans. *American Journal of Physiology* 1991; **261**: E457–65.

29. Beutler B, Milsark IW, Cerami A. Passive immunization against cachectin/tumor necrosis factor protects mice from lethal effect of endotoxin. *Science* 1985; **229**: 869–71.

30. Ziegler E, McCutchan JA, Fierer J *et al*. Treatment of gram-negative bacteremia and shock with human antiserum to a mutant *Escherichia coli. New England Journal of Medicine* 1982; **307**: 1225–30.

31. J5 Study Group. Treatment of severe infectious purpura in children with human plasma from donors immunized with *Escherichia coli* J5: a prospective double-blind study. *Journal of Infectious Diseases* 1992; **165**: 695–701.

32. Baumgartner J, Glauser MP, McCutchan JA *et al*. Prevention of Gram-negative shock and death in surgical patients by antibody to endotoxin core glycolipid. *Lancet* 1985; **i**: 59–63.

33. Calandra T, Glauser M, Schellekens J, Verhoef J, the Swiss-Dutch J5 Immuno-globulin Study Group. Treatment of Gram-negative septic shock with human IgG antibody to *Escherichia coli* J5. A prospective double-blind randomized trial. *Journal of Infectious Diseases* 1988; **158**: 312–19.

34. The Intravenous Immunoglobulin Collaborative Study Group. Prophylactic intra-venous administration of standard immune globulin as compared with core-lipopolysaccharide immune globulin in patients at high risk of postsurgical infection. *New England Journal of Medicine* 1992; **327**: 234–40.

35. Siber GR. Immune globulin to prevent nosocomial infections. *New England Journal of Medicine* 1992; **327**: 269–70.

36. Ziegler EJ, Fisher CJ, Sprung CL *et al*., the HA-1A Sepsis Study Group. Treatment of gram-negative bacteremia and septic shock with HA-1A human monoclonal antibody against endotoxin. A randomized, double-blind, placebo-controlled trial. *New England Journal of Medicine* 1991; **324**: 429–36.

37. Quezado ZMN, Natarison C, Hoffman WD. Looking back on HA-1A. *Archives of Internal Medicine* 1994; **154**: 2393.

38. McCloskey RV, Straube RC, Sanders C, Smith SM, Smith CR, the CHESS Trial Study Group. Treatment of septic shock with human monoclonal antibody HA-1A: a randomized, double blind, placebo-controlled trial. *Annals of Internal Medicine* 1994; **121**: 1–5.

39. Greenman RL, Schein RMH, Martin MA. A controlled trial of E5 murine mono-clonal IgM antibody to endotoxin in the treatment of gram-negative sepsis. *Journal of the American Medical Association* 1991; **266**: 1097–102.

40. Weiss J, Eisbach P, Shu C *et al*. Human bactericidal/permeability increasing protein and a recombinant NH_2-terminal fragment cause killing of serum-resistant gram-negative bacteria in whole blood and inhibit tumor necrosis factor release induced by the bacteria. *Journal of Clinical Investigation* 1992; **90**: 1122–30.

41. Fisher Jr. CJ, Marra MN, Palardy JE, Marchbanks CR, Scott RW, Opal SM. Human neutrophil bactericidal/permeability-increasing protein reduces mortality rate from endotoxin challenge: a placebo-controlled study. *Critical Care Medicine* 1994; **22**: 553–8.

42. Von der Möhlen MAM, Kimmings AN, Wedel NI. Inhibition of endotoxin-induced cytokine release and neutrophil activation in humans by use of recombinant bacter-icidal/permeability-increasing protein. *Journal of Infectious Diseases* 1995; **172**: 144–51.

43. Sprung C, Caralis PV, Marcial EH *et al*. The effects of high-dose corticosteroids in patients with septic shock. A prospective, controlled study. *New England Journal of Medicine* 1984; **311**: 1137–43.

44. The Veterans Administration Systemic Sepsis Cooperative Study Group. Effect of

high-dose glucocorticoid therapy on mortality in patients with clinical signs of systemic sepsis. *New England Journal of Medicine* 1987; **317**: 659–65.

45. Bone RC, Fisher CJ Jr, Clemmer TP, Slotman GJ, Metz CA, Balk RA. A controlled trial of high-dose methyl prednisolone in the treatment of severe sepsis and septic shock. *New England Journal of Medicine* 1987; **317**: 653–8.

46. Strieter RM, Remick PA, Ward PA *et al.* Cellular and molecular regulation of tumor necrosis factor production by pentoxifylline. *Biochemical Biophysical Research Communications* 1988; **155**: 1230–6.

47. Schade UF. Pentoxyfylline increases survival in murine endotoxin shock and decreases formation of tumor necrosis factor. *Circulatory Shock* 1990; **31**: 171–81.

48. Levi M, ten Cate H, Bauer KA *et al.* Inhibition of endotoxin-induced coagulation and fibrinolysis by pentoxifylline or by a monoclonal anti-tissue factor antibody in chimpanzees. *Journal of Clinical Investigation* 1994; **94**: 114–20.

49. Gerard C, Bruyns C, Marchant A *et al.* Interleukin 10 reduces the release of tumor necrosis factor and prevents lethality in experimental endotoxemia. *Journal of Experimental Medicine* 1993; **177**: 547–50.

50. Fernandez-Botran R. Soluble cytokine receptors: their role in immunoregulation. *FASEB Journal* 1991; **5**: 2567–74.

51. Van Zee KJ, Kohno T, Fischer E, Rock GS, Moldawer LL, Lowry SF. Tumor necrosis factor soluble receptors circulate in during experimental and clinical inflammation and can protect against excessive tumor necrosis factor α *in vitro* and *in vivo*. *Proceedings of the National Academy of Sciences, USA* 1992; **89**: 4845–9.

52. Girardin E, Roux-Lombard P, Grau GE, Suter P, Gallati H, the J5 Study Group. Imbalance between tumour necrosis factor-α and soluble TNF receptor concentrations in severe meningococcaemia. *Immunology* 1992; **76**: 20–3.

53. Ashkenazi A, Marsters SA, Capon DJ *et al.* Protection against endotoxic shock by a tumor necrosis factor receptor immunoadhesin. *Proceedings of the National Academy of Sciences, USA* 1991; **88**: 10535–9.

54. Fisher Jr. CJ, Agosti JM, Opal SE *et al.* Treatment of septic shock with the tumor necrosis factor receptor: Fc fusion protein. *New England Journal of Medicine* 1996; **334**: 1697–702.

55. Tracey KJ, Fong Y, Hesse DG *et al.* Anti-cachectin/TNF monoclonal antibodies prevent septic shock during lethal bacteraemia. *Nature* 1987; **330**: 662–4.

56. Hinshaw LB, Tekamp-Olson P, Chang ACK *et al.* Survival of primates in LD100 septic shock following therapy with antibody to tumor necrosis factor (TNF). *Circulatory Shock* 1990; **30**: 279-92.

57. Silva AT, Bayston KF, Cohen J. Prophylactic and therapeutic effects of a monoclonal antibody to tumor necrosis factor-α in experimental gram-negative shock. *Journal of Infectious Diseases* 1990; **162**: 421–7.

58. Fong Y, Tracey KJ, Moldawer LL *et al.* Antibodies to cachectin/tumor necrosis factor reduce interleukin 1β and interleukin 6 appearance during lethal bacteremia. *Journal of Experimental Medicine* 1989; **170**: 1627–33.

59. Zanetti G, Heumann D, Gérain J *et al.* Cytokine production after intravenous or peritoneal gram-negative bacterial challenge in mice. Comparative protective efficacy of antibodies to tumor necrosis factor-α and to lipopolysaccharide. *Journal of Immunology* 1992; **148**: 1890–7.

60. Abraham E, Wunderink R, Silverman H *et al.* Efficacy and safety of monoclonal antibody to human tumor necrosis factor α in patients with sepsis syndrome: a randomized, controlled, double-blind, multicenter clinical trial. *Journal of the American Medical Association* 1995; **273**: 934–41.

61. Carlet J, Cohen J, Andersson *et al.* INTERCEPT: an international efficacy and safety study of monoclonal antibody (MAb) to human tumor necrosis factor in patients with the sepsis syndrome. In *Program of the 34th Interscience Conference*

on Antimicrobial Agents and Chemotherapy. Orlando, Florida; 1994; **7**: Washington DC: American Society for Microbiology.

62. Libert C, Vink A, Coulie P *et al.* Limited involvement of interleukin-6 in the pathogenesis of lethal septic shock as revealted by the effect of monoclonal antibodies against interleukin-6 or its receptor in various murine models. *European Journal of Immunology* 1992; **22**: 2625–30.

63. Silva AT, Cohen J. Role interferon-γ in experimental gram-negative sepsis. *Journal of Infectious Diseases* 1992; **166**: 331–5.

64. Ohlsson K, Björk P, Bergenfeldt M, Hageman R, Thompson RC. Interleukin 1 receptor antagonist reduces mortality from endotoxin shock. *Nature* 1990; **348**: 550–2.

65. Fischer E, Marano MA, van Zee KJ *et al.* Interleukin-1 receptor blockade improves survival and hemodynamic performance in *Escherichia coli* septic shock, but fails to alter host responses to sublethal endotoxemia. *Journal of Clincal Investigation* 1992; **89**: 1551–7.

66. Fisher Jr. CJ, Dhairiant JFA, Opal SM *et al.* Recombinant human interleukin 1 receptor antagonist in the treatment of patients with sepsis syndrome. *Journal of the American Medical Association* 1994; **271**: 1836–43.

PART 3

Support of treatment-related complications

CHAPTER 7

Improved control of chemotherapy-induced emesis

EDITH A PEREZ————————————————————

INTRODUCTION

Information on patient quality of life is increasingly being sought to provide a more comprehensive evaluation of the outcome of cancer treatment. The prevention and management of chemotherapy-induced emesis greatly influence the quality of life of patients receiving chemotherapy. Cytotoxic chemotherapeutic agents may induce nausea and vomiting of variable intensity and duration. Both side-effects have been shown to be notable stressors for patients who undergo chemotherapy. Therefore, effective protection from nausea and vomiting associated with chemotherapy has been one of the most important goals of anti-emetic therapy.

In recent years, considerable progress has been made in managing chemotherapy-induced emesis.

Since the earliest reports of the ability of 5-hydroxytryptamine-3 (5-HT$_3$) receptor antagonists to block emesis associated with chemotherapy drugs, a variety of different compounds have been synthesized and developed for this purpose. The introduction of these agents has dramatically improved the management of chemotherapy-induced emesis.[1,2,3]

This review discusses several factors that have contributed to improved anti-emetic control, including new findings regarding the physiology of emesis, insight into the pathogenesis of chemotherapy-induced emesis, standardization of anti-emetic trial methodology, and the development and evaluation of intravenous and oral 5-HT$_3$ antagonists. In clinical studies performed to date, these agents have proven to be both effective and safe. In addition to a high degree of effectiveness, these agents are characterized by a low incidence of significant side-effects and the absence of extrapyramidal reactions. The current state of knowledge with respect to the serotonin antagonists as anti-emetics for patients receiving cytotoxic chemotherapy is summarized.

PHYSIOLOGY OF EMESIS

The mechanisms involved in chemotherapy-induced emesis are an area of active preclinical research. Studies in a variety of species have provided evidence that an intact abdominal visceral innervation is critical for the initiation of emesis following chemotherapy administration.[4–6] Therefore, the current hypothesis is that the primary site of emetogenesis of cytotoxic chemotherapy is in the gut wall, leading to activation of vagal afferents, which in time trigger central emetic pathways.

THE ROLE OF SEROTONIN IN CHEMOTHERAPY-INDUCED EMESIS

Serotonin (5-hydroxytryptamine) is a widely distributed neurotransmitter whose actions are mediated by 5-HT receptors.[7] Three main groups of 5-HT receptors have been characterized.[8–10] One of these, the type 3 (5-HT$_3$) receptor appears to play a key role in the emetic process.[11]

The initial clue identifying the role of the 5-HT$_3$ receptor in chemotherapy-induced emesis arose from speculation on the mechanism by which high-dose metoclopramide was able to prevent cisplatin-induced emesis. Unlike other dopamine D$_2$ receptor antagonists, high-dose metoclopramide had shown an unusually good ability to antagonize the emesis associated with cisplatin.[12] This led to the suggestion that an alternative mechanism, unrelated to D$_2$ receptor blockade, might be involved.[13] In fact, prior investigators had demonstrated that higher doses of metoclopramide, in addition to its antidopaminergic properties, were also weak 5-HT$_3$ antagonists.[14]

Miner et al. subsequently employed a selective 5-HT$_3$ antagonist, which had no capability to block D$_2$ receptors (dolasetron), in the ferret model, a system used to evaluate preclinical activity of new anti-emetics.[15]

Using this agent, they were able to completely inhibit the capacity of cisplatin to produce emesis in this experimental model. Costal et al. noted similar findings employing another selective 5-HT$_3$ antagonist, tropisetron.[16]

SELECTIVE 5-HT$_3$ ANTAGONISTS: MECHANISM(S) OF ACTION

The mechanisms of action by which 5-HT$_3$ antagonists exert their anti-emetic effects remain only partially defined. Both peripheral and central sites of action have been proposed (Fig. 7.1). Significant insight into the process of 5-HT$_3$ antagonist action has been gained from studies exploring the means by which chemotherapy produces emesis. There is considerable evidence that chemotherapy can damage small intestinal mucosa, resulting in the release of a number of neuroactive substances including serotonin.[17,18] The major storage site for serotonin in humans is the enterochromaffin cells of the small intestine.[19–23] Significant numbers of 5-HT$_3$ receptors have been identified on vagal afferents and other neurons within the gut.[11,14,24] Using the ferret model, Hawthorn et al.

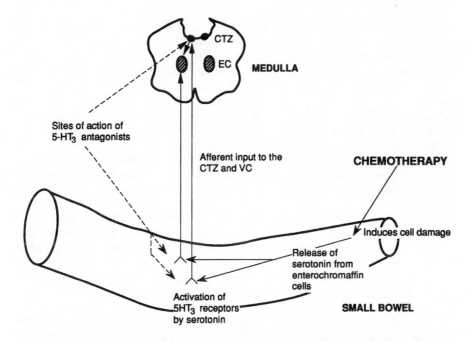

Fig. 7.1.   Model illustrating the sites of action of the 5-HT₃ receptor antagonists in blocking chemotherapy-induced emesis. VC, vomiting center; CTZ, chemoreceptor trigger zone.

were able to completely prevent emesis in response to cisplatin through a combination of bilateral nerve sectioning.[25] These observations combined with the results of prior studies led them to propose the following hypothesis: (1) cisplatin triggers the release of serotonin from enterochromaffin cells in the gut; (2) serotonin then binds to vagal and splanchnic 5-HT₃ receptors increasing afferent input to the vomiting center resulting in its activation; (3) 5-HT₃ receptor antagonists may prevent emesis by blocking the latter process.

5-HT₃ antagonists act by preventing the activation of 5-HT released from gut mucosal enterochromaffin cells (EC). Excessive release of 5-HT from such EC has been demonstrated to occur in response to cytotoxic drugs.[26] Additional sites of 5-HT₃ receptor activation, such as the nucleus tractus solitarius or the area postrema in the brainstem, may play a secondary role in emetogenesis. This hypothesis is partially supported by data from studies in the ferret, in which increases in c-*fos* oncogene expression in the area postrema and nucleus tractus solitarius have been seen after cisplatin administration,[27] which is potentially indicative of neuronal activation involved in the emetic response. The mechanisms by which cytotoxic drugs induce 5-HT release from EC are not clear, but may involve free radical generation and perhaps the involvement of cholinergic interneurons.[6,26]

The reported preclinical differences between 5-HT₃ receptor antagonists include structure, selectivity, potency, anti-emetic predictability, and duration of action.[4,5] Ondansetron is a carbazole derivative and exists as a racemate that contains two enantiomers, whereas granisetron is an indazole derivative that exists as a single molecular species without enantiomers. Van Wijngaarden *et al.*[28]

compared the binding profile of a range of 5-HT$_3$ receptor antagonists and reported different receptor specificity for different 5-HT$_3$ antagonists.[28] Using radioligand-binding techniques to measure the affinity of these agents, they demonstrated that ondansetron, granisetron and tropisetron have high affinity for 5-HT$_3$ receptors, but that ondansetron also has detectable binding (pK_i >5, where pK_i is the −log of the ligand concentration to yield 50 per cent receptor binding) at 5-HT$_{1B}$, 5-HT$_{1C}$, α_1-adrenergic, and opioid μ sites. In contrast, granisetron was shown only to bind to 5-HT$_3$ receptors, and tropisetron only to 5-HT$_3$ and 5-HT uptake receptors. In addition, the affinity of ondansetron for the 5-HT$_3$ receptor was 250–500 times greater than for other receptor types. In the case of granisetron and tropisetron, the selectivity ratios were greater than 1000:1. The functional (clinical) relevance of these findings has not yet been defined.

Recent studies reported by Gebauer *et al.*[29] have demonstrated the presence of 5-HT autoreceptors on the EC of the guinea pig. It appears that activation of a 5-HT$_4$ receptor on the EC suppresses the release of 5-HT, whereas activation of an EC 5-HT$_3$ receptor enhances the release. The investigators also reported different relative efficacies for the various 5-HT$_3$ antagonists on the afferent neuronal 5-HT$_3$ receptors and on the EC 5-HT$_3$ receptors. Ondansetron, granisetron and tropisetron all block vagal afferent 5-HT$_3$ receptors, whereas the EC 5-HT$_3$ receptor is blocked by granisetron or tropisetron, but not by ondansetron. There was a weak blocking activity of the EC 5-HT$_4$ receptor by tropisetron in this model.

ANTI-EMETIC TRIAL METHODOLOGY

The application of standardized study methodology has been instrumental in the recent progress made in anti-emetic therapy. Within the past 15 years, accurate and reliable methods of evaluating both nausea and vomiting have been developed.[30,31] This methodology includes both reproducible objective parameters, as well as subjective assessments from the patient. By general consensus, response criteria for acute emesis are defined as:

- Complete response − no episodes of retching or emesis
- Major response − two or fewer emetic episodes
- Minor response − three to five episodes
- Failure − more than five emetic episodes.

Subjective parameters include visual analog scales and patient diaries to assess nausea, and descriptive scales for measuring patient satisfaction with therapy. Accurate assessment of the side-effect profile of new anti-emetics is also an important component of this improved study methodology.

In a similar fashion to the study of new chemotherapeutic agents, a systematic program to evaluate investigational anti-emetics begins with phase I trials to determine safety and tolerance, then proceeding to phase II studies to establish efficacy, and finally phase III studies for comparison to standard therapy. The optimal design for phase III trials evaluating new anti-emetics is that of randomized, double-blind, parallel group studies. However, crossover group studied designs have sometimes been employed to provide direct patient comparisons of each treatment option, and to allow patient preference for one treatment or the other to be expressed. Using this organized approach, active new single agents are reliably identified, and rational combinations of anti-emetics can then be developed.

CLINICAL DEVELOPMENT OF SEROTONIN ANTAGONISTS

A number of selective 5-HT$_3$ antagonists have entered clinical evaluation as potential anti-emetic agents for chemotherapy-induced emesis (Table 7.1). Chemotherapy, and specifically cisplatin, results in two distinct patterns of emesis, the first a well-described and studied acute emetic, and the second a less well-recognized syndrome of delayed emesis (Table 7.2). By comparison to the acute emesis syndrome the pathogenesis of delayed emesis remains undefined.

After it was realized that 5-HT$_3$ receptor antagonists administered intravenously presented a distinct advantage over the more traditional agents used to treat chemotherapy-induced nausea and vomiting, anti-emetic prophylaxis with intravenous 5-HT$_3$ receptor antagonists during chemotherapy became well established.[32,33]

Whereas intravenous anti-emetic agents can effectively control chemotherapy-induced emesis, oral therapy may be more convenient and acceptable to patients. An effective oral 5-HT$_3$ receptor antagonist would allow administration in ambulatory and outpatient settings, which is particularly important for patients in whom the onset of emesis may be delayed, such as those receiving treatment with cyclophosphamide. Outpatient administration would also reduce the requirements for medical resources. The convenience of an oral drug would

Table 7.1 Selective 5-HT$_3$ antagonists

Ondansetron
Granisetron
Tropisetron
Dolasetron

Table 7.2 Chemotherapy-induced emesis

Acute	
Definition:	Within 24 h following chemotherapy
Incidence:	~ 100% of patients not receiving anti-emetic treatment
Pathogenesis:	Serotonin (5-HT$_3$) receptor
	Dopamine-2 receptor
Delayed	
Definition:	16–120 h following chemotherapy
Incidence:	20–93% of chemotherapy-treated patients
Pathogenesis:	Undefined
	No clear role for the 5-HT$_3$ receptor

benefit both patients and staff, translating into a reduction in the overall cost of chemotherapy and associated treatments. Patient- and drug-related factors should be considered when selecting patients for 5-HT$_3$ receptor antagonist therapy. Women are more prone to emesis than are men, as are younger patients.[34,35] In addition, emesis is more difficult to control in women.[36]

The chemotherapeutic regimen itself also directly affects the likelihood of nausea and vomiting. Chemotherapeutic drugs vary in their potential to cause emesis, with higher doses generally having increased emetogenic potential (Table 7.3).[37–39]

Although 5-HT$_3$ receptor antagonists achieve better emetogenic control than older anti-emetics in patients receiving moderately emetogenic chemotherapy,[40–42] the more costly 5-HT$_3$ receptor antagonists are best used in these patients only after weighing the risk factors for emetogenesis and the particular patient's ability to tolerate more traditional anti-emetic therapy. The 5-HT$_3$ receptor antagonists are almost never indicated to prevent emesis in patients being treated with chemotherapeutic regimens with a moderately low potential for emetogenicity, except for the rare individual who is intolerant of alternative drugs.

INTRAVENOUS AND ORAL SEROTONIN ANTAGONISTS: THEIR USE AS ANTI-EMETICS

Preclinical studies have demonstrated that control of emesis due to either chemotherapy or radiotherapy can be obtained with lower doses of granisetron than tropisetron (by a factor of two or three) or ondansetron (by a factor of eight to ten).[3] Both granisetron and tropisetron have a longer duration of action than ondansetron (twofold to threefold in animal models of emesis). The plasma half-life of granisetron in patients receiving chemotherapy has been reported to be 10.6 hours versus 4.0–4.5 hours for ondansetron. Considerable interpatient variability in plasma drug concentration has been reported. However, clinical data do not support any obvious relationship between the plasma kinetics of 5-HT$_3$ receptor antagonists and their anti-emetic effects.

A variety of studies highlight the overall efficacy and safety profile of the 5-HT$_3$ antagonists tested. Although retrospective analysis did suggest clinical differences among these agents,[43] review of these recently reported prospective randomized trials allows us to interpret more directly for any potential similarities or differences.

Despite the pharmacological differences described, no meaningful clinical differences have yet emerged with respect to efficacy between the available 5-HT$_3$ receptor antagonists in the prevention of chemotherapy-induced acute emesis. However, a study to demonstrate a true clinical difference of 10 per cent between two of the compounds with 80 per cent power would require 1000 patients, and if the clinical difference were only 5 per cent, then it would require a study of 3000 patients.

Table 7.3 Emetogenicity of commonly used chemotherapeutic agents[37–39]

Moderately low (<30%)	Moderate (30–60%)	Moderately high (60–90%)	High (>90%)
Altretamine	Asparaginase	Actinomycin D	Cisplatin
Androgens		Carmustine ≧100mg/m^2	Cytarabine >500 mg/m^2
Bleomycin		Cyclophosphamide ≧600 mg/m^2	Dacarbazine
Busulfan	Carboplatin	Dactinomycin	Ifosfamide >1.5 g/m^2
Chlorambucil	Carmustine <100 mg/m^2	Daunorubicin >50 mg/m^2	Mechlorethamine
Cladribine	Cyclophosphamide <600 mg/m^2	Lomustine	Streptozocin
Corticosteroids	Daunorubicin <50 mg/m^2	Methotrexate >200 mg/m^2	
Cytarabine ≦500 mg/m^2	Doxorubicin ≦50 mg/m^2	Procarbazine	
Docetaxel		Semustine	
Estrogen			
Etoposide	Hexamethylmelamine		
Fluorouracil			
Fludarabine	Idarubicin		
Hydroxyurea	Ifosfamide ≦1.5 g/m^2		
Melphalan			
Mercaptopurine	Methotrexate >500 mg/m^2		
Methotrexate ≦200 mg/m^2			
Mitomycin			
Mitoxantrone			
Paclitaxel			
Pentostatin			
Progestin			
Teniposide			
Thioguanine			
Thiotepa			
Topotecan			
Vinblastine			
Vincristine			
Vinorelbine			

Dosing issues

Using the 5-HT$_3$ receptor antagonist drugs at their lowest effective doses is one way to reduce the cost of such therapy. Initial dose-finding studies with granisetron, which compared 40 and 160 µg/kg doses, showed the lower dose to be optimal in preventing nausea and vomiting induced by moderately to highly emetogenic chemotherapy. Based on these results, many clinical efficacy trials conducted with granisetron have used the 40 µg/kg dose (or a simplified 3 mg regimen), and this remains the recommended dose in some countries.

The results from two randomized double-blind trials provided the basis for the United States' Food and Drug Administration (FDA) approval of a 10 µg/kg granisetron dose.[44,45] In a study comparing 2, 10 and 40 µg/kg doses of intravenous (IV) granisetron in 157 patients receiving highly emetogenic chemotherapy, the two higher doses were significantly more effective than the lowest dose.[44] However, the 40 µg/kg dose did not significantly increase anti-emetic control over the 10 µg/kg dose. In this study, complete responses (defined as no vomiting and no more than mild nausea) were attained in 30.8 per cent of patients treated with 2 µg/kg, 61.5 per cent of patients in the 10 µg/kg group, and 67.9 per cent of patients receiving the 40 µg/kg dose.

Similar results were obtained in the second dose-response study, which compared single doses of IV granisetron (5, 10, 20 and 40 µg/kg) in 353 patients stratified for high- or low-dose cisplatin therapy (Fig. 7.2).[45] Again, no signifi-

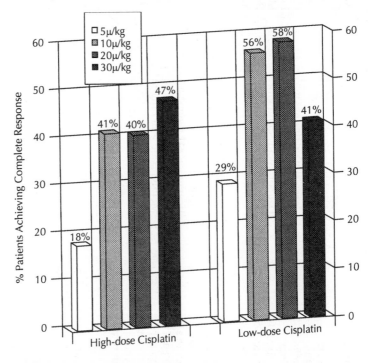

Fig. 7.2. Cisplatin: high- versus low-dose. Percentage of patients treated with high- and low-dose cisplatin who had a complete response (no vomiting, no use of rescue anti-emetics) to pretreatment with intravenous (IV) granisetron, 5, 10, 20, or 40 µg/kg.

cant therapeutic gain was achieved by increasing the dose of granisetron above 10 μg/kg in either stratum.

In the United States, the recommended dose of IV ondansetron for prophylaxis of cisplatin-induced nausea and vomiting is 0.15 mg/kg every 4 hours × 3 doses or a single 32 mg dose; in Europe the recommendation is 8 mg. Dose-finding studies in Europe and the United States that compared IV ondansetron (8 mg, 32 mg and three 0.15 mg/kg doses given 3 hours apart) showed inconsistent results. For example, Beck et al.[46] demonstrated that the 32 mg dose (used for moderately emetogenic regimens) was more effective in preventing nausea and vomiting associated with high dose cisplatin therapy.[46,47]

At their recommended doses, granisetron, ondansetron, tropisetron and dolasetron have proved to be effective in patients receiving highly emetogenic drugs. Some institutions have begun lowering 5-HT$_3$ receptor antagonist drug doses (particularly ondansetron) as a cost-saving measure in patients receiving chemotherapeutic drugs that have lower emetogenic potential. Although controlled clinical trials have not been done to establish the efficacy of these regimens, an open-label pilot study by Hesketh et al. supports the feasibility of titrating the 5-HT$_3$ receptor antagonist dose in combination with dexamethasone according to the emetogenic potential of the chemotherapeutic regimen without compromising anti-emetic control.[48]

In this trial, patients received a single dose of IV ondansetron in combination with dexamethasone, 20 mg IV, 30 min before administration of emetogenic chemotherapy. The ondansetron dose was stratified according to the emetogenic potential of chemotherapy – 32 mg if the chemotherapy was highly emetogenic, 24 mg if the emetogenic potential was moderately high, and 8 mg for moderately emetogenic chemotherapy. Complete response, defined as no emetic episodes, occurred in 38 of 53 (72 per cent) patients receiving highly emetogenic chemotherapy, 45 of 51 (88 per cent) patients given moderately highly emetogenic drugs, and 24 of 31 (77 per cent) patients treated with moderately emetogenic chemotherapy. However, complete absence of nausea was only reported by 51 per cent, 69 per cent, and 47 per cent of these three groups, respectively.

Optimizing oral therapy

Oral administration of the 5-HT$_3$ receptor antagonists may improve convenience and acceptability of treatment while at the same time reducing cost. Both granisetron and ondansetron are available in oral formulations. Oral granisetron can be used to prevent acute nausea and vomiting associated with moderately and highly emetogenic chemotherapy; oral ondansetron is effective only in patients receiving chemotherapeutic regimens with a moderate potential for emetogenicity. A variety of recent studies have been completed comparing the efficacy of different intravenous versus oral anti-emetics.

The efficacy of the recommended dose for oral granisetron, 1 mg b.i.d., was established in an international dose-finding study involving 930 patients receiving moderately emetogenic chemotherapy.[49] In this investigation, total control of emesis was achieved in 43.7 per cent of those who received 0.25 mg b.i.d., 53.6 per cent of those who received 0.50 mg b.i.d., 58.8 per cent of those who received 1 mg b.i.d., and 54.0 per cent of those who received 2 mg b.i.d.

Maximum efficacy at the 1 mg b.i.d. dose was achieved without any significant increase in adverse events, compared with the lower-dose regimens.

Oral granisetron has also been proved superior to conventional oral anti-emetic regimens in controlling nausea and vomiting associated with moderately emetogenic chemotherapy. Heron et al., for example, compared the following anti-emetic regimens:[50]

- Oral granisetron, 1 mg b.i.d. for 7 days
- Oral granisetron, 1 mg b.i.d. for 7 days, plus dexamethasone, a single 12 mg IV dose, prior to cisplatin
- IV dexamethasone, one 12 mg dose, plus metoclopramide in a 3 mg/kg loading dose followed by 4 mg/kg infusion on day 1 and oral metoclopramide, 10 mg t.i.d. on days 2–6.[50]

In this randomized, double-blind trial of 357 cisplatin-treated patients, monotherapy with oral granisetron was equivalent to the combination of metoclopramide plus dexamethasone in symptom control during the first 24 hours. The combination of oral granisetron and dexamethasone was significantly superior to either of the other two regimens. The rates of total control (no nausea, no vomiting) were 37.2 per cent for metoclopramide plus dexamethasone, 43.7 per cent for oral granisetron, and 54.7 per cent for oral granisetron plus dexamethasone.

Indirect comparison of data from the trial reported by Heron et al.[50] with historical results obtained in SmithKline Beecham-sponsored trials of IV granisetron indicate that oral granisetron, 1 mg b.i.d., is also comparable to the parenterally administered drug in reducing nausea and vomiting in patients receiving high-dose cisplatin (> 80 mg/day). At 24 hours after cisplatin administration, the mean overall complete response rate was 60.3 per cent among patients receiving IV granisetron, 40 µg/kg, and 52.1 per cent in patients treated orally.[51]

Recent findings have shown that oral granisetron (1 mg b.i.d.) is an effective anti-emetic.[52] The feasibility of modifying this regimen to a once-daily dose of 2 mg of oral granisetron has been investigated in a randomized, double-masked, parallel-group trial involving 64 centres in the United States.[53]

Of 700 chemotherapy-naive adult patients randomized to treatment (201 men, 499 women), three did not receive chemotherapy and were excluded from the analysis of efficacy. A total of 697 patients, among whom the most common malignancy was breast cancer, received both study drug and chemotherapy and were included in the intent-to-treat analysis of the data. The cytostatic agents and doses varied, but the most commonly used – either singly or in combination – were cyclophosphamide (73.7 per cent), doxorubicin (50.4 per cent), and 5-fluorouracil (38.7 per cent); carboplatin, methotrexate, etoposide, vincristine, and cisplatin were each given to 11–17 per cent of patients. Granisetron was given 1 hour before chemotherapy in all patients, and then 12 hours later in the group receiving 1 mg b.i.d.; the group receiving 2 mg once daily received placebo at this time.

During the 24 hours after administration of chemotherapy, no differences between the two groups could be detected in any of the outcome measures. Total control (no nausea, no vomiting, and no use of rescue anti-emetics) was achieved in at least 50 per cent of all patients; about 52 per cent had no nausea, and more than 76 per cent had no vomiting. The use of rescue anti-emetic medication was similar to the incidence of vomiting. Granisetron appeared to be more effective in men than in women, although no statistical comparisons were performed. Analysis of subsets of patients showed no difference in response with different cytostatic regimens.[54] It was concluded that a once-daily dose of oral granisetron (2 mg) was as effective as 1 mg b.i.d. in preventing nausea and vomiting associated with moderately emetogenic chemotherapy.

Perez *et al.* recently reported the results of a study evaluating the efficacy and safety of oral granisetron versus intravenous ondansetron in prevention of moderately emetogenic chemotherapy-induced nausea and vomiting.[55] This was a multicentre, double-blind, parallel-group study comparing the prophylactic efficacy and safety of 2 mg oral granisetron versus 32 mg IV ondansetron given once before cyclophosphamide- or carboplatin-based chemotherapy. Chemotherapy-naive patients (866 females, 219 males) received two 1 mg granisetron tablets ($n = 542$) or placebo at 60 min pre-chemotherapy, and a 15 min infusion of ondansetron ($n = 543$) or placebo at 30 min pre-chemotharapy. Dexamethasone or methylprednisolone were permitted. The primary efficacy end-point was total control (defined as no emesis, nausea or use of anti-emetic rescue medication) at 24 and 48 hours after start of chemotherapy. Secondary end-points were incidence of emesis and nausea (plus incidence of anti-emetic rescue) at 24 and 48 hours. Comparable efficacy was shown for all end-points ($P < 0.0001$) (Table 7.4).

Safety was assessed up to 11 days post-chemotherapy. Adverse experiences were similar in both groups, except for dizziness (5.4 per cent granisetron-versus 9.6 per cent ondansetron-treated patients; $P = 0.01$) and abnormal vision (0.6 per cent granisetron versus 4.2 per cent ondansetron-treated patients; $P < 0.001$). The authors concluded that granisetron tablets provided comparable efficacy to IV ondansetron in chemotherapy-naive patients receiving moderately emetogenic chemotherapy and that both agents were well tolerated.

A recently completed study performed in the United States compared the efficacy of 2 mg oral granisetron versus 32 mg intravenous granisetron in approximately 1000 chemotherapy-naive patients receiving cisplatin at ≥ 70 mg/m^2 (personal communication, C. Friedman, December 1996). Preliminary data are that the efficacies of oral granisetron and intravenous ondansetron in preventing nausea and vomiting at the doses and schedules used, are equivalent.

Another 5-HT$_3$ receptor antagonist that has been investigated in an oral-only

Table 7.4 Comparison of efficacy of oral granisetron versus IV ondansetron in prevention of nausea and vomiting

	24 hours		48 hours	
	Oral granisetron	*IV ondansetron*	*Oral granisetron*	*IV ondansetron*
Total control (%)	59.4	58.0	46.7	43.8
No emesis (%)	71.0	72.6	58.7	59.1
No nausea (%)	60.0	58.4	47.4	44.4

regimen is ondansetron. In many of the clinical trials, however, ondansetron was not compared with other anti-emetics or was compared only with placebo.[56] In addition, an initial intravenous dose was commonly used, making it difficult to separate the intravenous and oral effects. No clear evidence can be found in these trials that oral ondansetron is superior to conventional anti-emetic regimens.[56] A search of the literature, however, reveals ten trials that assessed the effectiveness of oral ondansetron used alone for control of acute emesis (Table 7.5). Three of these trials were uncontrolled,[57–59] two were placebo controlled,[60–61] and two compared ondansetron alone with combinations of ondansetron plus dexamethasone[62] or ondansetron plus the dopamine antagonist metopimazine.[63] The combination therapies showed superior efficacy. The remaining three trials compared oral ondansetron used as a single agent with conventional anti-emetic regimens[64–66] and showed it to be approximately equal in efficacy to metoclopramide. Indeed, one of these trials showed the combination of dexamethasone and metoclopramide to be superior to oral ondansetron.[66]

Nine of the ten trials of oral ondansetron for the prevention of acute emesis involved patients receiving moderately emetogenic chemotherapy. In the one study that enrolled patients due to receive cisplatin chemotherapy,[62] complete control of acute emesis (during the first 24–48 hours after cisplatin) was achieved in only 7 per cent of patients given oral ondansetron alone, although an additional 22 per cent reported only one or two episodes of emesis. Despite oral ondansetron being given at a dose of 8 mg three times daily, 78 per cent of the patients reported moderate or severe nausea in the 24–28 hours after cisplatin. Conclusions are difficult to draw, however, because this study was small, and cisplatin was administered on day 4 of chemotherapy, following other agents.

Delayed emesis

Delayed emesis, defined as emesis occurring more than 24 hours after chemotherapy administration, often affects patients receiving cisplatin, cyclophosphamide, doxorubicin, or ifosfamide.[67] It is usually less severe than acute emesis and peaks in intensity on the second to third days after chemotherapy. Vomiting can persist for several days thereafter, however. The mechanism of the delayed emetogenic response to antineoplastic drugs is unclear, but it may differ from that responsible for acute emesis.

Few data support the continued use of 5-HT$_3$ receptor antagonists to control delayed emesis. Some of the studies designed to evaluate the efficacy of these drugs for preventing acute emesis also reported emesis rates over succeeding days in the presence or absence of continued anti-emetic therapy. Because these studies did not consider the effect of acute emesis control or other prognostic factors on the risk of delayed emesis, the relevance of the findings is questionable.

These methodology problems were addressed in a large, placebo-controlled, double-blind trial by Navari *et al.* designed to evaluate the efficacy of oral ondansetron in controlling cisplatin-induced delayed emesis.[68] The results showed ondansetron significantly superior to placebo in reducing emesis rates for up to 5 days (Fig. 7.3). The advantage of ondansetron became progressively

Table 7.5 Summary of trials of oral ondansetron in the prevention of acute emesis (first 24 hours after chemotherapy)

Reference	No. of patients	Chemotherapeutic and anti-emetic regimens	Main results
Uncontrolled trials			
Marschner et al.[57]	40	Cyclophosphamide-epirubicin Ondansetron, 8 mg TID, for up to 10 cycles	77% Steady or better control of vomiting during whole treatment period; 60–100% control of nausea (none or mild)
Campora et al.[58]	29	CMF* Ondansetron, 8 mg TID	No emesis in 86%; no nausea in 62%
Rosso et al.[59]	54	Cyclophosphamide, ≥600 mg/m² in combination Ondansetron, 8 mg TID	No emesis in 89%; no nausea in 68%
Placebo-controlled trials			
Beck et al.[60]	318	Cyclophosphamide, ≥450 mg/m², plus methotrexate, ≥60 mg/m², or doxorubicin, ≥35 mg/m² Ondansetron, 1 mg, 4 mg, 8 mg, or placebo, all TID	No emesis in 19%, 57%, 65%, and 66% in the placebo, 1 mg, 4 mg and 8 mg ondansetron groups, respectively
Cubeddu et al.[61]	324	Cyclophosphamide, >500 mg/m², with doxorubicin, >40 mg/m², methotrexate, etoposide, 5-fluorouracil, mitozantrone, bleomycin, and/or vincristine Ondansetron, 1 mg, 4 mg, 8 mg, or placebo, all TID	No emesis in 12%, 37%, 64% and 66% in the placebo, 1 mg, 4 mg and 8 mg ondansetron groups, respectively
Comparative trials			
Smith et al.[62]	27	Vincristine, methotrexate (day 1), bleomycin (days 2, 3), and cisplatin, 100 to 120 mg/m² (day 4) Ondansetron, 8 mg TID, plus placebo; or ondansetron, 8 mg TID, plus oral dexamethasone	Ondansetron plus dexamethasone gave complete (no episodes) or major (1 to 2 episodes) control of emesis in 78% on days 4–5 of chemotherapy, compared with 30% with ondansetron plus placebo
Herrstedt et al.[63]	30	Moderately emetogenic Ondansetron, 8 mg BID, plus placebo; or ondansetron, 8 mg BID, plus metopimazine, 30 mg QID	No emesis in 47% with ondansetron alone and in 63% with ondansetron plus metopimazine; no nausea in 20% with ondansetron alone and in 40% with ondansetron plus metopimazine
Fraschini et al.[64]	Four series of 20 patients each	Cyclophosphamide–doxorubicin-based Ondansetron, 1 mg, 4 mg, 8 mg TID; or conventional regimen of intravenous lorazepam, metoclopramide, and diphenhydramine plus oral prochlorperazine	No emesis during 2 day study period in 35%, 55%, 65% and 85% in conventional anti-emetics group, and 1 mg, 4 mg and 8 mg ondansetron groups, respectively
Marschner et al.[65]	120	Cyclophosphamide–epirubicin Ondansetron, 8 mg TID, plus IV placebo; or metoclopramide, 60 mg IV, plus 20 mg orally TID	No emesis in 60% and 47% with ondansetron and metoclopramide, respectively; no nausea in 49% and 28% with ondansetron and metoclopramide, respectively
Levitt et al.[66]	164	CMF Ondansetron, 8 mg TID, plus IV placebo; or metoclopramide, 10 mg TID, plus dexamethasone, 10 mg IV	No vomiting in 82% and 89% with ondansetron and conventional regimen, respectively; significantly less nausea with conventional regimen than with ondansetron

TID = three times daily; BID = twice daily; QID = four times daily; IV = intravenously.
*Standard chemotherapy regimen of cyclophosphamide–methotrexate–5-fluorouracil.

smaller as the daily incidence of emesis in placebo-treated patients decreased over the course of the study, however. The authors concluded that continued use of ondansetron beyond day 3 for controlling cisplatin-induced delayed emesis should be questioned.

In this investigation, chemothrapy-naive patients were given IV ondansetron, 0.15 mg/kg × 3 doses, for control of actue emesis. Five hundred and thirty-eight patients who did not require rescue anti-emetic therapy were then randomized to three treatment regimens:

- Placebo on days 2–6
- Oral ondansetron, 8 mg b.i.d. on days 2 and 3, and placebo on days 4–6
- Oral ondansetron, 8 mg b.i.d. on days 2–6.

On days 2 and 3, a complete-plus-major response (no more than two emetic episodes) was achieved in significantly more ondansetron-treated patients than in those who received placebo (56 per cent versus 37 per cent). Analysis of data from subsequent days for patients who did not undergo rescue therapy earlier showed a complete-plus-major response among 94 per cent of ondansetron-treated patients on day 4 and 98 per cent on day 5, and among 85 per cent of placebo patients on day 4 and 88 per cent on day 5. By day 6, the complete-plus-major response rates exceeded 95 per cent in both the ondansetron and placebo groups.

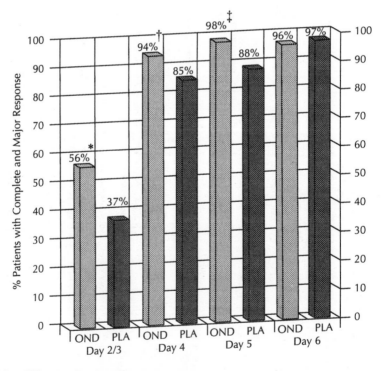

Fig. 7.3. Efficacy of oral ondansetron versus placebo. Control of delayed emesis, days 2–6, with ondansetron (OND) versus placebo (PLA). *P = 0.001; †P = 0.005; ‡P = 0.006. Reproduced from Navari *et al.* with permission.[68]

Combination therapy

Dexamethasone is well-accepted as an efficacious and safe anti-emetic. Some clinicians have questioned its use in cancer patients because of potential immunosuppression, metastases formation, and other adverse effects seen with chronic corticosteroid use.[69] However, a limited number of doses of dexamethasone are usually administered as part of an anti-emetic regimen, and adverse effects are very rarely documented with its intermittent use.

The benefit of adding dexamethasone to 5-HT$_3$ receptor antagonist therapy is considerable. Studies report an improvement in the control of nausea and vomiting with complete response rates from 9 per cent to 20 per cent greater than those observed with a 5-HT$_3$ receptor antagonist alone. Clearly, the benefits of adding dexamethasone to 5-HT$_3$ receptor antagonist therapy outweigh the risks of acute corticosteroid use. Therefore, combination therapy for the control of chemotherapy-induced nausea and vomiting is a logical choice given the potential synergistic effect, different mechanisms of action, and low incidence of adverse effects of both dexamethasone and 5-HT$_3$ receptor antagonists.[70,71]

Combination therapy with a 5-HT$_3$ receptor antagonist plus a corticosteroid is safe and effective for the management of chemotherapy-induced nausea and vomiting. With the addition of dexamethasone, complete response rates between 80 and 90 per cent are achieved in patients receiving moderately emetogenic chemotherapy and between approximately 60 and 70 per cent in most studies with cisplatin. With the improved efficacy and patient preference over traditional anti-emetics and the low incidence of adverse effects and cost of corticosteroids, combination therapy using a 5-HT$_3$ receptor antagonist plus dexamethasone represents a major improvement in the management of chemotherapy-induced nausea and vomiting and should be recommended in all patients receiving moderately high or highly emetogenic chemotherapy, unless medically contraindicated.

CONCLUSIONS

In conclusion, the 5-HT$_3$ antagonists are an effective and safe group of agents for the prevention of acute emesis induced by chemotherapy. They have demonstrated effective control of emesis over a wide range of doses and schedules with both cisplatin- and non-cisplatin-based chemotherapy regimens with a very favourable therapeutic ratio. Issues of appropriate method of administration, dosing and cost continue to be investigated. Recent data suggest equivalent efficacy of different intravenous 5-HT$_3$ receptor antagonists and of oral granisetron versus intravenous ondansetron in patients receiving moderately high or highly emetogenic chemotherapy. Preliminary data also suggest equivalent efficacy utilizing the oral preparation of dolasetron. Corticosteroids should be recommended as adjunctive therapy to 5-HT$_3$ receptor antagonists. Appropriate focus for future investigations with these agents will be to better define optimal dose and schedule, to further study their use in preventing delayed and anticipatory emesis, and to explore the potential utility of combining these agents with conventional anti-emetics.

REFERENCES

1. Perez EA, Hesketh PJ, Gandara DR *et al*. Serotonin antagonists in the management of cisplatin-induced emesis. *Seminars in Oncology* 1991; **18**: 73–80.
2. Perez EA, Gandara DR. Advances in the control of chemotherapy-induced emesis. *Annals of Oncology* 1992; **3**: S47–S50.
3. Andrews PLR, Bhandari P, Davey PT *et al*. Are all 5-HT$_3$ receptor antagonists the same? *European Journal of Cancer* 1992; **28**A: 52–56.
4. Andrews PLR, Davis CJ. The mechanism of emesis induced by anti-cancer therapies. In: Andrews PLR, Sanger GJ eds. *Emesis in Anticancer Therapy, Mechanisms and Treatment*. London: Chapman and Hall, 1993: 113–62.
5. Andrews PLR, Blower PR. The physiology of cytotoxic-induced emesis: New insights. Presented at a Satellite to the Seventh European Conference of Clinical Oncology Meeting, Jerusalem, Israel, November 1993: 14–17.
6. Torri Y, Mutoh M, Saito H *et al*. Involvement of free radical in cisplatin-induced emesis in *Suncus murinus*. *European Journal of Pharmacology: Environmental Toxicology and Pharmacology* 1993; **248**: 131–5.
7. Essman WB. Serotonin distribution in tissues and fluids. In: Essman WB ed. *Serotonin in health and disease: availability, localization and distribution*, vol. 1. New York: SP Medical & Scientific, 1978: 15–180.
8. Bradley PB, Engel G, Feniuk W *et al*. Proposals for the classification and nomenclature of funcional receptors for 5-hydroxytryptamine. *Neuropharmacology* 1986; **25**: 263–576.
9. Gaddum JH, Picarelli ZP. Two kinds of tryptamine receptor. *British Journal of Pharmacology* 1957; **12**: 323–8.
10. Peroutka SJ, Snyder SH. Multiple serotonin receptors: Differential binding of [^{3}H]-5-hydroxytryptamine [^{3}H] lysergic acid diethylamide and [^{3}H] spiroperidol. *Molecular Pharmacology* 1979; **16**: 687–99.
11. Richardson BP, Engel G, Donatsch P *et al*. Identification of serotonin M-receptor subtypes and their specific blockade by a new class of drugs. *Nature* 1985; **316**: 126–31.
12. Gralla RJ, Itri LM, Pisko SE *et al*. Antiemetic efficacy of high-dose metoclopramide: Randomized trials with placebo and prochlorperazine in patients with chemotherapy-induced nausea and vomiting. *New England Journal of Medicine* 1981; **305**: 905–9.
13. Miner WD, Sanger GJ. Inhibition of cisplatin-induced vomiting by selective 5-hydroxytryptamine M-receptor antagonism. *British Journal of Pharmacology* 1986; **88**: 497–9.
14. McRitchie B, McCledland CM, Cooper SM *et al*. Dopamine antagonists as antiemetics and as stimulants of gastric motility. In: Bennet A, Velo G eds. *Mechanisms of gastrointestinal motility and secretion*. New York: Plenum, 1984: 303–26.
15. Miner WD, Sanger GJ, Turner DH. Comparison of the effect of BRL 24924, metoclopramide and domperidone on cisplatin-induced emesis in the ferret. *British Journal of Pharmacology* 1986; **88**: 374.
16. Costall B, Domeney AM, Naylor RJ *et al*. 5-Hydroxytryptamine M-receptor antagonism to prevent cisplatin-induced emesis. *Neuropharmacology* 1986; **25**: 959–61.
17. Vermorken JB, Pinedo HM. Gastrointestinal toxicity of cis-diamminedichloroplatinum (II). *Netherlands Journal of Medicine* 1982; **25**: 275–9.
18. Gunning ST, Hogan RM, Tyers MB. Cisplatin induces biochemical and histological changes in the small intestine of the ferret. *British Journal of Pharmacology* 1987; **90**: 135.
19. Bertaccini G. Tissue 5-hydroxytryptamine and urinary 5-hydroxyindoleacetic acid after partial or total removal of the gastro-intestinal tract in the rat. *Journal of Physiology* (*London*) 1960; **153**: 239–49.

20. Robinson RG, Gershon MD. Synthesis and uptake of 5-hydroxytryptamine by the myenteric plexus of the guinea-pig ileum: A histochemical study. *Journal of Pharmacology and Experimental Therapy* 1971; **178**: 311–24.

21. Fozard JR. Neuronal 5 HT receptors in the periphery. *Neuropharmacology* 1984; **23**: 1473–86.

22. Dunbar AW, McClelland CM, Sanger GJ. BRL 24924: A stimulant of gut motility which is also a potent antagonist of the von-Bezold–Jarisch reflex in anaesthetized rats. *British Journal of Pharmacology* 1986; **88**: 319.

23. Resnick RH, Gray SJ. Distribution of serotonin (5-hydroxytryptamine) in the human gastrointestinal tract. *Gastrointestinal* 1961; **41**: 119–21.

24. Sanger GJ. Increased gut cholinergic activity and antagonism of 5-hydroxytryptamine M-receptors by BRL 24924: Potential clinical importance of BRL 24924. *British Journal of Pharmacology* 1987; **91**: 77–87.

25. Hawthorn J, Ostler KJ, Andrews PLR. The role of the abdominal visceral innervation and 5-hydroxytryptamine M-receptors in vomiting induced by the cytotoxic drugs cyclophosphamide and cisplatin in the ferret. *American Journal of Experimental Physiology* 1988; **73**: 7–21.

26. Schworer H, Racke K, Kilbinger H. Cisplatin increases the release of 5-hydroxytryptamine (5-HT) from the isolated vascularly perfused small intestine of the guinea-pig: Involvement of 5-HT$_3$ receptors. *Naunyn-Schmiedebergs Archives of Pharmacology* 1991; **344**: 143–9.

27. Reynolds DJM, Barber NA, Grahame-Smith DG *et al.* Cisplatin-evoked induction of c-*fos* protein in the brainstem of the ferret: The effect of cervical vagotomy and the anti-emetic 5-HT$_3$ receptor antagonist granisetron (BRL 43694). *Brain Research* 1991; **565**: 231–6.

28. Van Wijngaarden I, Tulp MTM, Soudijn W. The concept of selectivity in 5-HT receptor research. *European Journal of Pharmacology* 1990; **188**: 301–12.

29. Gebauer A, Merger M, Kilbinger H. Modulation by 5-HT$_3$ and 5-HT$_4$ receptors of the release of 5-hydoxytryptamine from the guinea pig small intestine. *Naunyn-Schmiedebergs Archives of Pharmacology* 1993; **347**: 137–40.

30. Gralla RJ, Clark RA, Kris MG, Tyson LB. Methodology in antiemetic trials. *European Journal of Cancer* 1991; **27**(1): 5–8.

31. Kris MG, Gralla RJ, Clark RA *et al.* Incidence, course, and severity of delayed nausea and vomiting following administration of high-dose cisplatin. *Journal of Clinical Oncology* 1985; **3**: 1379–404.

32. Bunce K, Tyers M, Beranek P. Clinical evaluation of 5-HT$_3$ receptor antagonists as anti-emetics. *Trends in Pharmacological Science* 1991; **12**: 46–8.

33. Smyth JF. New directions for anti-emetic research. *Annals of Oncology* 1994; **5**: 569–70.

34. Soukop M, McQuade B, Hunter E *et al.* Ondansetron compared with metoclopramide in the control of emesis and quality of life during repeated chemotherapy for breast cancer. *Oncology (Switzerland)* 1992; **49**: 295–304.

35. Roila F, Tonato M, Basurto C *et al.* Antiemetic activity of high doses of metoclopramide combined with methylprednisolone versus metoclopramide alone in cisplatin-treated cancer patients: A randomized double-blind trial of the Italian Oncology Group for Clinical Research. *Journal of Clinical Oncology* 1987; **5**: 141–9.

36. Tonato M, Roila F, Del Favero A. Methodology of antiemetic trials: A review. *Annals of Oncology* 1991; **2**: 107–14.

37. Tortorice PV, O'Connell MB. Management of chemotherapy-induced nausea and vomiting. *Pharmacotherapy* 1990; **10**: 129–45.

38. Gralla RJ. Treating emesis: An overview of agents. *Pharmacology and Therapeutics* 1991; **16**: 655–660.

39. Walton SC, Koenig TJ. Effectiveness and economy of low-dose ondansetron. *American Journal of Health System Pharmacology* 1995; **52**: 546–7.

40. Marty M, on behalf of the Granisetron Study Group. A comparative study of the use of granisetron, a selective 5-HT$_3$ antagonist, vs a standard antiemetic regimen of chlorpromazine plus dexamethasone in the treatment of cytostatic-induced emesis. *European Journal of Cancer* 1990; **26**: S28–S32.

41. Bonneterre J, Chevalier B, Metz R *et al*. A randomized, double-blind comparison of ondansetron and metoclopramide in the prophylaxis of emesis induced by cyclophosphamide, fluorouracil, and doxorubicin or epirubicin chemotherapy. *Journal of Clinical Oncology* 1990; **8**: 1063–69.

42. Kaasa S, Kvaløy S, Diactoa MA *et al*. A comparison of ondansetron with metoclopramide in the prophylaxis of chemotherapy-induced nausea and vomiting: a randomized, double-blind study. *European Journal of Cancer* 1990; **26**: 311–14.

43. Dilly S. Are granisetron and ondansetron equivalent in the clinic? *European Journal of Cancer* 1992; **28**A: S32–5.

44. Riviere A, on behalf of the Granisetron Study Group. Dose-finding study of granisetron in patients receiving high-dose cisplatin chemotherapy. *British Journal of Cancer* 1994; **69**: 967–71.

45. Navari RM, Kaplan HG, Gralla SM *et al*. Efficacy and safety of granisetron, a selective 5-hydroxytryptamine-3 receptor antagonist, in the prevention of nausea and vomiting induced by high-dose cisplatin. *Journal of Clinical Oncology* 1994; **12**: 2204–10.

46. Beck TM, Hesketh PJ, Madajewicz S *et al*. Stratified, randomized, double-blind comparison of intravenous ondansetron administered as a multiple-dose regimen vs two single-dose regimens in the prevention of cisplatin-induced nausea and vomiting. *Journal of Clinical Oncology* 1992; **10**: 1969–75.

47. Seynaeve C, Schuller J, Buser K *et al*. Comparison of the antiemetic efficacy of different doses of ondansetron, given as either a continuous infusion or a single intravenous dose, in acute cisplatin-induced emesis. A multicentre, double-blind, randomised, parallel-group study. *British Journal of Cancer* 1992; **66**: 192–7.

48. Hesketh PJ, Beck T, Uhlenhopp M *et al*. Adjusting the dose of intravenous ondansetron plus dexamethasone to the emetogenic potential of the chemotherapy regimen. *Journal of Clinical Oncology* 1995; **13**: 2117–22.

49. Hacking A, on behalf of the Granisetron Study Group. Oral granisetron – simple and effective: a preliminary report. *European Journal of Cancer* 1992; **28**A: S28–S32.

50. Heron JF, Goedhals L, Jordaan JP *et al*, on behalf of the Granisetron Study Group. Oral granisetron alone and in combination with dexamethasone: a double-blind randomized comparison against high-dose metoclopramide plus dexamethasone in prevention of cisplatin-induced emesis. *Annals of Oncology* 1994; **5**: 579–84.

51. Perez EA. Acute emesis: can oral treatment match IV? Presented at the Satellite Symposium: Emesis Control and Beyond. Satellite Symposium, 19 November, 19th ESMO Congress, 1992, Lisbon, Portugal.

52. Bleiberg HH, Spielmann M, Falkson G, Romain D. Antiemetic treatment with oral granisetron in patients receiving moderately emetogenic chemotherapy: A dose-ranging study. *Clinical Therapy* 1995; **17**: 38–51.

53. Ettinger D, Eisenberg P, Fitts D *et al*. A double-blind comparison of the efficacy of two dose regimens of oral granisetron in preventing acute emesis in patients receiving moderately emetogenic chemotherapy. *Cancer* 1996; **78** 144–51.

54. Johnsonbaugh RE, Mason BA, Friedman CJ, Fitts D. Oral granisetron is an effective anti-emetic in patients receiving moderately emetogenic chemotherapy. *Proceedings of the American Society of Clinical Oncologists* 1994; **13**: 437. Abstract.

55. Perez EA, Chawla SP, Kaywin PK *et al*. Efficacy and safety of oral granisetron versus IV ondansetron in prevention of moderately emetogenic chemotherapy-induced nausea and vomiting. *Proceedings of the American Society of Clinical Oncology* 1997; 149.

56. Cooke CE, Mehra IV. Oral ondansetron for preventing nausea and vomiting. *American Journal of Hospital Pharmacy* 1994; **51**: 762–71.
57. Marschner NW, Adler M, Jaenicke F *et al*. Langzeitergebnisse der antiemetischen Effectivät des 5-HT$_3$-Antagonisten Ondansetron. *Onkologie* 1990; **13**: 313–15.
58. Campora E, Olivia C, Mammoliti S *et al*. Oral ondansetron (GR 38032F) for the control of CMF-induced emesis in the outpatient. *Breast Cancer Research and Treatment* 1991; **19**: 129–32.
59. Rosso R, Campora E, Cetto G *et al*. Oral ondansetron (GR 38032F) for the control of acute and delayed cyclophosphamide-induced emesis. *Anticancer Research* 1991; **11**: 937–40.
60. Beck TM, Ciociola AA, Jones SE *et al*. Efficacy of oral ondansetron in the prevention of emesis in outpatients receiving cyclophosphamide-based chemotherapy. *Annals of Internal Medicine* 1993; **118**: 407–13.
61. Cubeddu LX, Pendergrass K, Ryan T *et al*. Efficacy of oral ondansetron, a selective antagonist of 5-HT$_3$ receptors, in the treatment of nausea and vomiting associated with cyclophosphamide-based chemotherapies. *American Journal of Clinical Oncology* 1994; **17**: 137–46.
62. Smith DB, Newlands ES, Rustin GJS *et al*. Comparison of ondansetron and ondansetron plus dexamethasone as antiemetic prophylaxis during cisplatin-containing chemotherapy. *Lancet* 1991; **338**: 487–90.
63. Herrstedt J, Sigsgaard T, Boesgaard M *et al*. Ondansetron plus metopimazine compared with ondansetron alone in patients receiving moderately emetogenic chemotherapy. *New England Journal of Medicine* 1993; **328**: 1076–80.
64. Fraschini G, Ciociolo A, Esparza L *et al*. Evaluation of three oral dosages of ondansetron in the prevention of nausea and emesis associated with cyclophosphamide–doxorubicin chemotherapy. *Journal of Clinical Oncology* 1991; **9**: 1268–74.
65. Marschner NW, Adler M, Nagel GA *et al*. Double-blind randomised trial of the antiemetic efficacy and safety of ondansetron and metoclopramide in advanced breast cancer patients treated with epirubicin and cyclophosphamide. *European Journal of Cancer* 1991; **27**: 1137–40.
66. Levitt M, Warr D, Yelle L *et al*. Ondansetron compared with dexamethasone and metoclopramide as antiemetics in the chemotherapy of breast cancer with cyclophosphamide, methotrexate and fluorouracil. *New England Journal of Medicine* 1993; **328**: 1081–4.
67. Ettinger DS. Preventing chemotherapy-induced nausea and vomiting: an update and a reviw of emesis. *Seminars in Oncology* 1995; **22**: 6–18.
68. Navari RM, Madajewicz S, Anderson N *et al*. Oral ondansetron for the control of cisplatin-induced delayed emesis: a large, multicenter, double-blind randomized comparative trial of ondansetron vs placebo. *Journal of Clinical Oncology* 1995; **13**: 2408–16.
69. Haid M. Steroid antiemesis may be harmful (letter). *New England Journal of Medicine*. 1981; **304**: 1237.
70. Kris MG. Rationale for combination antiemetic therapy and strategies for the use of ondansetron in combinations. *Seminars in Oncology* 1992; **19**: 61–6.
71. Smith DB, Newlands ES, Spruyt OW *et al*. Ondansetron (GR38032F) plus dexamethasone: Effective antiemetic prophylaxis for patients receiving cytotoxic chemotherapy. *British Journal of Cancer* 1990; **61**: 323–4.

CHAPTER 8

Treatment of malignancies and infectious complications in patients with HIV infection

UMBERTO TIRELLI————————————————————————————

INTRODUCTION

The acquired immunodeficiency syndrome (AIDS) was first reported in 1981 as a combined epidemic of *Pneumocystis carinii* pneumonia (PCP) and Kaposi's sarcoma (KS).[1-3]

This syndrome has emerged as the most important epidemic of our time. By the end of 1992, 611589 cases of AIDS have been reported worldwide.[4] The number of AIDS cases officially reported to the World Health Organization (WHO) represents probably only one third of the real total. Delay in reporting, under-reporting and inadequate means of diagnosis almost certainly contribute to this gross underestimation. The identification of the aetiological agent, human immunodeficiency virus (HIV), a human T-lymphotropic retrovirus, represents one of the most significant steps in AIDS research.[5-7] HIV may infect many human cells, including those in the brain, but is able to recognize the CD4+ lymphocyte surface molecule and has a strong affinity for this subset of lymphocytes. The selective cytopathic effect of HIV on CD4+ lymphocytes results in an imbalance in the usual ratio of CD4+ to CD8+ cells, with a decline in lymphocyte recognition and response to antigens. As the response to antigens by T lymphocytes is a prime initiator of the immune response, the lack of cellular immune response results in increased susceptibility to opportunistic infections and neoplasms, which an intact immune system will normally resist.

Diagnosis of AIDS was based on detection of antibodies to HIV, in combination with defects of cellular immunity (such as T lymphocyte abnormalities noted above) and the presence of characteristic opportunistic infections or neoplasms, specifically defined by the United States Centers for Disease Control (CDC) and including PCP, disseminated cytomegalovirus and others. In 1987, the CDC surveillance definition for AIDS was revised to emphasize HIV infection status through the inclusion of additional indicator diseases and acceptance of presumptive diagnosis of some indicator diseases.[8] In 1993 a new CDC classification was made available, including the CD4+ cell count (< 200/mm^3, or < 14 per cent of the total WBC count) and three other disease parameters as AIDS defining pathologies.[9]

The accumulated evidence strongly suggests the conclusion that transmission of HIV occurs only through blood, sexual activity and perinatal events.

ANTIRETROVIRAL THERAPY

Drugs that interfere with many of the steps in HIV replication have been developed. These drugs include inhibitors of reverse transcriptase, protease and regulatory protein, Tat. Inhibitors of reverse transcriptase can prevent the spread of infectious virus to new cells, but do not interfere with the replication of HIV genomes that are integrated into the host genome. Drugs such as zidovudine (also known as AZT), didanosine (dideoxyinosine or ddI), and zalcitabine (dideoxycytidine or ddC) delay the clinical progression of HIV infection, whereas others, such as stavudine (d4T) have favourable effects on certain surrogate markers of progression.[10–18] Newer agents such as Ro24-7429 (Tat inhibitor) and protease inhibitors, both interfering with events later in the replication and therefore affecting both acute and chronic infections,[19–23] and combinations are being evaluated in clinical trials.

Zidovudine (AZT, azidothymidine)

Zidovudine is a thymidine analogue that inhibits the replication of HIV *in vitro*. AZT is phosphorylated by cellular enzymes to a 5′-triphosphate form that interferes with a viral RNA-dependent DNA polymerase (reverse transcriptase) and chain elongation of the viral DNA, thereby inhibiting viral replication. Anaemia and neutropenia are the most frequent adverse reactions associated with zidovudine therapy. The low-dose regimen (500 mg/day) is more effective and better tolerated than the previously recommended higher dose (1000–1200 mg/day). Beginning zidovudine therapy before the onset of AIDS delays the progression of the disease, as manifested by the delayed onset of opportunistic infection and neurologic disease.[16,24,25] The preliminary results of a large European trial (the Concorde Trial) suggested that survival of HIV-infected patients was equivalent whether zidovudine therapy was begun early or late in the course of infection.[26] No definitive recommendation can be made on the basis of this study about the best time to institute zidovudine therapy. Current recommendations anyway in the USA are to begin therapy with AZT at a dose of 500–600 mg daily in all HIV-infected patients whose CD4+ cells count drops below 500/mm.[3,27] The most common and serious problem associated with long-term zidovudine therapy is waning efficacy over time.

Dideoxyinosine (ddI, didanosine)

Dideoxyinosine is the deaminated 3′-deoxy analogue of the physiologic deoxynucleoside, 2-deoxyadenosine. It inhibits HIV replication *in vitro* at concentrations of 1–10 μM, well below toxic levels.[28] Current preparations of didanosine include buffered chewable tablets taken in the fasting state and a powder for suspension with antacid. Didanosine was initially approved for use in patients with advanced HIV infection who were intolerant to zidovudine treatment or in whom zidovudine had failed. Nowadays the current opinion is that switching from AZT to ddI may be beneficial after a certain period of zidovudine therapy, although the optimal time for change in therapy is unclear. Pancreatitis is the most serious toxic effect of ddI and is occasionally fatal, but peripheral neuropathy is the principal dose-limiting side-effect. Elevations in serum uric acid have also been noted, as well as headache and diarrhoea.

Dideoxycytidine (ddC, zalcitabine)

Dideoxycytidine is the 3'-deoxy analogue of the physiologic deoxynucleoside, 2'-deoxycytidine. Even if several studies[29–31] indicated that ddC may have a limited role as a single drug for the treatment of HIV infection, encouraging observations prompted the evaluation of alternating and combination regimens of ddC and AZT[31,32] with the aim of reducing toxic effects while maintaining antiviral benefits. The clinical role of ddC will be more clearly defined when results became available from a number of phase II/III studies ongoing, evaluating ddC alone or in combination with AZT.

NEOPLASTIC COMPLICATIONS OF AIDS

HIV-related cancers are being seen in increasing numbers. The most frequent neoplasias are KS and non-Hodgkin's lymphomas (NHL), while other types of tumours occur at lesser frequencies. Overall, the natural history of cancers in HIV-infected patients is quite different from those of the general population. The aggressive course of tumours, leucopenia, opportunistic infections, and pre-existing AIDS-related problems make treatment extremely difficult.

Kaposi's sarcoma

KS is the commonest neoplasm in AIDS patients. This tumour develops predominantly in homosexual men and to a lesser extent in other risk groups. In the USA the proportion of AIDS cases presenting with KS decreased from nearly 50 per cent in 1981 to less than 20 per cent in 1987.[33] After an initial rapid increase in the frequency of AIDS-associated KS, the proportion of AIDS cases presenting with KS steadily declined in Europe, from 38 per cent in 1983 to 14 per cent in 1991.[34,35] As seen in the United States, such decline is unlikely to be an artefact due to the broadening of the CDC definition of AIDS and was consistently seen in each HIV transmission category.[36] The diminishing proportion of homosexual men in the total number of cases of AIDS and the fact that KS tends to appear in the most sexually active homosexuals, who were both the first to develop AIDS and those likeliest to manifest KS, may help to explain such a decline. Furthermore, KS represents an early clinical manifestation of HIV infection, which generally coexists with a still relatively well-preserved immune function. Whether the decrease is due to the reduction of at-risk homosexual behaviours, or to changes in the prevalence of other unknown agents or cofactors, it may provide further clues for understanding the aetiology of KS.

Kaposi's sarcoma is a tumour of vascular origin. Little was known of the nature of the malignant cells until a major breakthrough in the study of the cellular nature of KS came with the establishment of long-term culture of AIDS-associated KS-derived spindle cells.[37] KS is a multifocal neoplasm capable of arising simultaneously in multiple sites, as a possible consequence of the local production of unique growth factors. The cause of KS in patients with HIV infection is not known yet, but it is highly probable that a prevalently sexually transmitted infectious agent could be associated with KS in the presence of immunodeficiency.[35,36]

KS is usually characterized by multifocal, widespread lesions at the onset of illness. These lesions may involve skin, oral mucosa, lymph nodes and visceral organs such as the gastrointestinal (GI) tract, lung, liver and spleen. At 2 years, survival is more than 80 per cent in patients without opportunistic infections and less than 20 per cent in patients with opportunistic infections. The majority of patients show skin lesions that occur as flat or raised plaques ranging from a few millimetres to 2–3 cm and from blue-purple to red-brown. The Kaposi's lesions in patients may be quite subtle at onset. Clinicians caring for persons at risk for AIDS should consider any new skin lesions with suspicion. Lymph node involvement occurs frequently. However, the precise incidence of nodal involvement specifically due to KS is unknown because of the multiplicity of other processes involving the nodes in these patients. Visceral involvement, particularly in the GI tract, affects nearly half of the reported cases. Stomach, duodenum, colon and rectum may be involved simultaneously, or only one site may be involved at one time. However, GI involvement may be asymptomatic, and only in advanced disease it may result in bleeding, diarrhoea, weight loss, abdominal cramps or even rectal pain.

Although lung involvement is less frequent than GI tract, it may also exhibit different features in KS. In fact, KS lesions may be noted incidentally during bronchoscopy to evaluate a pneumonic process. Alternatively, lung involvement may result in radiographic abnormalities (bilateral, mixed interstitial and alveolar infiltrates or bilateral nodular infiltrates, pleural effusions) with symptoms of cough, dyspnoea and fever. Lesions from KS have been observed at autopsy in all organs including brain, pancreas, heart and blood vessels. These lesions remain generally asymptomatic, although in some cases patients present with headache or bowel obstruction.[38,39]

Despite the overall progressive course of KS, there may be a wide range of disease progression in different patients. A rapid course with short survival is seen in patients with opportunistic infections, systemic symptoms (fever, night sweats, or weight loss) and in those with significant depletion of CD4+ lymphocytes. Alternatively, prolonged survival with minimal disease has been noted in other patients with KS whose immune system is relatively intact. The overall prognosis in patients with KS appears to depend on the severity of immune suppression and HIV infection, rather than on the neoplastic proliferation and tumour load.[40]

No universally accepted classification exists for this disease. The most widely used staging classifications are those of Krigel and Mitsuyasu (Table 8.1).[38–41] Also Krown and co-workers have published criteria for evaluation of KS. This staging system offers uniform and precise critera for disease evaluation, response to treatment and clinical staging. It includes measures of extent of

Table 8.1   Two staging systems for Kaposi's sarcoma[38,41]

Krigel's staging system

Stage I	Cutaneous, locally indolent
Stage II	Cutaneous, locally aggressive or without regional lymph nodes
Stage III	Generalized cutaneous and/or lymph node involvement[a]
Stage IV	Visceral

Subtypes

A	No systemic symptoms
B	Systemic symptoms: weight loss (> 10% or fever (> 37.8°C, unrelated to an identifiable source of infection lasting > 2 weeks)

Mitsuyasu's staging system

Stage I	Limited cutaneous (< 10 lesions or one anatomic area)
Stage II	Disseminated cutaneous (> 10 lesions or more than one anatomic area)
Stage III	Visceral only (GI, LN)
Stage IV	Cutaneous and visceral, or pulmonary KS

Subtypes

A	No systemic symptoms
B	Fever > 37.8°C, unrelated to identifiable infection for 2 weeks or weight loss (> 10%)

Table 8.2   Recommended staging classification (Krown, Metroka and Wernz)[42]

	Good risk (0) (all of the following)	Poor risk (1) (any of the following)
Tumor (T)	Confined to skin and/or lymph nodes and/or minimal oral disease[a]	Tumor-associated oedema or ulceration Extensive oral KS Gastrointestinal KS KS in other non-nodal viscera
Immune system (I)	CD4+ cells > 200/µl	CD4+ cells < 200/µl
Systemic illness (S)	No history of OI or thrush No 'B' symptoms[b] Performance status > 70 (Karnofsky)	History of OI and/or thrush 'B' symptoms present Performance status < 70 Other related HIV-related illness (e.g. neurological disease, lymphoma)

[a] Minimal oral disease in non-nodular KS confined to the palate.
[b] 'B' symptoms are unexplained fever, night sweats, > 10% involuntary weight loss, or diarrhoea persisting for more than 2 weeks.
OI = opportunistic infection.

the disease, severity of immunodeficiency and presence of systemic symptoms (Table 8.2).[42]

The staging procedures to determine disease extent in KS are reported in Table 8.3. According to general opinion, full staging of KS is not required in all circumstances but only when indicated by symptoms and findings on physical

Table 8.3 Kaposi's sarcoma staging procedures

Complete physical examination (including rectal and oral examination)
Biopsy of skin lesions and/or LN
Chest X-ray
Gastroscopy and colon endoscopy (Bronchoscopy[a])
CT scan of abdomen
Laboratory studies: complete blood count, common serum chemistries, HIV serology,
CD4+ and CD8+ lymphocytes count

[a] In patients with abnormal chest X-ray.

examination or laboratory studies. It is clear, however, that the determination
and accurate documentation (e.g. photographs) of the disease extent is essential
for the evaluation of new possibly active drugs.

Therapy

As the natural course of KS disease progression is highly variable, evaluating the
long-term efficacy of systemic treatment was difficult. Instead, neither local nor
systemic treatment of KS was found to alter the ultimate course of the disease.
Both treatments may, however, result either in disappearance or reduction in size
of specific skin lesions and thereby alleviate the discomfort associated with the
disease, but no data show that treatment improves survival. Local modalities
include surgical excision, electrodessication and radiation therapy. However,
surgery is usually employed in order to obtain a diagnosis. KS is generally
very responsive to radiation therapy; good palliation can be obtained with doses
around 2000 cGy.[43] Most of the experience of radiation therapy has been
collected in cutaneous lesions of KS. Oral and pharyngeal lesions are equally
radiosensitive but successful control of these lesions is less frequent.

Table 8.4 shows the results of single and multiple chemotherapy agents in KS.
Overall, single chemotherapy agents may control the disease in approximately

Table 8.4 Single and multiple agents chemotherapy of epidemic Kaposi's sarcoma

Reference	Drug	Overall response rate (%)
Volberding et al.[51]	Vinblastine (VLB)	26
Mintzer et al.[49]	Vincristine (VCR)	61
Wernz et al.[52]	Bleomycin (BLM)	77
Laubenstein et al.[47]	VP16	76
Balker et al.[44]	VP16	0
Gill et al.[45]	Adriamycin (ADM)	53
Kaplan et al.[46]	VLB/VCR	43
Wernz et al.[52]	VLB/BLM	62
Laubenstein et al.[47]	ADM–BLM–VLB	86
Gill et al.[45]	ADM–BLM–VCR (ABV)	67
Minor [48]	VLB–VCR–methotrexate	81
Gill et al.[53]	ADM vs. ABV	48 vs. 88

30 per cent of patients, while combination chemotherapy produces responses in about 90 per cent of patients.[44–53]

The wide variation in response rates reflects patient selection rather than a significant difference in chemosensitivities. Although cytotoxic chemotherapy is effective in KS, it may further compromise immune response in AIDS patients. Many studies have confirmed the efficacy of high doses of alpha-2 recombinant interferon (IFN) followed by a maintenance regimen three times a week. Response rate to IFN in patients without opportunistic infections ranges from 30 per cent to 50 per cent; in contrast, if patients have a history of opportunistic infections and/or B symptoms, the response rate is lowered to 20 per cent.[54,55] In general, treatment with IFN is well-tolerated, but no decrease in the incidence of opportunistic infections could be observed. Combination of IFN with chemotherapy showed no benefit in comparison with any other agent alone. Encouraging results were obtained with the combination of IFN and AZT.[56–58] Moreover, the recent use of liposomal doxorubicin in phase II trials has shown promising results in terms of response rate and toxicity.[59,60]

In conclusion, no significant impact on survival has been demonstrated among patients with KS with the treatments available to date. Since optimal therapy of all stages is still in early phase of development, patients should be treated according to study protocols whenever possible. This is especially advisable for patients also receiving AZT, due to the possible overlapping myelotoxicity of this agent with antiproliferative agents. Even if a patient is not treated according to well-established treatment protocols, the general recommendations reported in Table 8.5 should be followed. Ultimately, the ideal treatment for the KS will be a combination of antiretroviral therapy to reverse the immunologic defects, chemotherapy to control tumour development and haemopoietic growth factors to ameliorate treatment toxicities.

Non-Hodgkin's lymphoma

There is an increase of NHL parallel to the time course of the AIDS epidemic. In all epidemiologic studies, the proportional morbidity has increased significantly above the levels observed in the pre-AIDS period, although less strikingly than KS. These tumours appear most frequently at the end stages of AIDS, at a time when the immune system is markedly impaired. As with ancillary care of

Table 8.5   Treatment of Kaposi's sarcoma by Krigel[38]

Extent of disease	Preferred treatment[a]
Localized	Surgical excision or radiation therapy
Indolent disseminated, cutaneous and/or lymphadenopathic	Immunotherapy and/or single-agent chemotherapy
Aggressive, disseminated or with systemic B symptoms	Combination chemotherapy

[a] Protocol therapies whenever possible.

opportunistic infections, patients with AIDS can be expected to survive longer, but HIV-related destruction of their T-cell immunity will continue. As a consequence of longer survival as well as better diagnosis, the incidence of lymphomas in AIDS patients will probably increase in the near future unless therapies are devised that halt or reverse the progressive immunodestruction of HIV.[33]

The majority of cases of HIV-related NHL consist of high-grade NHL, with a B-phenotype; the most common histologies are Burkitt's lymphoma, immunoblastic lymphoma and the otherwise not specified 'undifferentiated' lymphoma. Taking into account these as well as other epidemiological data, the Center for Disease Control (CDC) of Atlanta has produced a third definition of AIDS. According to the last definition, besides primary CNS-NHL, high-grade NHL with non B-, non T- or with B-phenotype is considered diagnostic of AIDS. This may occur in HIV-positive persons even in the absence of opportunistic infections and/or KS.[8]

Pathogenesis of these lymphomas has been linked to Epstein–Barr virus (EBV) latent infection of B lymphocytes and abnormal immune regulation of these infected cells. Oncogene activation in an EBV-infected cell may lead to malignant transformation.[61]

The clinical findings in patients with HIV-related lymphomas have been remarkably uniform in all reported series, and are summarized in Tables 8.6 and 8.7.[62–79] The prevalence of high-grade histotypes ranges from 60 per cent to 98 per cent of cases in the principal American case series and in 75–100 per cent of cases in the European case series. Widely disseminated disease is diagnosed at the time of initial presentation, with extranodal sites of disease described in 65–98 per cent of patients. Also common to all series is the description of unusual sites of lymphomatous disease. Lymphoma has been described in the myocardium, adrenals, earlobes, maxillae, gall bladder, orbit, rectum, and other such sites. Aside from these unusual sites of disease, most series have been consistent in the description of bone marrow involvement, occurring in approximately in 20–46 per cent of cases, GI tract involvement occurring in 7–45 per cent, and involvement of the CNS presenting either as primary CNS lymphoma, or as leptomeningeal lymphoma in patients with systemic disease. Primary CNS-HIV-related lymphoma shows an incidence ranging from 3 per cent to 36 per cent in the various series previously reported. The disease appears as a single or multiple lesion which is located preferably in the white paraventricular matter, in the basal ganglia, in the thalamus, in the corpus callosum and in the cerebral verms.[80]

To distinguish between CNS lymphoma involvement and opportunistic infections within the CNS is extremely difficult on purely clinical criteria in the absence of biopsy. The clinical and radiological characteristics are quite often similar. On the other hand, invasive diagnostic procedures such as stereotactic biopsy or open sky biopsy after craniotomy may present practical problems in patients with poor performance status and in a bad general condition. This consideration explains why an elevated number of cases of CNS involvement from NHL are diagnosed only at autopsy.

In one third of cases the onset of lymphomas is preceded by persistent generalized lymphadenopathy (PGL). Enlargement of pre-existent lymph nodes always requires a biopsy to exclude the suspicion of an evolution towards malignant lymphoma. Staging procedures in HIV-related lymphomas ideally

Table 8.6 Principal case series of HIV-related non-Hodgkin's lymphoma in the USA

Reference	No. patients	Risk group	Clinico-pathological characteristics
Ziegler et al.[79]	90	Homosexual men	High grade 62%, intermediate 28% Stages III–IV 58% Extranodal sites 98% (CNS, bone marrow, GI tract, mucocutaneous sites) Median survival 6 months
Di Carlo et al.[63]	29	Homosexual men 28 Polytransfused 1	High grade 28%, intermediate 45% Extranodal sites 90% Phenotypes B Median survival 6 months for intermediate and 3 months for high grade
Ioachim et al.[66]	31	Homosexual men 30 IV drug user 1	High grade 97% Extranodal sites 48% (CNS, GI tract, heart, testis, bladder, kidney) Low response rate to therapy
Levine et al.[70]	68	Homosexual men 59 IV drug users 6 Unknown 3	High grade 87% Stage IV 63% Extranodal sites: CNS 32%, GI tract 26%, bone marrow 25% Median survival < 1 year Opportunistic infections after intensive chemotherapy
Markowitz et al.[72]	8	Homosexual men 5 IV drug users 3	Stage IV 100% Severe cytopenia after conventional doses of chemotherapy Short survival
Knowles et al.[69]	89	Homosexual men 71 IV drug users 17	High grade 69% Stage III–IV 53% Extranodal sites 87% (GI tract, CNS, liver) Phenotypes B, polyclonality Median survival 5 months
Kaplan et al.[68]	84	Homosexual men 78 IV drug users 4 Heterosexuals 2	High grade 77% Stage III–IV 82% Extranodal sites (bone marrow 31%, liver 26%, CNS 12%) Median survival < 4.3 months
Egert & Beckstead[64]	31	Homosexual men 31	High grade 98% Stage I 68% (CNS 43%) Phenotypes B
Lowenthal et al.[71]	43	Homosexual men 41 IV drug users 2	Intermediate high grade 93% Stage IV 49% Extranodal sites 65% (bone marrow 46%, CNS 40%, lung 25%) Median survival 6 months

Table 8.7 Literature review of HIV-related non-Hodgkin's lymphoma in Europe

Reference	No. patients	Risk group	Clinico-pathological characteristics
Raphael et al.[76]	16	?	Immunoblastic lymphoma 69% Burkitt's lymphoma 19% Extranodal sites 69% (CNS, bone marrow, mucosae) Median survival 9 months
Skinhoj et al.[78]	3	Homosexual men 2 Hemophiliac 1	High grade 3/3 Stage III–IV 3/3
Jara et al.[67]	5	Homosexual men? IV drug user?	High grade 5/5 Stage III–IV 5/5 Reduced response rate to therapy
Huhn & Serke[65]	16	Homosexual men? IV drug users?	Intermediate–high grade 75% Stage II–IV 100% Extranodal sites 81% (CNS 38%, liver 31%, bone marrow 31%) Phenotypes B
Andrieu et al.[62]	92	Homosexual men 65 IV drug users 8 Heterosexuals 8 Polytransfused 6 Homosexual men– IV drug users 4 Unknown 8	High grade 96% Stage III–IV 52% CR after chemo- + radiotherapy 37% High mortality 54%
Schmid[77]	17	?	?
Oksenendler et al.[75]	53	Homosexual men? IV drug users?	High grade 100% Stage III–IV 58%
Italian Cooperative Group on AIDS-related tumours[74]	150	IV drug users 96 Homosexual men 31 Others 23	High grade 73% Stage III–IV 66%

should be superimposable on those used for non-Hodgkin's lymphomas in the general population. Although poor performance status and bad general conditions may be an obstacle to a thorough staging assessment, bone marrow biopsy, chest X-ray, CT scan of thorax and abdomen, gastrointestinal tract X-ray, ENT examination and lumbar puncture are recommended in all instances.

Therapy

The treatment of AIDS-associated NHL presents several problems. First, the majority of patients have advanced stage disease at initial presentation. Second, the high-grade lymphomas frequently involve the bone marrow and the CNS. Third, immunodeficiency and a history of previous opportunistic infections complicate the immunosuppressive chemotherapy. Fourth, the leucopenia commonly seen in patients infected with HIV makes the use of a conventional multi-agent chemotherapy regimen very difficult.

In the case series of Ziegler and co-workers, which reported results obtained with various combinations of chemotherapy regimens (CHOP, ProMACE MOPP, and M-BACOD with or without radiation therapy), complete remissions (CR) were less than 53 per cent, relapses were 54 per cent and median survival was only 6 months.[79] Comparable results in terms of response and survival have been reported by Lowenthal and co-workers with the same combination chemotherapy regimens. In these series patients achieved a 50 per cent CR rate; however, 41 per cent of relapses occurred after an average of 4 months (range 3–7).[71] With the combination chemotherapy regimen COMET-A (cyclophosphamide, vincristine, methotrexate, etoposide and intrathecal methotrexate), Kaplan and co-workers obtained CR in 58 per cent of cases with 31 per cent relapse rate.[68] These data can be superimposed on those obtained with the aforementioned conventional chemotherapy. In this case series unfavourable prognostic factors for survival were a low value of CD4+ lymphocyte, the presence of opportunistic infections, low performance status according to Karnofsky and the administration of high-dose cyclophosphamide (more than 1 g/m^2).

Within the French–Italian Cooperative Study Group a prospective study was initiated in two individualized groups of patients. Patients with previous history of opportunistic infections and poor performance status were treated with low-dose chemotherapy regimen. Patients without these factors were eligible for an intense and brief treatment with a slightly modified LNH84 regimen.[81] The aim of this study was to evaluate if this regimen could induce a similar complete response rate to standard NHL and to study the prognostic factors related to lymphoma and HIV infection.

In a prospective multicentre study, treatment outcomes were assessed in 141 cases of seropositive HIV-lymphomas submitted to aggressive chemotherapy.[82] Adult lymphoma patients with performance status < 3 and no active opportunistic infection were consecutively treated with three cycles of doxorubicin 75 mg/m^2, cyclophosphamide 1200 mg/m^2, vindesine 2 mg/m^2 × 2, bleomycin 10 mg × 2 and prednisolone 60 mg/m^2 × 5 (ACVBP). This treatment was followed by consolidation with high-dose methotrexate with leucovorin, ifosfamide, etoposide, asparaginase and cytarabine (LNH84). CNS prophylaxis with intrathecal methotrexate was routinely used and was followed by maintenance zidovudine. Ninety-three patients had high-grade lymphoma (59 Burkitt's type) and forty-eight intermediate grade. Stage III–IV was present in eighty-six patients, meningeal involvement found in twenty-nine cases and thirty had bone marrow infiltration. Sixty-two patients had more than two extranodal localizations. LDH levels were above the normal value in ninety-five cases. Median CD4+ lymphocytes count was 227/mm^3.

Eighty-nine patients (63 per cent) achieved CR, nineteen (13 per cent) partial remission, thirteen failed to respond and twenty (14 per cent) died during ACVBP courses, eight from progression of the disease. With a median follow-up of 28 months, median survival and disease-free survival are 9 and 16 months respectively. Median survival for non-responders was 5 months. In multivariate analysis four factors were strongly associated with shorter survival: (1) CD4+ < 100/mm^3, (2) performance status > 1, (3) immunoblastic lymphoma, (4) prior AIDS. In the absence of all risk factors probability of survival at 2 years was 50 per cent. Death was caused by lymphoma and AIDS. Twenty-three patients died of opportunistic infections in persisting CR. In a selected group of HIV-related lymphoma, intensive chemotherapy with LNH84 can yield a high complete response rate. For patients with CD4+ > 100/mm^3 and performance status < 2, probability of survival at 2 years was 50 per cent. Prolongation of survival is more related to the underlying immunodeficiency and only control of this parameter will improve the results of an effective antineoplastic regimen.

As far as patients with previous history of opportunistic infections and poor performance status are concerned, the French–Italian Cooperative Study Group included patients with poor prognosis AIDS-related non-Hodgkin's lymphoma together with those with performance status $\geq$ 3 and/or opportunistic infections in a prospective study with a 50 per cent reduced-dose combination chemotherapy regimen:[83] CHVmP-vincristine-bleo (cyclophosphamide 300 mg/m^2 IV day 1, doxorubicin 25 mg/m^2 IV day 1, teniposide 30 mg/m^2 IV day 1, prednisone 20 mg/m^2 orally days 1–5, vincristine 2 mg IV day 15, and bleomycin 10 mg IV day 15), given every 21 days for eight cycles, and concomitant zidovudine 500 mg orally per day. The aims of this combined treatment were both to reduce bone marrow toxicity and the infectious complications related to chemotherapy (with the low-dose chemotherapy regimen) and to control the HIV and the related infectious complications (with zidovudine therapy).

Thirty-seven patients entered this prospective study. When the diagnosis of NHL was made, 41 per cent of the patients had asymptomatic HIV infection, 27 per cent had ARC and 32 per cent already had a CDC-defined diagnosis of AIDS. The median CD4+ cell count was 35/mm^3. Only twenty-nine patients are evaluable for response, in that eight received only one cycle of chemotherapy. Fifteen out of twenty-nine (52 per cent) patients obtained an objective response, with only four (14 per cent) achieving a CR with a duration of 1, 4, 14 and 29+ months. The most common side-effect was bone marrow toxicity, with two toxicity-related deaths. Out of the twenty-one patients who actually received concomitant zidovudine treatment, only twelve (57 per cent) were able to receive the drug during chemotherapy. The other nine patients had to stop the antiretroviral treatment due to haematological toxicity. Nine (43 per cent) cases of opportunistic infections were observed. Out of the sixteen patients who did not receive zidovudine, in thirteen patients the reason was the presence of granulocytopenia at the diagnosis of NHL, while the other three patients refused the drug. Five (31 per cent) cases of opportunistic infections were observed.

In conclusion, this study revealed that patients with poor prognosis AIDS-related NHL did not benefit from a combined low-dose chemotherapy regimen and concomitant zidovudine treatment. We obtained a lower CR rate when compared with other published reports using conventional or low-dose chemotherapy. In addition, despite the low-dose chemotherapy regimen employed, we observed signficant bone marrow toxicity with two toxic deaths. Finally, the early association of zidovudine did not prevent a high (43 per cent) occurrence of opportunistic infections during or immediately after treatment.[84]

Treatment of HIV-related NHL with chemotherapy is associated with an increased risk of side-effects, in particular bone marrow toxicity. We compared[85] the toxicity and the cost of chemotherapy with G-CSF versus chemotherapy without G-CSF. We have analyzed thirty-seven consecutive patients treated with intensive chemotherapy regimens, nineteen patients from July 1989 to June 1991 without G-CSF and eighteen patients from July 1991 to September 1992 with G-CSF, 5 µg/kg per day SC starting 24 hours after chemotherapy for

13 days in all cycles. The chemotherapy regimens employed were the LNH84 regimen[81] and the CHOP-like regimen, CHVmP/VCR-BLM[83] given for 3–6 cycles. The analysis was performed only for the first three cycles of chemotherapy. The cost of 1 day of hospitalization in our division was about US$450. Patient characteristics and results of the study are summarized in Table 8.8.

The side-effects of G-CSF were uncommon and mild. We have shown that treatment with G-CSF significantly reduces the nadir WBC in patients with CD4+ ≥ 200, the mean delay between the chemotherapy cycles and the mean toxicity-related days of hospitalization. Therefore, by contrast with what one might expect, the cost of chemotherapy + G-CSF vs. chemotherapy alone did not increase; actually it decreased. In addition, a decreased incidence of mucositis was observed, although there is no positive impact on the overall response rate.

Table 8.8 Chemotherapy with and without G-CSF in HIV-related non-Hodgkin's lymphoma

	Without G-CSF	*With G-CSF*	*P value*
No. patients	19	18	
Median age (range)	36 (28–59)	32 (18–51)	
Male/female	17/2	15/3	
Histology (W.F.)			
G/H/I/J/K	2/4/–/12/1	3/1/1/8/5	
Stage			
I/II/III/IV	3/5/1/10	2/2/7/7	
Median CD4+ cell count/mm^3	235	120	
Results–toxicity			
Day of nadir WBC, mean (from chemotherapy start)	10.8 (± 2.8)	8.4 (± 1.5)	0.006[b]
Nadir WBC/mm^3, mean (all pts)	281 (± 248)	514 (± 439)	0.09[b]
Nadir WBC/mm^3, mean (pts with CD4+ ≥ 200)	410	1293	0.009[b]
Mean no. of chemotherapy cycles/pt	2.7 (± 0.7)	2.4 (± 0.8)	NS[b]
Pts with documented infections	11%[a]	8%	NS[c]
Pts with mucositis	47%	22%	0.08[c]
Cycles at full dose	88%	86%	NS[c]
Mean delay between the chemotherapy cycles (days)	9.0 (± 6.4)	4.0 (± 4.7)	0.01[b]
Results–response			
Overall response	88%	78%	0.22[c]
Results–cost			
Mean toxicity-related days of hospitalization	18.0 (± 13.2)	6.4 (± 9.1)	0.003[b]
Mean hospitalization + G-CSF cost/cycle	$3232 (± 2283)	$2282 (± 1345)	NS[b]

[a] Fatal in 1 patient.
[b] Mann–Whitney test.
[c] Fisher test chi-square.

In conclusion, G-CSF in addition to chemotherapy should be preferred in the treatment of patients with HIV-related NHL.

Hodgkin's disease

Hodgkin's disease (HD) is one of the most frequent neoplasias reported in patients with HIV infection after KS and NHL. Despite its high frequency it is not yet classified as an AIDS-defining criterion. Since HD occurs typically in young patients it is not clear whether cases described in the literature are the expression of an increase of the incidence of the disease or more probably the expression of a coincidence. However, the clinical syndrome of HD in HIV-infected patients is changing. There is a higher incidence (80–86 per cent) of stage III and IV disease. Additionally, an atypical pattern of spread of the disease with a dissemination without mediastinal and hilar involvement has been noted.[86] Histopathology is unusual as the majority of the cases are of mixed cellularity (56 per cent), followed by nodular sclerosis (34 per cent), and lymphocyte depletion (6 per cent). Treatment with standard chemotherapy (MOPP, MOPP + ABVD, ABVD) has resulted in long-term remissions, but chemotherapy is poorly tolerated and opportunistic infections have increased. Survival is shortened by refractory disease and AIDS-related complications.[69,71,73,87,88]

Since 1985, HD has been described in ninety-two Italian patients with HIV infection, with a significant increase of mixed cellularity and lymphocyte depletion subtypes and advanced stages at presentation in comparison with the general population of Italian HD patients.[89] Taking into consideration that the median CD4+ cell count at diagnosis of HD of the overall group is 249/mm^3, AZT is currently recommended in these patients. However, the combination of chemotherapy and AZT is difficult to perform, due to the related bone marrow toxicity. We compared[90] the outcome and, in particular, the occurrence of opportunistic infection in two consecutive groups of patients treated with chemotherapy with and without AZT. The first group of thirty-two patients was treated with chemotherapy alone (MOPP or MOPP + ABVD), the second group of seventeen patients was treated with chemotherapy (EBV: epirubicin 70 mg/m^2 IV day 1, bleomycin 10 mg/m^2 IV day 1 and vinblastine 6 mg/m^2 IV day 1) and AZT (500 mg/day orally from the beginning of chemotherapy or after three cycles of chemotherapy). Only thirteen patients of the latter group were evaluable for this study, in that four did not receive AZT therapy because of severe granulocytopenia at HD diagnosis (in two patients) and refusal in the other two patients. Table 8.9 reports the treatment outcome in the two groups of patients.

While the median CD4+ cell count and median follow-up in the two groups of patients can be superimposed, only one opportunistic infection occurred in the group of patients treated with chemotherapy + AZT in comparison with sixteen opportunistic infections observed in the twenty-eight evaluable patients treated with chemotherapy without AZT (8 per cent vs. 57 per cent, $P = 0.003$). The combined treatment also seems feasible and quite tolerable, with no toxic deaths and a large number of patients being able to receive the scheduled therapy. Therefore, our data demonstrated that the addition of AZT as antiretroviral therapy to chemotherapy decreases the occurrence of opportunistic infections during chemotherapy or follow-up in patients with HD and HIV infection.

Table 8.9   Chemotherapy with and without AZT in patients with HD and HIV infection

	Chemotherapy	Chemotherapy + AZT	P value
No. of evaluable pts	32	13	
Median CD4+ cell count/mm^3 (range)	275(29–842)	166(26–1100)	
Mean no. of chemotherapy cycles/pt	4.7($\pm$ 1.5)	5.4($\pm$ 1.1)	0.08[a]
Complete remission rate	56%	61%	0.25[b]
Pts with grade 3 and 4 haematological toxicity	52%	66%	0.21[b]
Pts with opportunistic infections	57%	8%	0.003[b]
Median follow-up in months (range)	12 (1–64)	11 (3–36)	

[a] Mann–Whitney test.
[b] Fisher test chi-square.

Anogenital neoplasia

Patients with chronic immunosuppression are at increased risk of tumours associated with human papilloma virus (HPV). For example, women who have undergone renal transplantation have shown a 100-fold increase in the incidence of vulvar carcinoma and a 14-fold increase in cervical cancer respectively.[91,92] Patients with HIV infection are at increased risk of developing HPV-associated cancers due to the fact that these individuals have a high rate of HPV infection. However, HPV-associated cancers may take many years to develop and it is possible that, due to the longer survival of patients with HIV infection owing to the improvement in medical therapy, the incidence of these tumours could significantly increase in future years. To date, only HPV types 16, 18 and 31 have been strongly correlated with the development of invasive cervical cancer.[93,94]

Vermund and co-workers[95] investigated the relationship between HPV, HIV and the development of cervical intraepithelial lesions in ninety-six high-risk women (fifty-one of whom were HIV seropositive) in the Bronx, New York. Thirty-seven (39 per cent) had cervicovaginal lavage specimens that were positive for HPV infection. Among the fifty-one HIV-infected women, twenty-seven (53 per cent) of the cervicovaginal samples contained HPV DNA, whereas only ten (22 per cent) of forty-five HIV-seronegative women were infected with HPV ($P < 0.005$). Seventeen of fifty-one (33 per cent) HIV-seropositive women had Papanicolau smear abnormalities demonstrating squamous intraepithelial lesions, compared with only six of forty-five (13 per cent) HIV-seronegative women ($P < 0.05$). The authors concluded that symptomatic HIV-infected women with HPV infection were at much higher risk for squamous intraepithelial lesions than any other subgroup, because the immunosuppression related to the HIV infection exacerbates HPV-mediated cervical abnormalities. They also suggested that yearly Papanicolau smear and gynaecologic examinations should be offered for women at high risk for HIV and for those with symptomatic HIV infection or with CD4+ cell counts less than 200/mm^3 every 6 months.

Maiman and co-workers[96] examined thirty-two HIV-seropositive women by cervical cytology, colposcopically directed biopsy and T-cell function. Analysis of cytologic specimens revealed one (3 per cent) woman with cytologic evidence of cervical intraepithelial neoplasia (CIN) and another two (6 per cent) with inflammatory atypia. Thirteen women (41 per cent) had CIN on colposcopically directed biopsy (seven had CIN 1 and six had CIN 2–3), fourteen (44 per cent) had cervicitis and one woman had both CIN and cervicitis.

All five patients with AIDS had histologically confirmed CIN, compared with 30 per cent (8 of 27) of non-AIDS patients ($P < 0.05$). Patients diagnosed with CIN had significantly lower CD4+ cell counts than those without CIN ($221/mm^3$ vs. $408/mm^3$; $P < 0.06$). Polymerase chain reaction detected HPV DNA in seven of twelve CIN specimens available for analysis, compared with none of seventeen patients who were histologically negative for CIN.

Smith and co-workers[97] studied forty-three HIV-seropositive women cytologically, colposcopically and histologically to detect the incidence of lower genital tract neoplasia, and its relationship to the degree of immunosuppression due to HIV infection. Twelve women (27 per cent) had an abnormal Papanicolau smear (three Koilocitotic atypia, four CIN 1, three CIN 2, one CIN 3 and one invasive cervical carcinoma). Colposcopically, three women had CIN 1, two CIN 2 and one CIN 3. Moreover, they also found a case of vaginal intraepithelial neoplasia and three cases of vulvar intraepithelial neoplasia.

Twenty-seven patients (63 per cent) had evidence of HPV infection and a significant correlation ($P < 0.005$) was found between clinical immunosuppression and abnormalities on cytology and histology.

Schwartz and co-workers[98] reported a case of squamous cell carcinoma of the cervix in a patient with HIV infection who, despite adequate treatment, died of rapid disease progression. Based on all these reports, invasive cervical cancer has been included in the 1993 CDC classification as an AIDS-defining pathology.[9]

Moreover Giorda and co-workers[99] reported a rapid evolution of disease and poor prognosis in a young HIV-seropositive patient with vulvar cancer and associated vulvar condylomas. Studies from the USA have demonstrated a high prevalence of anal intraepithelial neoplasia (AIN) in HIV-positive homosexual and bisexual persons, particularly in those with advanced HIV infection and anal condylomata.[100,101] As observed with cervical cancer, HPV DNA (types 16, 18 and 31) has been demonstrated within anal cancer tissues.[102,103]

Recently, Lorenz and co-workers[104] retrospectively reported six cases of squamous cell carcinoma of the anus in homosexual men seen at the University of California, San Francisco between 1985 and 1988. Five patients already had AIDS at the time of the diagnosis and only two of them were alive after 1 year following treatment. The authors concluded that in their experience these tumours were very aggressive and their outcome was very poor. Svensson and co-workers[105] reported a case of a homosexual man with an anal fistula and a subsequent histological diagnosis of squamous cell carcinoma.

Safavi and co-workers[106] reported that among seventy-five consecutive surgical procedures on patients with HIV infection, the squamous cell carcinoma was diagnosed in three cases (4 per cent). Recently, Palefsky and co-workers[107] reported that men with group IV HIV disease have a high prevalence of anal HPV infection, a rapid rate of progression of anal disease and are at high risk of developing invasive anal cancer.

Other tumours

Van Ginkel and co-workers[108] recently reported the development of multiple primary melanomas in an HIV-positive homosexual man. Another case of melanoma developing in an HIV-2-infected homosexual man with multiple sexual contacts in Africa is described by Merkle and co-workers.[109]

We described a case of squamous cell carcinoma and a basalioma of the skin, with a poor outcome in the first patient.[110]

A case of acute myelomonoblastic leukaemia in a homosexual man is reported by Murthy and co-workers[111] who provided data indicating that HIV may infect myelomonoblasts *in vivo*. Puppo and co-workers[112] described a similar case of acute non-lymphoid leukaemia in an intravenous drug using HIV-positive woman. Lee and co-workers[113] reported the case of a young black woman with AIDS who developed a squamous cell carcinoma of the umbilicus, a very rare urachal cancer. Remick and co-workers[114] reported a case of infiltrating ductal adenocarcinoma of breast in a 26-year-old HIV-infected woman. The authors stated that despite favourable biologic prognostic parameters the patient had disseminated carcinoma. Aricò and co-workers[115] described seven cases of malignant tumours resulting from the analysis of 338 HIV-positive subjects enrolled in the Italian Registry for HIV infection in children. These tumours included four cases of NHL and a case of KS, a hepatoblastoma, and an acute B-cell lymphoblastic leukaemia. Only the child who had hepatoblastoma is alive in complete remission after 4 years from the diagnosis. McLoughlin and co-workers[116] reported the first case of disseminated gastrointestinal leiomyosarcoma in a child, as well as Ross and co-workers[117] who reported a primary hepatic leiomyosarcoma. The relationship of these last pediatric cases to HIV is unclear, but, because these tumours are not generally associated with immunodeficiency, immunosuppression alone may not be enough to explain their occurrence. The multiple disseminated nature of the leiomyosarcoma suggests a role of circulating transforming growth factor secondary to HIV infection, similar to the pathogenesis of KSD.[118]

OPPORTUNISTIC INFECTIONS

The appearance of an opportunistic infection may be the first sign of underlying HIV infection. It is often present atypically in HIV-infected patients, frequently in the form of disseminated disease and characterized by a high density of organisms.[119] Conventional treatments are often inadequate since infections tend to persist in HIV patients and usually require long-term suppressive therapy. Typically, the infections may be either viral, bacterial, protozoal or fungal in origin.

Viral infections

Cytomegalovirus (CMV), a member of the human herpes family of viruses, infects directly through mucous membrane contact or via tissue or blood transfusion. Clinical features depend on the site of infection. CMV can cause retinitis, colitis, pneumonitis, oesophagitis, hepatitis and adrenalitis.[120,121] Recovery of

CMV on culture only is not adequate to diagnose acute infection. Histologic demonstration of virus in tissue, visualization by endoscopy of ulcers found to contain virus, or demonstration of virus by special strains or culture of broncho-alveolar lavage is necessary; retinitis can be diagnosed by ophthalmologic findings alone.

Ganciclovir has been shown to arrest the progression of disease due to CMV and sometimes it can cause regression of disease, especially chorioretinitis, but lesions progress with discontinuation of therapy, necessitating prolonged maintenance therapy.[122–124] Haematological toxicity frequently necessitates dose reduction or discontinuation of therapy.[125] Because AIDS patients often have low blood cell counts due to their underlying disease or treatment with zidovudine, this toxicity is often problematical. Primary prophylaxis for clinical illness due to CMV is not practical, given the high prevalence of subclinical CMV infection in HIV-infected individuals, the toxicities and difficulties in administration of available agents.[126] Metroka and Josefberg[127] reported results on efficacy and tolerance of high-dose acyclovir as prophylaxis for CMV.

Recently, another drug, foscarnet, has been made available for the treatment of CMV disease. Foscarnet is a pyrophosphate analogue that inhibits various viral DNA polymerases, including the reverse transcriptase of HIV.[128] In addition to its action on CMV, the use of foscarnet in patients with AIDS has been reported to be associated with declines in HIV culture positivity and in the circulating levels of the HIV core antigen p24.[129] Foscarnet appears to have considerably less bone marrow toxicity than that seen with ganciclovir, suggesting that simultaneous therapy with zidovudine and foscarnet can be tolerated. Some studies[130–132] demonstrated that foscarnet is effective in the treatment of CMV retinitis and may prolong survival of HIV-infected patients with CMV retinitis.

As with CMV, the prevalence of herpes simplex virus (HSV) infection in AIDS risk groups is extremely high. Ulcerative disease in an HSV-positive individual is considered an AIDS-defining diagnosis.[8] HSV types 1 and 2 and varicella-zoster virus (VZV) typically infect epithelial and nerve tissues. Herpes simplex occurs in repeated attacks as an acute disease marked by grouped vescicles on erythematous bases, often on the border of the lips, anus or genitals. Herpes zoster is an acute reactivation of virus residing in the nerve roots near the base of the spine. Symptoms are vescicular dermatitis associated with neuralgia. The diagnosis of HSV infection is usually clinical, but as HSV grows easily and rapidly in cell culture, such culture should be performed to confirm the diagnosis. The diagnosis of VZV infections, which are almost always cutaneous, is usually an obvious one and rarely requires viral isolation or biopsy. Perianal ulcers, proctitis and other HSV-related syndromes can be treated with acyclovir and recurrence prevented by daily acyclovir maintenance.[120] Severe mucocutaneous disease, due to acyclovir-resistant HSV infections, can be treated with foscarnet.[133] Treatment of severe VZV infection may require hospitalization and intravenous acyclovir.

Epstein–Barr virus has been reported to be associated with HIV-infected patients or as a cause of oral hairy leucoplakia, lymphadenopathy, B-cell lymphoma and intestitial pneumonitis.[134,135] There is currently no effective therapy for EBV infection.

Bacterial infections

Mycobacterium tuberculosis infection is increasingly being reported in AIDS patients, particularly among those from areas where tuberculosis (TB) is prevalent. TB occurs in an estimated 4 per cent of AIDS cases.[136] Patients often present with extrapulmonary, particularly lymphatic, involvement and atypical disseminated disease. The clinical presentation of TB depends on the degree of immunosuppression.[137] The tuberculosis skin test is not reactive in most cases of TB with AIDS. Culture of sputum, blood or tissue biopsy is necessary for confirmation of TB. Patients with AIDS and TB usually respond to standard anti-TB therapies such as isoniazid and rifampicin for at least 6 months augmented with pyrazinamide, ethambutol or streptomycin during the first 2 months. The drugs used should be determined by sensitivities of the isolates. The CDC has recommended that HIV-seropositive patients with latent *M. tuberculosis* infection receive isaniazid preventative therapy.[136]

Mycobacterium avium complex (MAC) infections are the commonest disseminated bacterial infections in AIDS.[138] Symptoms of MAC infection are non-specific. Fever, maliase and weight loss are the commonest. Diarrhoea, malabsorption and abdominal pain are symptomatic of gastrointestinal involvement. Lymphatic involvement may be seen as lymph node enlargement and splenomegaly. Anaemia, leucopenia and thrombocytopenia may result from bone marrow infection. Blood culture techniques are most sensitive for diagnosis of MAC; however, culture time may be 1–7 weeks. MAC is typically treated with a combination of bactericidal and bacteriostatic drugs, since no single drug is effective against all strains. Clarithromycin, amikacin, ciprofloxacin, clofazamine, ethambutol, and rifampicin are commonly used agents in combination therapy. Therefore, it is not possible to recommend a regimen for treatment or suppression other than to suggest a combination of agents to which the particular isolate demonstrates susceptibility *in vitro*.[126] Rifabutin has also been demonstrated to be effective both in the treatment and prophylaxis of MAC infection in AIDS patients.[139,140] Future investigations will be necessary to guide clinicians in its appropriate management.

Other bacteria are a common source of serious infection in patients with HIV infection. *Streptococcus pneumoniae* and *Haemophilus influenzae* or other streptococci cause 2–10 per cent of AIDS-related pneumonias.[141] In the 1993 CDC classification, recurrent pneumonia (two or more episodes within a 1-year period), with or without a bacteriologic diagnosis, is included in the AIDS case definition criteria.[9] Salmonellae, shigellae and campylobacteria are common causes of enteritis.[142] Standard antimicrobial therapies are generally effective for bacterial infections in AIDS. Further studies will be necessary to clarify if persons with these conditions will benefit from special approaches.

Protozoal infections

Pneumocystis carinii pneumonia (PCP) is the commonest opportunistic infection and has been estimated to occur in 80–85 per cent of patients with AIDS at some point of their illness.[143] Clinical presentation may be sudden with rapid onset of hypoxia and respiratory failure, or more gradual, with breathlessness, non-productive cough and fever. *Pneumocystis carinii* can also involve extrapulmonary sites such as liver and skin. The diagnosis of PCP is made by microsopic examinations of induced sputum, bronchoalveolar lavage, or trans-bronchial biopsy.[144,145] An indirect immunofluorescent assay using monoclonal anti-pneumocystis antibodies is also used.[146] Co-trimoxazole is the first-line treatment for acute PCP; intravenous pentamidine is frequently used as the second-line treatment. The major disadvantages of co-trimoxazole is the high rate[147,148] of adverse reaction in patients with HIV infection and neutropenia, that can be a major problem if concomitant AZT is used. Pancreatitis may be a cumulative dose-dependent toxicity of pentamidine, and must be watched for if using ddI as an antiretroviral at the same time.

Approximately 80 per cent of patients with PCP recover fully from their first episode of pneumonia. In patients in whom these agents failed, a salvage regimen of trimetrexate and leucovorin has been shown to be promising.[149] Dapsone is also used in patients that are intolerant to co-trimoxazole.[150]

Recently, atovaquone a non-sulphonamide therapy for the treatment of PCP has been made available: it has been shown to be effective and well-tolerated in patients who are intolerant to co-trimoxazole.[151] Zidovudine decreases the frequency of subsequent episodes of PCP.[152] Recurrent infection and relapse are common in AIDS-related PCP. Aerosolized pentamidine is approved for prophylaxis of PCP and the US Public Health Service has issued guidelines for PCP prophylaxis in people with HIV infection.[153]

Toxoplasmosis associated with AIDS has become one of the commonest causes of encephalitis.[154,155] Symptoms include neurological abnormalities such as headache, motor changes, seizures, sensory loss, tremor, blindness, personality changes, confusion, disorientation and coma. Computed tomography (CT) scanning reveals the diagnostic solitary or multiple focal lesions in most cases, but magnetic resonance imaging (MRI) is more sensitive. Antibody detection does not give definitive diagnosis because most cases of *Toxoplasma* encephalitis are a reactivation of latent infection. Brain biopsy can give a definitive diagnosis, but therapy is usually begun after a presumptive diagnosis based on CT scan or MRI.[156] Should a single lesion be observed by MRI scanning, other diagnoses such as lymphoma and, less commonly, tuberculoma, cryptococcoma or Kaposi's sarcoma should be pursued.[144] Pyrimethamine in combination with sulphadiazine is the first line of treatment for toxoplasma encephalitis. If treatment is begun with a presumptive diagnosis, clinical and CT scan response are usually seen within 10 days. Without lifelong maintenance therapy, recurrence rates reach 80%. Pyrimethamine and sulphadiazine therapy is associated with a high incidence of toxicity including bone marrow suppresssion and sulphadiazine allergy. Clindamycin in combination with pyrimethamine is also used for the treatment of *Toxoplasma* encephalitis.[157] Further studies to determine the best regimens for secondary prophylaxis are necessary. For patients seropositive for toxoplasmosis, further studies will be necessary to determine whether prophylaxis regimens exist where the potential protective benefits outweigh the risk of adverse effects.[126]

Isosporiasis is an enteric coccidiosis caused by *Isospora belli* and in patients with AIDS usually causes a chronic watery diarrhoea, which may be intermittent and may be difficult to distinguish clinically from other diarrhoeal illness. It is diagnosed by finding the organism on microscopic examination of the stool.[158] Isosporiasis usually responds within 1 week to treatment with oral co-trimoxazole.[159]

Lower dose co-trimoxazole or sulphadoxine/pyrimethamine suppressive treatment has been recommended to prevent recurrence.

Cryptosporidium is a protozoan parasite which is a common cause of enteritis in patients with AIDS. Symptoms of cryptosporidiosis include watery diarrhoea, abdominal cramping pain and weight loss. Diagnosis is by identification of oocystis on faecal smear.[160] There is currently no treatment available for cryptosporidial enteritis.

Microsporidia are parasites that have been determined to be pathogenic in humans and may be responsible for some cases of colitis in AIDS. Microsporidia are difficult to detect because they do not stain well and require electron microscopy for identification.[161] There is no known treatment for microsporidiosis.

Fungal infections

Candidiasis is the most frequent mycotic opportunistic infection in HIV patients. The most important species clinically is *Candida albicans* although other species may cause the same syndromes. Oral candidiasis occurs in nearly all AIDS patients at some point in their illness and is characterized by frequent recurrences after treatment.[162] *Candida albicans* infection can also affect the oesophagus, vaginal mucosa, gastrointestinal tract and skin. Oesophagitis in particular is the second commonest manifestation of *Candida* infection in AIDS, characteristically causing retrosternal pain. The diagnosis is based on clinical appearance or on the recovery of pathogenic fungi from direct cultures of specimens.

There are many agents effective against candidiasis, including nystatin, clotrimazole, ketoconazole, fluconazole and itraconazole.[163–165]

Cryptococcosis occurs in 6–13 per cent of AIDS patients, with more than two thirds of cases presenting meningoencephalitis.[166,167] Symptoms of cryptococcal meningitis include fatigue, fever, headache, personality changes and seizures. Pulmonary infection may be asymptomatic or appear with lobar or interstitial pneumonitis and pleural effusion; disseminated disease may involve virtually any organ system. Analysis of cerebrospinal fluid (CSF) often shows a heavy burden of organisms with a markedly positive India-ink slide and very high CSF cryptococcal antigen titres. In addition to CSF evaluation, patients with extraneural sites of infection should have specimens obtained for histology and culture when appropriate (skin, bone, lung, blood and urine).

Initial choice of therapy remains amphotericin B with or without oral flucytosine. Suppressive therapy is necessary. Fluconazole at high dose has been approved for treatment and maintenance of cryptococcal meningitis.[168] Itraconazole may also be useful in preventing relapse.[169] It is still matter of discussion whether amphotericin B or fluconazole is the treatment of choice.

Histoplasma capsulatum is a fungus that has been recognized with increasing frequency in patients with HIV infection. In AIDS patients, disseminated disease is the primary clinical presentation.[170,171] Presenting symptoms are non-specific and include fever, chills, sweats, weight loss, vomiting and diarrhoea. Pneumonitis with diffuse or patchy reticulonodular infiltrate is also common. Diagnosis of histoplasmosis depends on documenting the organisms in clinical specimens by culture or histopathology. Amphotericin B followed by maintenance therapy with either amphotericin B or ketoconazole are the standard therapies for histoplasmosis. Relapses are common.

Coccidiomycosis is endemic to the south-western United States and Central America. Reports suggest that patients with HIV infection are at increased risk for disseminated coccidiomycosis.[172] Symptoms are non-specific. Pulmonary involvement is common and disseminated infection may involve kidneys, spleen lymph nodes, brain and thyroid. Diagnosis is based on detection of the organism by examination or culture of bronchoscopically obtained specimens. The infection may respond to treatment with amphotericin B, but relapse may occur rapidly upon discontinuation of therapy.

Acknowledgements

This work was supported by the Istituto Superiore di Sanità, AIDS project 1995 and by the Associazione Italiana per la Ricerca sul Cancro, Milan, Italy. The author would also like to thank Domenico Errante, Giampiero Di Gennaro, Massimo Boccalon, Guglielmo Nasti, Marcello Tavio and Emanuela Vaccher, for their assistance.

REFERENCES

1. Gottlieb MS, Schroff R, Schanker HM *et al*. *Pneumocystis carinii* pneumonia and mucosal candidiasis in previously healthy homosexual men. Evidence of a new acquired cellular immonodeficiency. *New England Journal of Medicine* 1981; **305**: 1425–31.
2. Hymes K, Cheung T, Green JB *et al*. Kaposi's sarcoma in homosexual men. *Lancet* 1981; **ii**: 598–600.
3. Friedman-Keen AE, Laubenstein L, Marmor M *et al*. Kaposi's sarcoma and pneumocystis pneumonia among homosexual men. New York and California. *Morbidity and Mortality Weekly Report* 1981; **30**: 305–8.
4. World Health Organization. Acquired immunodeficiency syndrome (AIDS) data as at 31 December 1992. *WHO Weekly Epidemiology Record* 1993; **68**: 9–10.
5. Gallo RC, Salahuddin SZ, Popovic M *et al*. Frequent detection and isolation of cytopathic retroviruses (HTLV-III) from patients with AIDS and at risk for AIDS. *Science* 1984; **224**: 500–3.
6. Montagnier L, Dauguet C, Axler C *et al*. A new type of retrovirus isolated from patients presenting with lymphadenopathy and AIDS: structural and antigenic relatedness with equine infectious anemia virus. *Annals of Virology (Institut Pasteur)* 1984; **135E**: 119-34.
7. Barré-Sinoussi F, Chermann JC, Rey F *et al*. Isolation of a T-lymphotropic retrovirus from a patient at risk for acquired immunodeficiency syndrome (AIDS). *Science* 1983; **220**: 868–70.
8. World Health Organization. Acquired immunodeficiency syndrome (AIDS), 1987 revision of CDC/WHO cases definition for AIDS. *WHO Weekly Epidemiology Record* 1988; **63**: 1.
9. Centers for Disease Control. 1993 revised classification system for HIV infection and expanded surveillance case definition for AIDS among adolescent and adults. *Morbidity and Mortality Weekly Report* 1993; **41**: 1–13.

10. Richman DD, Fischl MA, Grieco MH *et al.* The toxicity of azidothymidine (AZT) in the treatment of patients with AIDS and AIDS-related complex: a double-blind, placebo-controlled trial. *New England Journal of Medicine* 1987; **317**: 192–7.
11. Yarchoan R, Perno CF, Thomas RV *et al.* Phase I studies of 2′,3′-dideoxycytidine in severe human immunodeficiency virus infections as a single agent and alternating with zidovudine (AZT). *Lancet* 1988; **1**: 76–81.
12. Fischal MA, Richman DD, Causey DM *et al.* Prolonged zidovudine therapy in patients with AIDS and advanced AIDS-related complex. *Journal of the American Medical Association* 1989; **262**: 2045–10.
13. Brett-Smith H, Griffith B, Mellors J *et al.* Effect of D$_4$T on HIV viremia. *VIII International Conference on AIDS, Amsterdam*, 1992: abstract POB 3011.
14. Yarchoan R, Mitsuya H, Thomas RV *et al.* *In vitro* activity against HIV and favourable toxicity profile of 2′,3′-dideoxyinosine. *Science* 1989; **245**: 412–5.
15. Dudley MN, Graham KK, Kaul E *et al.* Pharmacokinetics of stavudine in patients with AIDS or AIDS-related complex. *Journal of Infectious Diseases* 1992; **166**: 480–5.
16. Hamilton JD, Hartigan PM, Simberkoff MS *et al.* A controlled trial of early versus late treatment with zidovudine in symptomatic human immunodeficiency virus infection – results of the Veterans Affairs Cooperative Study. *New England Journal of Medicine* 1992; **326**: 437–43.
17. Kahn JO, Lagakos SW, Richman DD *et al.* A controlled trial comparing continued zidovudine with didanosine in human immunodeficiency virus infection. *New England Journal of Medicine* 1992; **327**: 581–7.
18. Vella S, Giuliano M, Pezzotti P *et al.* Survival of zidovudine-treated patients with AIDS compared with that of contemporary untreated patients. *Journal of the American Medical Association* 1992; **267**: 1232–6.
19. Roberts NA, Martin JA, Kinchington D *et al.* Rational design of peptide-based HIV proteinase inhibitors. *Science* 1990; **248**: 358–61.
20. Craig JC, Duncan IB, Hockley D *et al.* Antiviral properties of Ro 31–8959, an inhibitor of human immunodeficiency virus (HIV) proteinase. *Antiviral Research* 1991; **16**: 295–305.
21. Hsu M-C, Schutt AD, Holly M *et al.* Inhibition of HIV replication in acute and chronic infections *in vitro* by a tat antagonist. *Science* 1991; **254**: 1799–802.
22. DeBouck C. The HIV-1 protease as a therapeutic target for AIDS. *AIDS Research Human Retroviruses* 1992; **8**: 153–64.
23. Rosen CA. HIV regulatory proteins: potential targets for therapeutic intervention. *AIDS Research Research Human Retroviruses* 1992; **8**: 175–81.
24. Fischl MA, Richman DD, Hansen N *et al.* The safety and efficacy of zidovudine (AZT) in the treatment of subjects with mildly symptomatic human immunodeficiency virus type 1 (HIV) infection: a double blind, placebo-controlled trial. *Annals of Internal Medicine* 1990; **112**: 727–37.
25. Volberding PA, Lagakos SW, Koch MA *et al.* Zidovudine in asymptomatic human immunodeficiency virus infection: a controlled trial in persons with fewer than 500 CD4-positive cell per cubic millimeter. *New England Journal of Medicine* 1990; **322**: 941–9.
26. Aboulker JP, Swart AM. Preliminiary analysis of the Concorde trial. *Lancet* 1993; **341**: 889–90.
27. Hirsch MS, D'Aquila RT. Therapy for human immunodeficiency virus. *New England Journal of Medicine* 1993; **328**: 1686–95.
28. Mitsuya H, Broder S. Inhibition of the *in vitro* infectivity and cytopathic effect of human T-lymphotropic virus type III/lymphadenopathy-associated virus (HTLV-III/LAV) by 2′,3′-dideoxynucleosides. *Proceedings of the National Academy of Sciences, USA* 1986; **83**: 1911–5.
29. Merigan TC, Skowron G, Bozzette S *et al.* Circulating p24 antigen levels and

responses to dideoxycytidine in human immunodeficiency virus (HIV) infections: a phase I and II study. *Annals of Internal Medicine* 1989; **110**: 189.

30. Merigan TC. ddC Study Group of the AIDS Clinical Trials Group of the NIAID: safety and tolerance of dideoxycytidine as a single agent. *American Journal of Medicine* 1990; **88**(Suppl. 5B): 11S.

31. Skowron G, Merigan TC. Alternating and intermittent regimens of zidovudine (3'-azido-3'deoxythymidine) and dideoxycytidine (2',3'-dideoxycytidine in the treatment of patients with acquired immunodeficiency syndrome (AIDS) and AIDS-related complex. *American Journal of Medicine* 1990; **88**(Suppl. 5B): 20S.

32. Yarchoan R, Perno CF, Thomas RV *et al.* Phase I studies of 2',3'-dideoxycytidine in severe human immunodeficiency virus infection as a single agent and alternation with zidovudine (AZT) *Lancet* 1988; **1**: 76.

33. Biggar RJ. Cancer in acquired immunodeficiency syndrome: an epidemiological assessment. *Seminars in Oncology* 1990; **17**(3): 251.

34. European Centre for the Epidemiological Monitoring of AIDS: AIDS Surveillance in Europe. *Quarterly Report* no. 31, 30 September 1991.

35. Beral V, Peterman AT, Berkelman RL *et al.* Kaposi's sarcoma among persons with AIDS: a sexually transmitted infection? *Lancet* 1990; **335**: 123–8.

36. Couturier E, Ancelle-Park RA, De Vincenzi I *et al.* Kaposi's sarcoma as a sexually transmitted disease (letter). *Lancet* 1990; **335**: 1105.

37. Nakamura S, Salahuddin SZ, Biberfeld P *et al.* Kaposi's sarcoma cells: long term culture with growth factor from retrovirus infected CD4+ T cells. *Science* 1988; **242**(4877): 425.

38. Krigel RL, Friedman-Kien AE. Kaposi's sarcoma in AIDS: diagnosis and treatment. In: De Vait V, Hellman S, Rosenberg SA eds. *AIDS etiology, diagnosis, treatment and prevention.* Philadelphia: JB Lippincott, 1988: 245–61.

39. Safai B. Pathology and epidemiology of epidemic Kaposi's sarcoma. *Seminars in Oncology* 1987; **14**(2) (Suppl. 3): 7.

40. Chachova A, Krigel R, Lafleur F *et al.* Prognostic factors and staging classification of patients with epidemic Kaposi's sarcoma. *Journal of Clinical Oncology* 1989; **7**(6): 724.

41. Mitsuyasu RT. Clinical variants and staging of Kaposi's sarcoma. *Seminars in Oncology* 1987; **14**(2 Suppl. 3): 17.

42. Krown S, Metroka C, Wernz JC. Kaposi's sarcoma in the acquired immunodeficiency syndrome: a proposal for uniform evaluation, response and staging criteria. *Journal of Clinical Oncology* 1989; **7**: 1201.

43. Hill DR. The role of radiotherapy for epidemic Kaposi's sarcoma. *Seminars in Oncology* 1987; **14**(2 Suppl): 19.

44. Balker PJM, Danner SA, Lange JMA *et al.* Etoposide for epidemic Kaposi's sarcoma: a phase II study. *European Journal of Cancer and Clinical Oncology* 1988; **24**(6): 1047.

45. Gill P, Deyton LR, Rorich M *et al.* Treatment of epidemic Kaposi's sarcoma (EKS) with vincristine, bleomycin and low dose adriamycin. *Blood* 1986; **68**(Suppl. 1): abstract 126a.

46 Kaplan L, Abrams D, Volberding PA. Treatment of Kaposi's sarcoma in acquired immunodeficiency syndrome with an alternating vincristine vinblastine regimen. *Cancer Treatment Reports* 1986; **70**: 1121.

47. Laubenstein LJ, Krigel RL, Odajuk CM. Treatment of epidemic Kaposi's sarcoma with etoposide or a combination of doxorubicin and vinblastine. *Journal of Clinical Oncology* 1984; **2**: 1115.

48. Minor DR. Vinblastine–methotrexate, vincristine chemotherapy for epidemic Kaposi's sarcoma. *Proceedings of the American Society for Clinical Oncology* 1988; **7**(4): abstract 16.

49. Mintzer DM, Real FX, Jovino L *et al.* Treatment of Kaposi's sarcoma and throm-

bocytopenia with vincristine in patients with the acquired immunodeficiency syndrome. *Annals of Internal Medicine* 1985; **102**: 200.

50. Volberding PA. The role of chemotherapy for epidemic Kaposi's sarcoma. *Seminars in Oncology* 1987; **14**(2) (Suppl. 3): 23.

51. Volberding PA, Abrams DI, Conant M *et al.* Vinblastine therapy for Kaposi's sarcoma in the aquired immunodeficiency syndrome. *Annals of Internal Medicine* 1985; **103**: 335.

52. Wernz J, Laubenstein L, Hymes K *et al.* Chemotherapy and assessment of response in epidemic Kaposi's sarcoma with bleomycin/velban. *Proceedings of the American Society for Clinical Oncology* 1986; **5**: abstract 4.

53. Gill PS, Rarick M, McCutchan JA *et al.* Systemic treatment of AIDS-related Kaposi's sarcoma: results of a randomized trial. *American Journal of Medicine* 1991; **90**: 427.

54. Groopman JE, Scadden DT. Interferon therapy for Kaposi's sarcoma associated with the acquired immunodeficiency syndrome (AIDS). *Annals of Internal Medicine* 1989; **110**(5): 335.

55. Mitsuyasu RT, Groopman JE. Biology and therapy of Kaposi's sarcoma. *Seminars in Oncology* 1984; **11**: 53.

56. Kovacs JA, Deyton L, Davey L *et al.* Combined zidovudine and interferon-α therapy in patients with Kaposi's sarcoma and the acquired immunodeficiency syndrome (AIDS). *Annals of Internal Medicine* 1989; **111**: 280.

57. Krown SE, Gold J, Niedzwiecki D *et al.* Interferon-α with zidovudine: safety, tolerance and clinical and virologic effects with the acquired immunodeficiency syndrome (AIDS). *Annals of Internal Medicine* 1990; **112**: 812.

58. Fischl MA. Antiretroviral therapy in combination with interferon for AIDS-related Kaposi's sarcoma. *American Journal of Medicine* 1991; **90**(Suppl. 4A): 2.

59. Goebel FD, Bogner JR, Spathling S *et al.* Quantitative ultrasound volume measurement serves as non-invasive method to follow response of cutaneous Kaposi's sarcoma lesions to doxil therapy. *Proceedings of the American Society for Clinical Oncology* 1993; **12**(51): abstract 7.

60. Northfelt DW, Martin FT, Kaplan LD *et al.* Pharmacokinetics (PK), tumor localization (TL), and safety of doxil (liposomal doxorubicin) in AIDS patients with Kaposi's sarcoma (AIDS-KS). *Proceedings of the American Society for Clinical Oncology* 1993; **12**(51): abstract 8.

61. List AF, Grego FA, Vogler LB. Lymphoproliferative disease in immunocompromized hosts: the role of Epstein–Barr virus. *Journal of Clinical Oncology* 1987; **5**(19): 1673.

62. Andrieu JM, Raphael M, Binet JA *et al.* HIV-associated NHL in France. *XIII Congress of ESMO*, Lugano 9, 1988: abstract 5.

63. Di Carlo EF, Amerson LB, Metroka CE *et al.* Malignant lymphomas and the acquired immunodeficiency syndrome. *Archives of Pathology and Laboratory Medicine* 1986; **110**: 1012.

64. Egert DA, Beckstead JH. Malignant lymphomas in the acquired immunodeficiency syndrome. Additional evidence for a B-cell origin. *Archives of Pathology and Laboratory Medicine* 1988; **112**: 602.

65. Huhn D, Serke M. Malignant lymphomas and HIV infection. In: *AIDS-related neoplasias. Recent results in cancer research.* Berlin: Springer-Verlag, 1988: 63–8.

66. Ioachim NL, Cooper MC, Hellman GC. Lymphomas associated with the acquired immunodeficiency syndrome (AIDS): a study of 35 cases. *Cancer Detection and Prevention* 1987; Suppl. 1: 557.

67. Jara C, Flores E, Alfonso PG *et al.* Presentation of 7 patients with human immunodeficiency virus infection and associated neoplasms. *Proceedings ECCO-4*, Madrid, 1987: abstract 1000.

68. Kaplan LD, Abrams DI, Feigal E *et al.* AIDS-associated non-Hodgkin's lymphoma in San Francisco. *Journal of the American Medical Association* 1989; **261**(15): 719.
69. Knowles DM, Chamulak GA, Subar M *et al.* Lymphoid neoplasia associated with the AIDS. The New York Medical Center Experience with 105 patients (1981–1986). *Annals of Internal Medicine* 1988; **108**: 744.
70. Levine AM, Sullivan-Halley J, Pike MC *et al.* Human immunodeficiency virus-related lymphoma-prognostic factors predictive of survival. *Cancer* 1991; **68**: 2466–72.
71. Lowenthal DA, Straus DJ, Campbell SW *et al.* AIDS-related lymphoid neoplasia. The Memorial Hospital Experience. *Cancer* 1986; **61**: 2325.
72. Markowitz M, Alonso G, Spicehandler D *et al.* HIV-related lymphoma: a recent experience. *IV International Conference on AIDS, Stockholm 326* 1988: abstract 7607.
73. Monfardini S, Tirelli U, Vaccher E *et al.* for the GICAT. Malignant lymphomas in patients with or at risk for AIDS. *Journal of the National Cancer Institute* 1988; **80**: 855.
74. Monfardini S, Vaccher E, Foà R *et al.* for the GICAT. AIDS-associated non-Hodgkin's lymphomas in Italy: intravenous drug users vs. homosexual men. *Annals of Oncology* 1990: **1**: 203.
75. Oksenhendler E, Molina TH, Gisselbrecht C *et al.* Non-Hodgkin's lymphomas (NHL) and human immunodeficiency virus (HIV) infection. *III International Symposium on Immunobiology in Clinical Oncology, Nice 161*, 1989: abstract 342: 25.
76. Raphael M, Tulliez M, Bellefqih S *et al.* Les lymphomas et le SIDA. *Annals of Pathology* 1986; **6**: 278.
77. Schmid E. AIDS-related neoplasias in Switzerland. *Proceedings ECCO-4, Madrid*, 1987: abstract 1000.
78. Skinhoj P, Ersball J, Nissen NI. Human immunodeficiency virus (HIV) associated non-Hodgkin's lymphomas in Denmark: report of three cases. *European Journal of Haematology* 1987; **38**: 71.
79. Ziegler JL, Beckstead AJ, Volberding PA *et al.* Non-Hodgkin's lymphomas in 90 homosexual men. *New England Journal of Medicine* 1984; **311**: 565.
80. Gill PS, Levine AM, Meyer PR *et al.* Primary central nervous system lymphoma in homosexual men. *American Journal of Medicine* 1985; **78**: 742.
81. Coiffier B, Gisselbrecht C, Herbrecht R *et al.* LNH-84 regimen: a multicenter study of intensive chemotherapy in 737 patients with aggressive malignant lymphoma. *Journal of Clinical Oncology* 1989; **8**(7): 1018–26.
82. Gisselbrecht C, Lepage E, Tirelli U *et al.* for the French–Italian Cooperative Study Group. Human immunodeficiency virus-related lymphoma treatment with intensive combination chemotherapy. *Proceedings of the American Society for Clinical Oncology* 1993: abstract 1227.
83. Carde P, Meerwaldt JH, van Glabbeke M *et al.* Superiority of second over first generation chemotherapy in a randomized trial for stage III–IV intermediate and high-grade non-Hodgkin's lymphoma (NHL): the 1980–1985 EORTC trial. *Annals of Oncology* 1991; **2**: 431–5.
84. Tirelli U, Errante D, Oksenhendler E *et al.* for the French–Italian Cooperative Study Group. Prospective study with combined low-dose chemotherapy and zidovudine in 37 patients with poor-prognosis AIDS-related non-Hodgkin's lymphoma. *Annals of Oncology* 1992; **3**: 843–7.
85. Tirelli U, Errante D, Tavio M *et al.* Treatment of HIV-related non-Hodgkin's lymphoma (NHL) with chemotherapy (CT) and granulocyte-colony stimulating factor (G-CSF): reduction of toxicity and of days of hospitalization with concomitant overall reduction of the cost. *IXth International Conference on AIDS, Berlin*, 1993: abstract WS-B16–2.

86. Riothmann S, Tourani JM, Andrieu JM. HIV-associated Hodgkin's disease: report of 45 cases. *European Journal of Cancer* 1991; Suppl 2: 13 (abstract).

87. Serrano M, Bellas C, Campo E *et al.* Hodgkin's disease in patients with antibodies to human immunodeficiency virus. A study of 22 patients. *Cancer* 1990; **65**: 2248–54.

88. Ree HJ, Strauchen JA, Amjad AK *et al.* Human immunodeficiency virus-associated Hodgkin's disease: clinicopathologic studies of 24 cases and preponderance of mixed cellularity type characterized by the occurrence of fibrohistiocytoid stromal cells. *Cancer* 1991; **67**: 1614–21.

89. Tirelli U, Errante D, Vaccher E *et al.* Hodgkin's disease in 92 patients with HIV infection: the Italian experience. *Annals of Oncology* 1992; **3** (Suppl. 4): S69–72.

90. Errante D, Tirelli U, Milo D *et al.* Chemotherapy (CT) with and without zidovudine (AZT) for Hodgkin's disease (HD) and HIV infection: a comparison in 49 patients (PTS). *IXth International Conference on AIDS, Berlin*, 1993: abstract PO-B13–1611.

91. Penn I. Cancers of the anogenital region in renal transplant recipients: analysis of 65 cases. *Cancer* 1986; **58**: 611–16.

92. Penn I. Tumors of the immunocompromised patient. *Annual Review of Medicine* 1988; **39**: 63–73.

93. Reid R, Geenberg M, Jenson AB *et al.* Sexually transmitted papillomaviral infections. The anatomic distribution and pathologic grade of neoplastic lesions associated with different viral types. *American Journal of Obstetrics and Gynecology* 1987; **156**: 212–22.

94. Pfister H. Relationship of papillomaviruses to anogenital cancer. *Obstetrics and Gynecology Clinics of North America* 1987; **14**: 349–61.

95. Vermund SH, Kelley KF, Klein RS *et al.* High risk of human papillomavirus infection and cervical squamous intraepithelial lesions among women with symptomatic human immunodeficiency virus infection. *American Journal of Obstetrics and Gynecology* 1991; **165**(2): 392–400.

96. Maiman M, Tarricone N, Vieria J *et al.* Colposcopic evaluation of human immunodeficiency virus-seropositive women. *Obstetrics and Gynecology* 1991; **78**: 84–8.

97. Smith JR, Botcherby M, James M *et al.* Influence of HIV on lower genital tract neoplasia. In: Giraldo G, Salvatore M, Piazza M, Zarrilli D, Beth-Giraldo E eds. *Biomedical and social development in AIDS and associated tumors.* Antiobiot. Chemother. Basel: Karger, 1991; **43**: 150–5.

98. Schwartz LB, Carcangiu ML, Bradham L *et al.* Rapidly progressive squamous cell carcinoma of the cervix coexisting with human immunodeficiency virus infection: clinical opinion. *Gynecology and Oncology* 1991; **41**: 255–8.

99. Giorda G, Vaccher E, Volpe R *et al.* An unusual presentation of vulval carcinoma in a HIV patient. *Gynecology and Oncology* 1992; **44**: 191–94.

100. Frazer IH, Medley G, Crapper RM *et al.* Association between anorectal dysplasia, human immunodeficiency virus in homosexual men. *Lancet* 1986; **ii**: 657–60.

101. Palefsky JM, Gonzales J, Creenblatt RM *et al.* Anal intraepithelial neoplasia and anal papillomavirus infection among homosexual males with group IV HIV disease. *Journal of the American Medical Association* 1990; **263**: 2911–16.

102. Beckmann AM, Daling RJ, Sherman KJ *et al.* Human papillomavirus infection and anal cancer. *International Journal of Cancer* 1989; **43**: 1042–9.

103. Palefsky JM, Holly EA, Gonzales J *et al.* Detection of human papillomavirus DNA in anal intra-epithelial neoplasia and anal cancer. *Cancer Research* 1991; **51**: 1014–19.

104. Lorenz HP, Wilson W, Leigh B *et al.* Squamous cell carcinoma of the anus and HIV infection. *Diseases of the Colon and Rectum* 1991; **34**(4): 336–8.

105. Svensson C, Kaigas M, Liabrink E *et al*. Carcinoma of the anal canal in a patient with AIDS. *Acta Oncologica* 1991; **30**(8): 986–7.

106. Safavi A, Gottesman L, Dailey TH. Anorectal surgery in the HIV+ patient: update. *Diseases of the Colon and Rectum* 1991; **34**(4): 299–304.

107. Palefsky JM, Holly EA, Ahn DK. Progression of anal cytologic changes in men with group IV HIV disease. *IX International Conference on AIDS, Berlin*, 6–11 June 1993: q60, abstract WS-B17–6.

108 Van Ginkel CJW, Sang RTL, Blaaungeers JLG *et al*. Multiple primary malignant melanomas in an HIV-positive man. *Journal of the American Academy of Dermatology* 1991; **24**: 284–5.

109. Merkle T, Braun-Falco O, Froschl M *et al*. Malignant melanoma in Human Immunodeficiency Virus Type 2 infection. *Archives of Dermatology* 1991; **127**: 266–7.

110. Tirelli U, Troiano T, Spina M *et al*. Skin carcinoma in 2 patients with HIV infection. *European Journal of Cancer* 1991; **27**(9): 1184.

111. Murthy AR, Ho D, Goetz MB. Relationship between acute myelomonoblastic leukemia and infection due to human immunodeficiency virus. *Review of Infectious Diseases* 1991; **13**: 254–6.

112. Puppo F, Scudeletti M, Murgia L *et al*. Acute myelomonocytic leukemia in an HIV-infected patient. *AIDS* 1991; **6**(1): 136–7.

113. Lee BT, Lefor AT, Didolkar MS. Squamous cell carcinoma of the umbilicus associated with Acquired Immunodeficiency Syndrome. *Journal of Surgical Oncology* 1991; **47**: 67–9.

114. Remick SC, Harper GR, Abdullah NA *et al*. Metastatic breast cancer in a young patient seropositive for Human Immunodeficiency Virus. *Journal of the National Cancer Institute* 1991; **83**(6): 447–8.

115. Aricò M, Caselli D, D'Argenio P *et al*. for the Italian Multicenter Study on Human Immunodeficiency Virus Infection in Children. Malignancies in children with human immunodeficiency virus type 1 infection. *Cancer* 1991; **68**: 2473–7.

116. McLoughlin LC, Nord KS, Joshi VV *et al*. Disseminated leiomyosarcoma in a child with acquired immune deficiency syndrome. *Cancer* 1991; **67**: 2618–21.

117. Ross JS, Del Rosario A, Bui HX *et al*. Primary hepatic leiomyosarcoma in a child with the acquired immunodeficiency syndrome. *Human Pathology* 1992; **23**(1): 69–72.

118. Chadwick EG, Connor EJ, Hanson IC *et al*. Tumors of smooth-muscle origin in HIV-infected children. *Journal of the American Medical Association* 1990; **263**: 3182–4.

119. Glatt AE, Chirgwin K, Landesman SH. Treatment of infections associated with human immunodeficiency virus. *New England Journal of Medicine* 1988; **318**: 1439–45.

120. Jacobson MA, Mills J. Serious cytomegalovirus disease in the acquired immunodeficiency syndrome. *Annals of Internal Medicine* 1988; **108**: 585–94.

121. Armstrong D, Gold JWM, Dryjanski J *et al*. Treatment of infections in patients with the acquired immunodeficiency syndrome. *Annals of Internal Medicine* 1985; **103**: 738–43.

122. Holland GN, Sidakaro Y, Kreiger AE *et al*. Treatment of cytomegalovirus retinopathy with ganciclovir. *Ophthalmology* 1987; **94**: 815–23.

123. Laskin OL, Caderberg DM, Mills J. Ganciclovir for the treatment and suppression of serious infections caused by cytomegalovirus. *American Journal of Medicine* 1987; **83**: 201–7.

124. Rolston K, Rodriguez S, Carvajal F *et al*. Therapy of cytomegalovirus infections with ganciclovir. *Vth International Conference on AIDS, Montreal*, 1989: 129 (abstract).

125. Drew WL, Buhles W, Erlich KS. Herpesvirus infections (cytomegalovirus, herpes

simplex virus, varicella zoster virus): how to use ganciclovir (DHPG) and acyclovir. *Infectious Diseases Clinics of America* 1988; **2**: 495–509.

126. Klein RS. Phrophylaxis of opportunistic infections in individuals infected with HIV. *AIDS* 1989; **3**(Suppl. 1): S161–73.

127 Metroka CE, Josefberg H. Usefulness of high dose acyclovir as prophylaxis for CMV. *VIth International Conference on AIDS, San Francisco* 1990: abstract 2111.

128. Sandstrom EG, Kaplan JC, Byngton RE *et al*. Inhibition of human T-cell lymphotropic virus type III *in vitro* by phosphonoformate. *Lancet* 1985; **1**: 1480–2.

129. Bergdahl S, Sonnerborg A, Larsson A *et al*. Declining levels of HIV p24 antigen in serum during treatment with foscarnet (letter). *Lancet* 1988; **1**: 1052.

130. Palestrine AG, Polis MA, De Smet MD *et al*. A randomized, controlled trial of foscarnet in the treatment of cytomegalovirus retinitis in patients with AIDS. *Annals of Internal Medicine* 1991; **115**: 665–73.

131. SOCA in collaboration with ACTG. Mortality in patients with the Acquired Immunodeficiency Syndrome treated with either foscarnet or ganciclovir for cytomegalovirus retinitis. *New England Journal of Medicine* 1992; **326**: 213–20.

132. Polis M, de Smet MD, Baird BF *et al*. Increased survival of a cohort of patients with acquired immunodeficiency syndrome and cytomegalovirus retinitis who received sodium phosphonoformate (foscarnet). *American Journal of Medicine* 1993; **94**: 175–80.

133. Erlich KS, Mills J, Chatis P *et al*. Acyclovir-resistant herpes simplex virus infections in patients with the acquired immunodeficiency syndrome. *New England Journal of Medicine* 1989; **320**: 293–6.

134. Okano M, Thiele G, Davis J *et al*. Epstein–Barr virus and human diseases: recent advances in diagnosis. *Clinical Microbiology Reviews* 1988; **1**: 300–12.

135. Greenspan J, Greenspan D, Lennette E *et al*. Replication of Epstein–Barr virus within the epithelial cells of oral 'hairy' leukoplakia, an AIDS-associated lesion. *New England Journal of Medicine* 1985; **313**: 1564–71.

136. Centers for Disease Control. Tuberculosis and human immunodeficiency virus infection: recommendations of the Advisory Committee for the elimination of tuberculosis. *Morbidity and Mortality Weekly Report* 1989; **38**: 236–50.

137. Chaisson R, Slotkin G. Tuberculosis and human immunodeficiency virus infection. *Journal of Infectious Diseases* 1989; **159**: 96–100.

138. Young LS. *Mycobacterium avium* complex infection. *Journal of Infectious Diseases* 1988; **157**: 863–7.

139. O'Brien RJ, Geiter LJ, Lyle MA. Rifabutin (ansamycin LM 427) for the treatment of pulmonary *Mycobacterium avium* complex. *American Review of Respiratory Disease* 1990; **141**: 821–6.

140. Siegal FP, Borenstein M, Gehan K *et al*. Rifabutin may delay the onset of Mycobacterium avium complex infection in patients with AIDS. In: *Final Program and Abstract of the Sixth International Conference on AIDS, San Francisco*, 20–24 June 1990: ThB518.

141. Chaisson RE. Bacterial pneumonia in patients with human immunodeficiency virus infection. *Seminars in Respiratory Infection* 1989; **4**: 133–8.

142. Chaisson RE. Infections due to encapsulated bacteria, salmonella, shigella and campylobacter. *Infectious Disease Clinics of North America* 1988; **2**: 475–84.

143. Mills J. *Pneumocystis carinii* and *Toxoplasma gondii* infection in patients with AIDS. *Review of Infectious Diseases* 1986; **8**: 1001–11.

144. Buckleu RM, Braffman MN, Stern JJ. Opportunistic infections in the acquired immunodeficiency syndrome. *Seminars in Oncology* 1990; **17**: 335–49.

145. O'Brien RF, Quinn JL, Miyhahara BT *et al*. Diagnosis of pneumocystis carinii by induced sputum in a city with moderate incidence of AIDS. *Chest* 1989; **95**: 136–8.

146. Fortun J, Navas E, Marti-Belda P *et al*. *Pneumocystis carinii* pneumonia in HIV-

infected patients: diagnostic yeld of induced sputum and immunofluorescent stain with monoclonal antibodies. *European Respiratory Journal* 1992; **5**(6): 665–9.

147. Kovacs JA, Hiemenz JW, Macher AM *et al*. *Pneumocystis carinii* pneumonia: a comparison between patients with the acquired immunodeficiency syndrome and patients with other immunodeficiencies. *Annals of Internal Medicine* 1984; **100**: 663–71.

148. Small CB, Harris CA, Friedland GH *et al*. The treatment of pneumocystis carinii pneumonia in the acquired immunodeficiency syndrome. *Archives of Internal Medicine* 1985; **145**: 837–40.

149. Allegra CJ, Chabner BA, Tuazon CU *et al*. Trimetrexate for the treatment of pneumocystis carinii pneumonia in patients with the acquired immunodeficiency syndrome. *New England Journal of Medicine* 1987; **317**: 978–85.

150. Opravil M, Heald A, Lazzarin A *et al*. Dapsone–pyrimethamine (DP) vs aerosolized pentamidine (AP) for combined prophylaxis of PCP and toxoplasmic encephalitis (TE). *IX International Conference on AIDS, Berlin*, 1993: PO-B10–1429.

151. Dohn M, Weinberg W, Rosenstock J *et al*. Atovaquone vs. pentamidine for PCP in patients with AIDS. *IX International Conference on AIDS, Berlin*, 1993: PO-B10–1421.

152. Fischl MA, Richman DD, Grieco MH *et al*. The efficacy of azidothymidine (AZT) in the treatment of patients with AIDS and AIDS-related complex. *New England Journal of Medicine* 1987; **317**: 185–91.

153. Centers for Disease Control. Guidelines for prophylaxis against *Pneumocystis carinii* pneumonia for persons infected with HIV. *Morbidity and Mortality Weekly Report* 1989; **38** (Suppl. 5).

154. Luft BJ, Remington JS. Toxoplasmosis of the central nervous system. In: Remington JS, Swartz MN eds. *Current clinical topics in infectious diseases*, vol. 6. New York: McGraw-Hill, 1985: 315–58.

155. Levy RM, Bredescen DE, Rosenblum ML. Neurological manifestations of the acquired immunodeficiency syndrome (AIDS): experience of UCSF and review of the literature. *Journal of Neurosurgery* 1985; **621**: 475–95.

156. Post MJD, Sheldon JJ, Hensley GT *et al*. Central nervous system disease in acquired immunodeficiency syndrome: prospective correlation using CT, MR Imaging and pathologic studies. *Radiology* 1986; **158**: 141–8.

157. Rolston K, Hoy J. Role of clyndamycin in the treatment of central nervous system toxoplasmosis. *American Journal of Medicine* 1987; **83**: 551–4.

158. De Hovitz JA, Pape JW, Boncy M *et al*. Clinical manifestations and therapy of *Isospora belli* infection in patients with acquired immunodeficiency syndrome. *New England Journal of Medicine* 1986; **315**: 87–90.

159. Pape JW, Verdier RI, Johnson WD Jr. Treatment and prophylaxis of Isospora belli infection in patients with the acquired immunodeficiency syndrome. *New England Journal of Medicine* 1989; **320**: 1044–7.

160. Soave R, Danner RL, Honig CL *et al*. Cryptosporidiosis in homosexual men. *Annals of Internal Medicine* 1984; **100**: 504–511.

161. Shadduck JA, Greeley E. Microsporidia and human infections. *Clinical Microbiology Reviews* 1989; **2**: 158–65.

162. Phelan JA, Saltzman BR, Friedland GH *et al*. Oral findings in patients with the acquired immunodeficiency syndrome. *Oral Surgery, Oral Medicine, Oral Pathology* 1987; **64**: 50–56.

163. De Wit S, Weerts D, Goosens H *et al*. Comparison of fluconazole and ketoconazole for oropharyngeal candidiasis in AIDS. *Lancet* 1989; **i**: 746–8.

164. Chave JP, Cajot A, Bille J *et al*. Single dose therapy for oral candidiasis with fluconazole in HIV infected adults: a pilot study. *Journal of Infectious Diseases* 1989; **159**: 806–7.

165. Inamatsu T, Mori T, Watanabe K *et al*. Treatment of deep-seated candidosis with

itraconazole: multi-centre study in Japan. *Symposium on Trends in the Management of Systemic Fungal Infections*, Nijmegen, The Netherlands, 5–7 September 1991 (abstract).

166. Zuger A, Louie E, Holzman RS *et al.* Cryptococcal disease in patients with the acquired immunodeficiency syndrome. *Annals of Internal Medicine* 1986; **104**: 234–40.

167. Eng RH, Bishburg E, Smith SM *et al.* Cryptococcal infections in patients with acquired immunodeficiency syndrome. *American Journal of Medicine* 1986; **81**: 19–23.

168. Sugar AM, Saunders C. Oral fluconazole as suppressive therapy of disseminated cryptococcosis in patients with acquired immunodeficiency syndrome. *American Journal of Medicine* 1988; **85**: 481–9.

169. Viviani MA, Tortorano AM, Langer M *et al.* Experience with itraconazole in cryptococcosis and aspergillosis. *Journal of Infections* 1989; **18**: 151–65.

170. Huang CT, McGarry T, Cooper S *et al.* Disseminated histoplasmosis in the acquired immunodeficiency syndrome. Report of five cases from a non endemic area. *Archives of Internal Medicine* 1987; **147**: 1181.

171. Mandell W, Goldberg DM, Neu HC. Histoplasmosis in patients with the acquired immunodeficiency syndrome. *American Journal of Medicine* 1986; **81**: 974.

172. Bronnimann DA, Adam RD, Galgiani JN *et al.* Coccidiomycosis in the acquired immunodeficiency syndrome. *Annals of Internal Medicine* 1987; **106**: 372–9.

PART 4

Psychological support

CHAPTER NINE

Psychological support for cancer patients and their medical carers

ANGELA HALL

INTRODUCTION

Cancer has been described as 'the standardised nightmare of our society'.[1] Of those population surveys that have been carried out in the last 25 years, cancer is perceived with most alarm and considered more serious than any other disease,[2] though in fact, there is a 5-year recurrence-free survival rate of 46 per cent for women and 35 per cent for men. Cancer seems almost benign in comparison with stroke where 40 per cent die within 6 months, and myocardial infarction, where 35 per cent of patients are dead within 1 month of their heart attack. However, in contrast to other chronic diseases, patients with cancer have special difficulties, attributable to the particular qualities of the disease. Cancer comes in many forms, some of which are entirely curable, whilst others at the other end of the spectrum are invariably fatal. Its course can be unpredictable and uncontrollable. The aetiology of many cancers is still rather poorly understood and many people have found that cancer is a stigmatizing disease, exacerbated by confusion about cause and the attribution of responsibility.

There is little doubt that many cancer sufferers need help in coming to terms with the major problems associated with the knowledge of having a potentially life-threatening disease and with the effects of treatments to be faced. This chapter looks at two general types of psychological support for patients. First, counselling, carried out in the main by health-care professionals and secondly, self-help, carried out by patients themselves. In addition, caring for cancer patients can be highly stressful: the remainder of the chapter is concerned with the under-recognized need for support of the health-care professionals themselves.

COUNSELLING

Most people have known someone who has died in a painful and undignified manner from cancer. Receiving the diagnosis triggers fearful images of one's own death and the manner of dying. For most patients the diagnosis represents a crisis in their lives: a point from which life will never seem or be the same again.

Patients' needs vary, not only between individuals at the time of initial diagnosis and treatment but also at different points in the illness trajectory. Many crave information. There may be a terrible sense of isolation and lack of support. A feeling of powerlessness is common, often combined with a need to take control and influence positively the outcome of the disease.

At the outset, it should be pointed out that counselling by no means represents the only form of psychological help available to patients. Maggie Watson[3] provides an excellent overview both of problem-specific psychological treatment methods and of treatment methods for specific diagnostic groups. In addition, her introduction discusses the professionalization of psychosocial oncology as a subspecialism of oncology: a multidisciplinary specialism whose skills may be practised by oncologists, nurses, psychiatrists, psychologists and social workers. Counselling is only one part of the remit of psychosocial oncology, but has been practised for long enough in this country for a start to be made on the evaluation of its worth.

What is counselling? In the broadest sense of the word, it means, quite simply, helping. This assumes that at least two people are involved, that the aim is for one person to help the other and that there is, at the very least, a minimal agreement about the nature of their interaction. Counselling activities range across a broad spectrum, from the qualities and skills necessary for communicating effectively at one end through to specialist professional help at the other. Considering the former, few doctors have undergone training in counselling, nor will it be advocated that they should necessarily do so. Even for those who take a particular interest in the area, it is unrealistic to expect hospital clinicians to find sufficient time to see their patients specifically for counselling sessions. However, the abilities of doctors to help their patients to understand and cope effectively with their problems, facilitating changes that may be necessary to bring these about, are intrinsic to good communication. In this way, communication and counselling skills are seen as synonymous. The significance of this assertion is highlighted in a recent study conducted by Slevin *et al.*,[4] evaluating patients' attitudes towards different sources of emotional support, which was defined as involving '. . . spending time with another person, listening and talking about problems and concerns in a way that is helpful and reassuring'. Patients rated emotional support from senior doctors at least as highly as that from their family, and more important than any other source. One effect of acquiring these skills is that doctors are then able to identify patients who may be in need of the specialist help provided by those with professional training and expertise. Studies show that between one quarter and one third of all cancer patients have significant psychological distress and that the majority accept counselling if offered.

Counselling is available through several different routes. It may be provided in hospital within specialist units or by specialist nurses or offered by patient-volunteers. It is becoming increasingly available as part of the services of primary health care practices. It may be sought privately by patients. It may be offered individually or on a group basis, face to face or via the telephone (Marcus *et al.*).[5] However, particularly within the hospital setting, there is great variation in the skills, abilities and level of training of those offering the counselling. Many of those who purport to offer counselling have been selected on the basis of being seen as kindly and well-motivated: the reality of the work

demands much more than a sympathetic shoulder to cry on. Many nurse-coun-
sellors recognize the need for training, but find that study-leave time and funding
are not forthcoming. A national survey carried out by Fallowfield and Roberts[6]
paints a disquieting picture of counsellors who are often 'overworked, under-
trained, under-resourced and insufficiently supervised'. In the survey 289 potential responders with responsibility for counselling cancer patients were identified
for inclusion and a response rate of 82 per cent was obtained. Only 25 per cent
had any recognized counselling qualification; 75 per cent did not belong to any
professional counselling organization. Less than half of the respondents claimed
to use any theoretical model and many expressed contrary and conflicting goals
in their work. An example is given of those counsellors who felt that improvement and normalization were *their* goals for their patients. This often meant
encouraging patients to adopt a 'fighting spirit', or face death 'bravely' or
respond to life as 'normal'. The authors point out that 'such stereotypes of
"good" adjustment to cancer can impose an immense burden on already psy-
chologically compromised individuals'.

In a world where there is competition for scarce resources, is there evidence
for the efficacy of oncology counselling? Those doctors who work with well-
qualified counsellors would assert that the service provided is invaluable, providing patients with the time that is in such short supply within the medical
profession. However, resource providers require more than anecdotal evidence
for need. In a comprehensive review published in 1983, Watson[7] concluded that
'the evidence relating to the benefits gained by patients is equivocal'. However,
the weakness did not necessarily lie in counselling itself, but rather in the
methodology of many studies which purported to evaluate its efficacy. Common
flaws included the absence of control or comparison group, absence of standardized, objective measures and the potential for bias introduced by intervention
and assessment being carried out by the same person. However, a more recent
review by Massey *et al.*[8] includes studies that 'have increasingly supported the
value of a range of psychosocial interventions to provide emotional support in
cancer patients'. Methodology has clearly become much more sophisticated; in
particular, emphasis has been placed on the development of appropriate outcome
measures. Because clinical anxiety and depression are such common sequelae of
a diagnosis of cancer and its treatment, early studies tended to look for large
differences in psychiatric morbidity between counselled and non-counselled
groups. However, failure to detect such differences does not necessarily indicate
that counselling does not have any benefit, but rather that psychiatric morbidity
is too blunt an instrument to detect it.

Increasingly, studies using different kinds of outcome show benefit to those
receiving counselling. Using individual crisis intervention counselling, Capone
et al.[9] found that counselled women with gynaecological cancer had better self-
image and had returned both to work and to prediagnosis levels of sexual
functioning more quickly than the non-counselled group. Linn *et al.*[10] also
used crisis intervention counselling with men with late-stage disease in five
different sites – lung, colon, stomach, pancreas and prostate. Although there
was no difference in terms of survival between counselled and control groups,
the former had improved perceived quality of life, feelings of internal control
and self-esteem. In a study by Cain *et al.*[11] women with gynaecological
cancer were randomized to one of three interventions: standard counselling or

'structured thematic counselling' which had a strong informational component, discussing diet, exercise, sex, emotional and physical problems. The women were assigned either on a group or on an individual basis. The women who received the information-structured approach, whether as a group or individually, were less anxious and depressed, had fewer sexual problems, better knowledge of their illness and reported better relationships with their care givers than those who received standard counselling.

These studies form only a fraction of relevant examples: the range of studies that have used psychological interventions in cancer care, including counselling, has been comprehensively and critically reviewed in a recent paper by Fawzy *et al.*[12] The authors point out that the precise nature of the interventions is unclear, given that the terms 'therapy', 'psychotherapy' and 'counselling' are so often used synonymously. However, it appeared from all the studies reviewed that 'the critical component of these interventions was the support and emotional engagement of the patient, regardless of which term was used'. Based on this review and their own clinical and research experience, the authors agree with the conclusion of Massey *et al.*,[8] that patients with cancer may benefit from a variety of intervention programmes. Interestingly, Fawzy *et al.* have been able to identify which kind of interventions seem to offer the greatest potential benefit to patients at different points in the disease trajectory. For patients who are newly diagnosed and/or have a good prognosis, a short term, structured, psychoeducational group intervention is proposed, to promote illness-related problem-solving skills and encourage active coping and participation in decision-making. For patients with metastatic disease, weekly group support programmes based on those developed by Spiegel *et al.*[13] are proposed, focusing on daily coping, pain management and the existential issues related to death and dying.

The meta-analysis of controlled outcome studies of psychosocial interventions published by Meyer and Mark in 1995[14] lends further weight to the argument that counselling, whether narrowly or broadly defined, should be offered as part of the illness management plan to all patients. More research is needed to ascertain which are the most effective interventions and whether different combinations may produce greater benefits for different kinds of patient.

SELF-HELP

There is abundant research evidence that cancer patients who have good social support, particularly close confiding ties, have lower levels of psychological distress. However, it should not be assumed that patients always receive the support that they need, even from an apparently close family. This quote from a 48-year-old woman with breast cancer makes the point:

> They are very good about helping with practical things, but I can't talk to anyone in the family about my real fears for the future. They just take the line that I've had the operation and the radiotherapy and now everything is back to normal, but *I* don't feel normal.

Another woman in the same study raised a slightly different difficulty:

> I know my husband and daughters are worried, so I think if I talked to them about *my* worries it would make it even worse for them, so I try to keep as cheerful as possible to keep *their* spirits up.

The aim of a study by Peters-Golden[15] was to examine perceived social support in 100 women with breast cancer and anticipated social support in 100 disease-free women. Fifty-six per cent of the healthy women said that they would avoid contact with someone they knew who had cancer. In contrast 72 per cent of the breast cancer patients reported that they were treated differently after people knew that they had cancer: 52 per cent found that they were 'avoided' or 'feared', 14 per cent felt that they were 'pitied'. Only 3 per cent thought that people were 'nicer' to them than previously. One half of the patients found that the support they received was inadequate for their needs, although there is no indication of how many of this group felt that they were avoided. In the face of this kind of evidence, it is easy to understand why some patients find the self-help group a haven.

The very existence of self-help groups has two implications. The first is that they exist to fulfil the needs that the health-care system does not meet (Taylor *et al.*[16]). The second is that they meet needs that the professionals cannot fulfil: in other words, they work because of people's needs to meet with others who have gone through the same experience. This was the view of Dr Vicky Clement-Jones, founder of BACUP, who said 'I realised that other patients could give me something unique which I could not obtain from my doctors and nurses, however caring'.[17] This statement identifies the core difficulty in evaluating the effectiveness of self-help groups. Most active members find questions about their group's effectiveness difficult to comprehend: they know *their* group works, so they have little interest in cooperating with any objective scientific attempt at validation. Those for whom self-help groups do not work either do not join one at all, or drop out very quickly, as demonstrated in the following quote from a woman following surgery for stage I breast cancer:

> I went with an open mind, I really did. But everyone seemed to have had recurrence of their cancer and that was all they talked about. On the second visit, I mentioned that I had a pain in my other breast and one of them turned to me and said 'Ooh, that'll be your recurrence starting up!' I was horrified . . . I never went back.

It is clear then that, by definition, self-help groups work for those who choose to belong.

What do we understand by a self-help group? Stephen Lock, in an interesting editorial on the subject[18] has arrived at a definition: 'A self-help group is a voluntary organisation usually of peers, who have come together for mutual help and support, in satisfying a common need, overcoming a common handicap or life-disrupting problem and bringing about desired social or personal change, or both.' In a wide-ranging study, Levy[19] identified four different types of group based upon purpose and composition. For our purposes, self-help groups belong to type II groups

> composed of members who share a common status or predicament which entails some degree of stress, and the aim of these groups is generally the amelioration of this stress through mutual support and the sharing of coping strategies and advice. There is no attempt to change their status; that is taken as more or less fixed and the problem for these members is how to carry on in spite of it.

Despite the enormous variety in both their purpose and composition, groups seem to share certain features which define and differentiate them from other forms of support. Support groups are set up and sanctioned by the members of the group themselves, rather than by an external agency. They may be initiated by professionals, but are then taken over by the group and are composed of members who share a common experience and its attendant problems. The primary and explicit purpose of the group is to provide help and support for the members in coping with their problems and in improving psychosocial functioning. The members' own effort, knowledge and skills are the primary source of help for the group: professionals who participate do so only at the invitation of the group. The structure of the group and the way in which it functions are under the control of the members though they may seek professional guidance about theoretical/philosophical frameworks.

Levy was interested in identifying the processes that were most prevalent in self-help groups in order to provide the foundation for a general theory of psychological intervention,

> because self-help groups tend to be pragmatically oriented and relatively free of the theoretical dogma to which most professionals are bound, it seems reasonable to assume that the techniques and approaches found to be used by them are likely to be those which have proven their effectiveness in the hands of laymen . . . the study of the activities of these groups holds the promise of leading to improvements in professional practice as well as enhancing the natural support systems that exist in everyday life.[19]

He described various processes that operate within self-help groups that are also found in other forms of psychological intervention and believed that those found to be the most prevalent may provide the foundation for a general theory that he was looking for. These include the exchange of normative and instrumental information and advice and looking for solutions to problems through finding alternative perceptions of circumstances and expanding the range of possible actions that may be taken. In addition, there was support for changes in attitude towards oneself and one's own behaviour. Members of the group provide powerful reinforcement for individuals coming to see themselves as capable of exerting control over their own behaviours and circumstances. Self-help groups were also important for reducing or eliminating a sense of isolation or uniqueness, through the process of comparison. Finally, bearing in mind the introductory comments about stigma, for many members suffering from what Goffman called 'spoiled identities',[20] the groups provide an opportunity to build a new identity and thus a new base from which to face the world. What is interesting about these processes is that they include all the elements of good counselling practice. This is what cancer sufferers want and need and can find from each other, in the absence of counselling provision in their own hospitals.

Levy[19] made two other interesting observations. The first was that membership of most groups cut right across social class. The common purpose or problems faced by members overrode differences in socioeconomic status, education and occupation; moreover interaction appeared easy. Secondly, with the exception of AA, the membership of all the groups observed was exclusively or predominantly female. In terms of cancer itself, the disease is more prevalent among men than among women. It would seem then that men are either less able to admit publicly their need for help and/or they do not see self-help groups as likely to be effective in meeting their needs.

In the UK, the most comprehensive source of information about the activities of self-help groups for cancer patients is the Cancerlink National Survey of Cancer Support and Self-Help Groups (1992).[21] Cancerlink acts as a resource to all independent cancer support and self-help groups which are set up on an autonomous basis: the survey identified 274 groups in 1988 and 350 in 1992, revealing a steady increase over the last decade. Of particular interest in the context of this chapter are two of their key findings. First, 'Groups, particularly the larger ones, are keen to obtain professional support and involvement, but there appears to be very little increase in the amount of professional involvement since our last survey in 1988.' Secondly, 'Despite considerable efforts by groups to encourage professionals working in partnership with them, results have been poor.' The professionals whom groups particularly wanted to involve were hospital doctors, general practitioners, district and Macmillan nurses. This contrasts with a survey of doctors conducted by Lock,[18] which found that 64 per cent of his sixty-four respondents perceived self-help groups as 'useful' or 'very useful' and 59 per cent would advise their patients to go to group meetings.

Although writing as long ago as 1976, Mantell *et al.* [22] were already exploring the areas in which these tensions and contradictions lie between patients and health-care professionals. They found 'a substantial amount of resentment among patients against professionals who derive their knowledge from "books" rather than from living with cancer. This may conceal an arrogance towards supervision that is threatening to the professional.' On the other hand, they also identified resistance from some health care professionals: 'Self-help is seen as a challenge to professionals' expertise and institutional maintenance. . . . Professionalisation of the lay person is perceived by some as threatening to the health professional–patient relationship.' In a later paper[23] Mantell also found claims that professional involvement can lead to dominance and thus weaken the autonomy and identity of members. It is clear that real effort needs to be made in order to break down this mutual antagonism, given the great scope that the self-help movement has to complement the work of the medical profession, including the potential for a more political role as identified by Lock.[18] Jertson[24] suggests that 'the professional should function as a facilitator, stimulating and guiding the group's organisation and perhaps withdrawing once it has achieved an effective and efficient level of operation.' In addition though, groups may need and welcome access to doctors for both information and encouragement. It is not inconceivable that much of the antagonism is purely the result of failure in communication.

SUPPORT FOR MEDICAL STAFF

In a thoughtful chapter, Roger Higgs[25] points out that the skills of self-care start with a paradox. All health professionals should be, or are training to be, experts in how to look after people. As experts they should be able to apply those same ideas to themselves, but manifestly do not: 'few studies have been made of self care for the health professional. But the impression of doctors, nurses and social workers risking their physical, psychological and social health is apparent everywhere.' A particular problem faced by oncologists is that the climate in medical school and in hospital-based training is inimical to self-care. A Canadian psychiatrist, Vincent[26] commented that during their training, doctors develop a great capacity for postponing immediate gratification in favour of long-term gains, an exaggerated commitment to work and a view that overvalues medical technology and undervalues the person's own needs and relationships. Doctors have been conditioned in a system that fosters the production of single-minded workaholics, emotionally highly controlled and with a tremendous capacity for hard work. In addition, Delvaux *et al.*[27] pointed out that it is often argued that oncologists find dealing with death and dying inherently stressful because of the conflict between the curative goals upon which most general training is based and the palliative/supportive goals of cancer care. Maguire[28] felt that the only way that staff poorly trained in communication skills can protect themselves from the stress of caring for cancer patients is by the use of distancing tactics, which as Higgs[25] points out, 'risks at a deeper level a dangerous splitting of our emotional responses'.

Early work on stress was extremely confusing, given that the term was used interchangeably to describe the stimulus, the experience and the response. Kasl and Cooper[29] clarified the issue by offering an understanding based on the concept of stress as an interactional rather than a univariate concept. The stress response is the subjective experience that is felt when the perceived environmental demands (stressors) exceed the individual's perception of their resources to meet those demands. Work in general can be considered as a stressor, without regard to the particular requirements of any one job. There is now a considerable research literature exploring occupational stress, from which Cooper[30] has identified six major categories of work-related stressor. This type of classification can be very helpful for anyone who is trying to disentangle the threads that make up their professional existence. The six categories of work-related stressor are as follows:

1. Factors intrinsic to the job (such as physical working conditions, shift work, work over/underload and job satisfaction).
2. Role in the organization (including role ambiguity and role conflict and conflicts stemming from organizational boundaries).
3. Career development (including under/overpromotion, lack of security and thwarted ambition).
4. Relationships at work (including the nature of relationships and social support from colleagues, boss and subordinates).
5. Organizational structure and climate (including job politics, lack of effective consultation and lack of participation in the decision-making process).
6. Work pressures on the family (including conflict between organization and family demands, conflicts between husband's and wife's careers, insufficient leisure/vacation time).

It should not be assumed that all stress is necessarily detrimental. It was Murray Parkes[31] who said 'Crisis can lead to the stars as well as to the grave'. Substituting stress for crisis, there are many people who apparently thrive in situations that for others will lead only to a harmful outcome, both for themselves and those around them. In an excellent paper, Cull[32] points out that stress is a function not only of the characteristics of the work setting and the challenge of the work, but the attributes of the individuals concerned. The notion of 'personality hardiness' has been identified by Kobasa and Kash[33] as an individual source of stress-resistance. Three characteristics – commitment, control and challenge – have been demonstrated as significant stress-resistance resources.

> The combination of a sense of commitment to self and the various areas of one's life, an attitude that one has influence over what occurs and a sense of challenge in the face of a changing environment has proven to interact with stressful life events in such a way as to lower mental and physical illness scores.[33]

High scores on a hardiness scale are thought to prevent excessive arousal in an individual. Studies of nurses have demonstrated a negative correlation between hardiness score and the chronic stress leading to burnout. The authors are currently conducting a similar study with oncologists.

Roberts,[34] in exploring the value of the concept of burnout refers to the original work by Freudenberger[35] who described a syndrome of exhaustion, disillusionment and withdrawal. He concludes that it is merely a new name for an old problem, but provides a useful guide to burnout signs and symptoms:

- Emotional changes include loss of humour, a persistent sense of failure, guilt and blame and frequent anger, resentment and bitterness.
- Among behavioural changes is found clock-watching, increasing resistance to going to work, postponing patient contact and increasing social isolation.
- Physical symptoms include tiredness, sleep disorders, frequent minor ailments and absenteeism and accident proneness.
- Finally, cognitive symptoms include increasing thoughts of leaving the job, an inability to concentrate, rigid thinking, increasing distrust and patient stereotyping.

In a sympathetic paper, Mount[36] considers the effects of chronic stress in oncologists and gives an expanded version of aids to diagnosing burnout. Either paper is well worth reading for anyone who suspects that they may be vulnerable to this condition. The first step in dealing effectively with burnout is an awareness of the problem developing.

Until recently the extent of burnout in clinical oncology had never been quantitatively assessed. However, a study by Whippen and Canellos[37] aimed to redress the balance by sending a questionnaire to 1000 randomly chosen subscribers of the *Journal of Clinical Oncology*. There was a 60 per cent response rate with 85 per cent of the responses received in the first 2 weeks. Nearly all the respondents spent a median of 70–79 per cent of their time devoted to patient care and 60 per cent described themselves as medical oncologists, 14 per cent were unspecified with the rest divided between radiology, paediatrics, surgery and gynaecology. Of the 598 respondents, 56 per cent felt some degree of burnout in their professional lives, with no significant association between speciality and burnout. The greater the amount of time spent in direct patient care, the higher the incidence of burnout. This replicates the finding of Bates and Moore[38] that the greatest stress amongst health professionals is experienced by those involved directly in patient care with a high level of responsibility.

Insufficient personal and/or vacation time was the most frequently chosen reason by 57 per cent to explain the existence of burnout. However, 53 per cent felt that continuous exposure to fatal illness was a factor and 56 per cent felt frustration and a sense of failure. The quantity of time devoted to symptomatic or palliative care rather than active therapy, particularly for medical oncologists, was perceived as excessive, as most respondents felt that time spent away from patients was desirable. In their discussion, the authors felt it difficult to escape the conclusion that many practitioners felt they were working too hard in a frustrating type of practice that may not have met the expectations on which they based their choice of oncology as their specialism. Paradoxically though, the great majority felt that their career *had* met their expectations from training. 'In the best light burnout can be seen not as a condemnation of the professional activity per se, but rather a reflection of the total quantity of the emotional stresses of practice, which dominate the majority of professional time in the practice of oncology.'

A similar survey has been conducted by Ramirez *et al.*[39] among all non-surgical oncologists in the United Kingdom, with a response rate of 83 per cent. Levels of burnout were broadly comparable with those of the normative data from the American study. Within the study group, clinical oncologists described significantly higher levels of work-related distress than medical oncologists or palliative care specialists. The factors that emerged most strongly as determinants of burnout were (1) perceived work overload, (2) dealing with patient suffering, and (3) being single. Of particular interest was the finding that 44 per cent of the doctors considered themselves inadequately trained in communication and 80 per cent felt that they had received insufficient training in management skills. There was a strong association between those who felt they were inadequately trained in these respects with the stressors of work overload and dealing with patient suffering. In other words, overload *was* an issue, but so was inadequate training in communication skills. Putting resources into reducing workload will not make the problem go away if there is not a parallel commitment to proper communication and management skills training for doctors.

Several authors mentioned in this chapter have suggested ways of combatting chronic stress and burnout for oncologists: the most comprehensive come from Mount.[36] He discusses at some length the following strategies:

- The encouragement of increased awareness of stress in self and colleagues.
- The clarification of appropriate goals and priorities.
- Encouragement of appropriate limit setting, including ways of ensuring personal space, both at and from work.
- The mobilization of collaborative input.
- The clarification of team roles and organizational patterns.
- The establishment of team support meetings and favourable working conditions.
- Exercise.
- The clarification and working through of previously unresolved psychodynamic issues.

Adopting even a few of these strategies can radically alter how stressors are perceived and responded to.

CONCLUSION

The theme of this chapter has been the provision of support for cancer patients and those who care for and about them. It seems to the author that the common factor emerging from the different sections is communication – between patients and doctors, patients and counsellors, patients and other patients and between doctors and their colleagues. It is likely that the most effective means of helping patients is to provide proper training in communication skills for *all* members of the health-care team. This will enable them to elicit and ameliorate distress, not only from those for whom they are caring, but from those with whom they work. Good communication can transform the experience of the disease for both patient and professional.

REFERENCES

1. Rosser JE, Maguire R. Dilemmas in general practice: The care of the cancer patient. *Social Science and Medicine* 1982; **16**: 323–31.
2. Knopf A. Changes in women's opinions about cancer. *Social Science and Medicine* 1976; **10**: 191–5.
3. Watson M ed. *Cancer patient care: psychosocial treatment methods.* Cambridge: BPS Books and Cambridge University Press, 1991.
4. Slevin ML, Nichols SE, Downer SM, Wilson P, Lister TA, Arnott S, Maher J, Souhami RL, Tobias JS, Goldstone AH, Lody M. Emotional support for cancer patients: what do patients really want? *British Journal of Cancer* 1996; **74**: 1275–79.
5. Marcus AC, Cella D, Sedlacek S, David Crawford E, Crane LA, Garrett K, Quigel C, Gonin R. Psychosocial counselling of cancer patients by telephone: a brief note on patient acceptance of an outcall strategy. *Psycho-Oncology* 1993; **2**: 209–14.
6. Fallowfield LJ, Roberts R. Cancer counselling in the United Kingdom, *Psychology and Health* 1992; **6**: 107–17.
7. Watson M. Psychosocial intervention with cancer patients: A review. *Psychological Medicine* 1983; **13**: 839–46.
8. Massey MJ, Holland JC, Straker N. Psychotherapeutic interventions. In: Holland JC, Rowland JH eds. *Handbook of psychooncology: psychological care of the patient with cancer.* Oxford: Oxford University Press, 1989: 455–69.
9. Capone MA, Good RS, Westie S, Jacobsen AF. Psychosocial rehabilitation in gynaecologic oncology patients. *Archives of Physical Medicine and Rehabilitation* 1980; **61**: 128–32.
10. Linn MW, Linn BS, Harris R. Effects of counselling for late-stage cancer patients. *Cancer* 1982; **49**: 1048–55.
11. Cain En, Kohorn EI, Quinlan DM, Latimer K, Schwartz PE. Psychosocial benefits of a cancer support group. *Cancer* 1986; **57**: 183–9.
12. Fawzy IF, Fawzy NW, Arndt LA, Pasnau RO. Critical review of psychosocial interventions in cancer care. *Archives of General Psychiatry* 1995; **52**: 100–13.
13. Spiegel D, Bloom JR, Kraemer HC, Gottheil E. Effect of psychosocial treatment on survival of patients with metastatic breast cancer. *Lancet* 1989; **ii**: 888–91.
14. Meyer TJ, Mark MM. Effects of psychosocial interventions with adult cancer patients: a meta-analysis of randomized experiments. *Health Psychology* 1995; **14**: 101–8.
15. Peters-Golden H. Choice or chance: Further evidence on illness and responsibility for health. *Social Science and Medicine* 1985; **20**(10): 483–91.
16. Taylor SE, Falke RL, Shoptaw SJ, Lichtman RR. Social support, support groups and the cancer patient. *Journal of Consulting Clinical Psychology* 1986; **54**: 608–15.
17. Clement-Jones V. Cancer and beyond: the formation of BACUP. *British Medical Journal* 1985; **291**: 1021–3.

18. Lock S. Self-help groups – the fourth estate in medicine? *British Medical Journal* 1986; **293**: 1596–600.
19. Levy LH. Self-help groups: types and psychological processes. *Journal of Applied Behavioural Science* 1976; **12**: 310–22.
20. Goffman E. *Stigma: notes on the management of spoiled identity.* Englewood Cliffs, NJ: Prentice Hall, 1963.
21. CancerLink. *Celebrating groups: the results of a national survey of cancer support and self-help groups.* London: CancerLink, 1992.
22. Mantell JE, Alexander ES, Kleiman MA. Social work and self-help groups. *Health and Social Work* 1976; **1**: 86–100.
23. Mantell JE. Cancer patient visitor programs: a case for accountability. *Journal of Psychosocial Oncology* 1983; **1**(1): 45–58.
24. Jertson JM. Self-help groups. *Social Work* 1975; **20**: 144–5.
25. Higgs R. Looking after yourself. In: Corney R ed. *Developing communication and counselling skills in medicine.* London: Tavistock/Routledge, 1991: 137–45.
26. Vincent MO. The sequelae of stress. *Canadian Medical Association Meeting*, Sasha-town, Saskatchewan, 1982.
27. Delvaux N, Razavi D, Farvacques C. Cancer care – a stress for health professionals. *Social Science and Medicine* 1988; **27**(2): 159–66.
28. Maguire P. Barriers to psychological care of the dying. *British Medical Journal* 1985; **29**: 1711–13.
29. Kasl SV, Cooper CL *Stress and health: issues in research methodology.* Chichester: John Wiley & Sons, 1987.
30. Cooper CL. Identifying stressors at work: recent research developments. *Journal of Psychosomatic Research* 1983; **2**: 369–76.
31. Murray Parkes C. Psychosocial transitions: a field for study. *Social Science and Medicine* 1971; **5**: 101–15.
32. Cull A. Studying stress in caregivers: art or science? *British Journal of Cancer* 1991; **64**: 981–4.
33. Kobasa SCO, Kash KM. Stress in oncology staff: measurement and management. In: Holland J, Massie M, Lesho L eds. *Current concepts in psychooncology and AIDS.* New York: Memorial Sloan-Kettering Cancer Centre, 1987: 137–43.
34. Roberts GA. Burnout: psychobabble or valuable concept? *British Journal of Hospital Medicine* September 1986: 194–7.
35. Freudenberger HJ. Staff burnout. *Journal of Social Issues* 1974; **30**: 159–65.
36. Mount B. Dealing with our losses. *Journal of Clinical Oncology* 1986; **4**(7): 1127–34.
37. Whippen DA, Canellos GP. Burnout syndrome in the practice of oncology: results of a random survey of 1000 oncologists. *Journal of Clinical Oncology* 1991; **9**(10): 1916–20.
38. Bates FM,. Moore BN. Stress in hospital personnel. *Medical Journal of Australia* 1975; **15**: 765–9.
39. Ramirez AJ, Graham J, Richards MA *et al.* Work-related distress among senior oncologists and palliative care specialists. *British Journal of Cancer* 1995; **71**: 1263–69.

CHAPTER TEN

Supportive therapy of elderly cancer patients

MARCELLO DE CICCO AND UMBERTO TIRELLI

INTRODUCTION

Recent years have been distinguished by remarkable successes in the treatment of some malignant tumors. Acute leukemias, lymphomas and testicular cancers are now curable even in their advanced stages with the use of aggressive combination chemotherapy alone or in association with radiation therapy. Unfortunately, however, the improved efficacy of antitumor treatments is often associated with a higher frequency of undesirable side-effects for the patient.

Only recently have the problems of the quality of life and the precise role of supportive care of the oncological patient been brought to the fore and addressed. Prevention and control of nausea, vomiting, diarrhea, infections, hyperthermia, deterioration in nutritional status and control of pain are certainly very important aspects of supportive care. However, an optimal supportive care program must also include evaluation of psychosocial aspects; that is, the prevention and control of all clinical symptoms, both physical and psychological, from the initial diagnosis, through treatment to the terminal phase of the illness. It is therefore clear that supportive care of oncological patients is a complex problem that requires a multidisciplinary approach involving physicians, nurses, psychologists, volunteers and family members.

In this chapter, we will concentrate on just two aspects of supportive care: control of pain and nutritional problems in oncological patients, with specific reference to elderly patients.

GENERAL CONCEPTS REGARDING ELDERLY PATIENTS

Physiological aspects

The elderly patient normally requires supportive care due to the physiological decline of different organs and apparatus linked to the aging process *per se*.[1] Instead, the elderly patient with cancer always needs supportive care for the effects of the tumor itself or for the antineoplastic therapies employed.

In the past, the elderly patient was rarely exposed to aggressive antitumor treatments owing to the widely held belief that, in contrast to the younger adult, the elderly patient could not tolerate the multiorgan and multisystem injury caused by such therapies.

Today, elderly patients constitute a significant fraction of the oncological population and with the refinement of diagnostic techniques and antitumor treatments, many of them are treated with more aggressive therapies. Therefore, it is important that we understand the physiological changes caused by aging and the impact that these may have on response of antitumor treatments if we are to deliver optimal supportive care to the elderly oncological patient. These changes are characterized by a large individual variability and may be influenced by nutritional status, lifestyle and presence or absence of chronic illness. Modifications of body composition include a global reduction of thin corporeal mass (muscles), total corporeal water, seroalbumin and a relative increase of body fat mass.[2] These changes, associated with progressive decrease in cardiac index, compromised plasma blood flow, glomerular filtration rate and hepatic blood flow, with pharmacokinetic implications.[3,4]

The hardening and the rigidity of many tissues contribute to the reduction of the regional blood flow caused by the increase in peripheral resistance.[5] Other parameters which cause a decline in elderly patients are pulmonary vital capacity and global respiratory function, hematopoietic reserve and the quota of bone calcium.[3,6] The skin experiences significant structural changes, with a decrease of subcutaneous fat and thinning of the epidermis and dermis with loss of elasticity, consequently reducing its efficacy as a protective barrier against exogenous agents.[7]

Until recently, this general decline in the functions of the main vital organs of the elderly patient presupposed a reduction in the therapeutic standards of antitumor treatments. Similarly, many drugs administered to elderly patients for non-malignant pathologies have a lower therapeutic value[8] and often major surgery is considered risky.[9] Therefore, the real impact of physiological changes in the elderly on the response of antitumor treatments is not easily determined.

Chemotherapy in the elderly

From data reported in the literature about the use of chemotherapy, it is not clear whether response and toxicity are different in the elderly compared to the younger patient.[10–12] Nevertheless, we must consider that, even if the data produced by these studies are interesting, their clinical utility is questionable as the subjects selected for a chemotherapeutic treatment are those with the best performance status, and therefore are different from the general elderly population with cancer. Moreover, it is possible that many researchers, as well as many publishers, hesitate to publish unfavorable results of uncontrolled trials.

It is evident that chemotherapeutic agents activated in the liver will be less therapeutically effective in the presence of a reduced liver function. In the same way, drugs excreted by the kidney will cause greater toxicity with the decline of the renal function. Cardiotoxic drugs may worsen a pre-existent myocardiopathy, causing a secondary reduction in a hepatorenal perfusion. Therefore, the hematological, gastrointestinal, hepatic, renal, central and peripheral nervous system and cutaneous (vesicant agents) toxicities of chemotherapy can be greatly accentuated in elderly cancer patients with decreased, even partial, function of major vital organs. The results of chemotherapy treatment can be optimized by a complete and individual evaluation of important physiological parameters, their correction in the case of pathological alterations, the selection of chemotherapy regimens more appropriate to the type of tumor and to the clinical condition of the patient, and finally adequate, consistent supportive care.

Radiotherapy in the elderly

For many cancers in elderly patients, radiotherapy is widely used with curative as well as palliative aims. Even if the sophisticated techniques utilized in the administration of radiotherapy permit a greater therapeutic benefit, important physical and sometimes psychological problems are caused by its use, particularly in elderly patients. Cutaneous and mucosal damage subsequent to radiotherapy involves a high risk of infection as a result of alteration in the function of the protective barrier of these tissues. This is prolonged in the elderly patient due to the lesser capacity to repair the tissue damage.[13]

The frequent anatomical and functional alterations of the digestive mucosae following radiotherapy can create major nutritional disturbance by producing or increasing, if pre-existing, protein–calorific malnutrition.[14]

The elderly patient treated with wide-field radiotherapy is not able to adequately recover from the hematological toxicity (myelodepression) secondary to the radiotherapy *per se* or secondary to a compromised bone marrow cellularity from previous or concomitant chemotherapy.[3] Prolonged anemia, neutropenia and thrombocytopenia provoke intense fatigue and a high risk of infection and hemorrhage. The toxicities of radiotherapy have an unfavorable impact on the psychological status of the patient. Supportive and emotional care to prevent or control the undesirable effects of radiotherapy are important to reduce morbidity and mortality and to improve the quality of life of elderly cancer patients.

Surgery in the elderly

Surgery represents the best, and often the only possible treatment for many solid tumors in elderly cancer patients. In radical cancer surgery, the reduction in function of vital organs caused by aging and the inability to tolerate post-operative stress due to an important pre-existent single or multiorgan weakness must always be borne in mind.

During surgery, cutaneous integrity is interrupted with an increase in risk of infection, many lymphatic and blood vessels are incised promoting further peripheral and regional circulatory deficits of vital organs and stasis that can lead to hypovolaemia and facilitate infectious processes.

However, the major stress of surgery concerns the cardiopulmonary apparatus. The risk of respiratory complications is especially high in elderly patients with chronic obstructive airways disease and reduced ventilatory capacity. Reduced renal function can cause difficulties in the maintenance of the delicate hydroelectrolytical balance with disastrous consequences on cardiorespiratory activity.

Post-operative hypoalimentation following digestive tract surgery can worsen pre-existent malnutrition in the elderly cancer patients, thus causing prolonged

Table 10.1 Basic concepts to consider in surgical patients with cancer

Pre-operating evaluation of vital organs function
Restabilizing of underlying physiological abnormalities
Active pulmonary toilette
Choice of the most appropriate surgical technique
Peri-operating maintenance of a correct hydroelectrolytical balance
Prevention, prompt identification and correction of post-operating complications
Adequate analgesic and nutritional support
Early mobilization
Recourse to family and friends for psychological support

delay in the processes of tissue repair which already have been compromised by the relative deficit of the loco-regional blood circulation.[14]

Post-operative pain is a cause of hemodynamic and metabolic stress,[15,16] prevents adequate pulmonary ventilation and expectoration[17] and delays mobilization of the patient. Immobility secondary to pain and weakness in operated or non-operated elderly patients predisposes to decubitus ulcers and to venous stasis, with risk of venous thrombosis and pulmonary embolism. Therefore, post-operative elderly patients are at a higher risk of developing respiratory complications, thrombophlebitis, thromboembolism, renal insufficiency, hydroelectrolytical disturbances, urinary tract infections and delirium (confusional states).

Table 10.1 summarizes some of the precautionary measures necessary when an elderly cancer patient must undergo surgery.

In conclusion, the physiological modifications of aging, their impact on the response to antitumor therapies whether chemotherapy, radiotherapy or surgery, and their alteration of protective mechanisms indicate and stress the need for intensive programs of medical and paramedical supportive care.

TREATMENT OF CANCER PAIN IN ELDERLY PATIENTS

General concepts

According to the data of Bonica,[18] 7 200 000 new cases of tumor are registered annually in the world, with an estimated prevalence of 15 000 000 cases. Pain is one of the most unpleasant symptoms that characterize the course of a neoplastic disease and is of prime importance in its incidence and clinical relevance.

If all stages of the disease are considered, 50 per cent of cancer patients feel pain, whereas in the advanced and terminal stages, this percentage increases to 75 per cent.[18]

In cancer patients, pain, especially chronic, has a specific destructive character because it is associated with the prospect of a short life expectancy, the irreversibility of the disease, and the inability of the physicians to cure the illness. It is very difficult for the patient to overcome the fears and anxieties associated with a diagnosis of cancer. If this difficulty is associated with cancer pain, it is not surprising that the patient develops psychological decompensations, that can contribute to the origin and maintenance of organic pain.[19]

In an elderly patient, all the physical and psychological factors related to cancer pain are exaggerated.[20] The idea that sensitivity to pain, as well as the sensitivity of the sensory organs, reduces with age, has not been substantiated by a series of experimental researches on the subject.[21,22] Instead, it has been confirmed that the percentage of 'pre-existent pain' increases with age.[22]

An elderly patient with chronic pain shows emotional instability and neurosis in a significantly higher percentage when compared to patients of the same age without pain.[23] A study of terminal elderly patients has demonstrated that pain had greater negative impact on psychological well-being than any other of the factors evaluated.[24] Moreover, poverty, low social status, and solitude foster a psychological response that increases the pain experienced by the elderly patient. Psychological support that improves the capacity of the patient to overcome the fear of pain, sometimes the predominant aspect of the illness, must be part of the medical treatment of pain. Furthermore, the medical and paramedical staff that help cancer patients must have a clear idea of pain, its etiology, its pathogenesis and its treatment.

An understanding of the etiology of pain is essential in order to plan its treatment. Pain, in cancer patients, is correlated with tumor, antitumor therapies, neoplastic cachexia and, especially in the elderly, with non-cancerous organic diseases.

Table 10.2 outlines specific pain syndromes in cancer patients. Pain is the direct result of tumor, antitumor therapies and other morbid conditions in 78 per cent, 19 per cent and 3 per cent respectively of cancer inpatients.[25]

Types of pain

Most cancer patients with pain present with two or more etiologies and/or types of pain.[25,26] In elderly cancer patients, the amount of pain correlated with chronic diseases secondary to aging accounts for the etiological multiplicity of pain. Therefore, pain can be classified according to its pathogenetic mechanisms which also helps in selecting the most appropriate treatment. Three types of pain can be distinguished: nociceptor pain, neuropathic pain and dysregulatory or reactive pain.[27]

Nociceptor pain is due to the stimulation of specific nociceptive nerve endings, whose neural sensor promptly indicates potential damage or the presence of disease. Pain due to bone metastasis, or hyperdistension of encapsulated organs (e.g. the liver) are typical examples of this kind of pain. Prostaglandins, bradykinin or H^+ ions are the most frequent pain mediators liberated at the site of neoplastic disease, with the function of exciting and sensitizing nociceptors.[28] Analgesic drugs of the peripheral and anti-inflammatory type have their major site of action at this level, interfering with the biochemistry of pain mediators and the neural excitation of nociceptors.

Neuropathic pain derives from damage to sensitive nerve fibres that discharge in an abnormal way causing pain.[29] The afferent excitation originates from sites nearer to the nerve than to the nociceptor which therefore is bypassed by the stimulus. Damage to nerve fibres can be caused by a direct and prolonged nerve compression due to tumor, surgical sectioning of the nerve or interference in the nerve biochemistry by chemotherapy or radiotherapy.

Local or generalized neuropathic pain due to any of the above situations is

Table 10.2   Pain syndromes in patients with cancer

Pain syndromes due to tumor infiltration/compression
Tumor infiltration of abdominal organs
  Distension of encapsulated organs (e.g. the liver, the kidney)
  Distension of hollow organs (e.g. the GI tract)
  Tumor-induced necrosis in solid organs (e.g. the pancreas)
  Tumor infiltration and inflammation of serous mucosae

Tumor infiltration of soft tissues
Tumor-induced occlusions of blood vessels
Tumor-induced occlusions of lymphatics

Tumor infiltration of bone
  Base of skull syndromes (e.g. clivus metastases)
  Vertebral body syndromes (e.g. C_2, C_7-T_1, metastases)
  Sacral syndrome

Tumor infiltration of nerve
  Peripheral nerve (e.g. peripheral neuropathy)
  Plexus (e.g. brachial or lumbar plexopathy)
  Spinal root
  Spinal cord
  Compression of central nervous system
  Epidural spinal cord compression
  Intracranial pressure

Pain syndromes due to cancer therapy
Post-surgery syndromes
  Post-thoractomy syndrome
  Post-mastectomy syndrome
  Post-radical neck syndrome
  Phantom limb syndrome

Post-chemotherapy syndromes
  Peripheral neuropathy
  Steroid pseudorheumatism
  Aseptic necrosis of bone (e.g. femoral head)
  Post-herpetic neuralgia

Post-irradiation syndromes
  Radiation fibrosis of brachial and lumbar plexus
  Radiation myelopathy
  Radiation-induced second primary tumors
  Radiation necrosis of bone

Pain syndromes due to neoplastic cachexia
  Paraneoplastic syndromes
  Myofascial syndrome

Pain syndromes not due to cancer or to cancer therapy
  Cervical and lumbar osteoarthritis
  Osteoporosis
  Headache
  Diabetic neuropathy
  Thoracic and abdominal aneurysms

Data modified from Foley.[25]

usually not very responsive to anti-inflammatory analgesics and opioid drugs.[30] Other drugs that interfere with an abnormal nerve excitability, such as the tricyclic antidepressives and anticonvulsants, are more helpful in relieving neuropathic pain.

Dysregulatory pain includes various types of chronic pain secondary to inappropriate (efferent) nerve control in the skeletomotor system (e.g. muscle spasm) or in the sympathetic system (e.g. reflex sympathetic dystrophy). Painful syndromes caused by abnormal mechanisms of control can be globally defined as 'paraneoplastic painful syndromes'. Somatic or sympathetic nerve blocks, by means of local anesthetics, with or without associated peripheral and central analgesic medication, are indicated in these cases in order to interfere with the dysregulatory control signals.

Thus, a systematic etiologic and pathogenetic evaluation of pain leads to a more rational approach to its treatment in the cancer patient.

Methods of treatment of pain

Before starting any pain treatment, it is necessary to fully inform the patient and their family about the diagnosis, prognosis and therapeutic strategy. This kind of approach reduces anxiety, insecurity and the isolation of the patient and promotes a situation of mutual cooperation and trust in alleviating the pain. Another major point to stress in the treatment of cancer pain is the need for collaboration between the family doctor, the oncologist and the specialist for the diagnosis and the treatment of pain.

For simplicity, the strategies for the treatment of cancer pain can be divided into three groups: [31]

- *Group I*: palliative surgery, radiotherapy, chemotherapy and hormone therapy to remove or reduce the tumor mass that is responsible for the pain.
- *Group II*: therapy with analgesic drugs, psychotherapy, physiotherapy and neurostimulation techniques.
- *Group III*: invasive procedures such as spinal analgesia with opiates, temporary local analgesia with local anesthetics, long-lasting local analgesia with neurolytic agents and radiofrequency, neurosurgical procedures.

The best therapeutic strategy should aim at a rapid reduction in pain and then its continuous control. The choice of treatment depends fundamentally on the etiopathogenesis of the pain and the selection of less traumatic techniques which, for prolonged treatments, are easily manageable for the patient.

Group I therapy

Cancer pain should be treated, first of all, with antitumor procedures and, if necessary, with analgesic therapy for the rapid control of the pain. Radiotherapy for the bone metastasis, chemotherapy in certain haematological and lymphatic neoplasms,[32] surgery for marrow compression, intestinal obstruction and pathological fractures, and hormone therapy in the breast and prostate neoplasms[33] can play a major role in the control of neoplastic pain even for prolonged periods. Nevertheless, in the elderly patient, palliative antitumor treatment

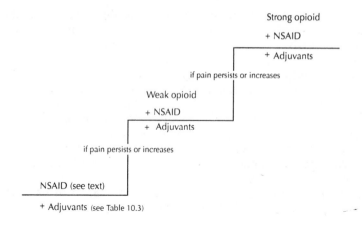

Fig. 10.1.   WHO's analgesic ladder for relief of cancer pain.

with analgesic intent should be considered after careful evaluation of the possible undesirable effects of the therapies.

Group II therapy

The administration of analgesic drugs is the most convenient and common method of treatment when specific antitumor therapy is no longer efficacious or advisable. The guidelines for the pharmacological treatment of pain are those developed by the 1986 WHO Conference in Geneva,[34] which are based on a scale with three levels. Each level specifies the most suitable analgesic and adjuvant drugs for the intensity of pain referred by the patient (Fig. 10.1).

Analgesics should be administered to the patient orally, at regular intervals according to the duration of action of the drug, and at personalized doses. Every pain therapy program should start off with drugs of the first level, that is, analgesics with peripheral effect decreasing neural pain signals (nociceptor pain) such as the non-steroid anti-inflammatory (NSAID) and antipyretic drugs. These agents are particularly useful in bone pain secondary to bone metastasis. In this category, acetylsalicylic acid and paracetamol are the drugs of first choice according to the WHO. Nevertheless, other NSAIDs such as the propionic acid derivatives (ibuprofen, flurbiprofen, naproxen), indomethacin, tolmenthin, piroxicam, diclofenac and ketoralac are often preferred and initially used in many countries. Slow-release preparations of NSAIDs allow the interval of drug administration to be prolonged, which is often preferred by patients.

Elderly patients are more subject to the toxic effects of these analgesics due to the low levels of serum albumin which bind NSAID and due to adverse pharmacological interactions with concomitant antihypertensives, antibiotics, anticoagulants and other drugs. Serious adverse effects of NSAIDs reported in the elderly have included liver failure, GI dysfunction, phototoxicity, headache, confusion, sodium and fluid retention.[35] Paracetamol is particularly hepatotoxic, especially in the presence of a pre-existing hepatopathy. Therefore, prior to the administration of NSAIDs to elderly patients, the pharmacokinetics of the chosen drug and the general fitness of the patient must be carefully considered.

Drugs of the second level of the WHO scale, consisting of a combination of NSAIDs with weak opioid drugs such as codeine, dextropropoxyphene and tramadol are indicated when NSAIDs alone do not produce sufficient analgesia or this is obtained with major toxic effects. The peripheral analgesic effect of NSAIDs and the central effect of opioid drugs mutually potentiate each other, thereby producing a higher level of analgesia. The drug of first choice is codeine, with dextropropoxyphene and tramadol as good alternatives for patients particularly sensitive to the emetic effect of codeine. However, dextropropoxyphene at high doses can produce hallucinations and mental confusion.

Drugs at the third level on the pharmacological scale become necessary when the second level drugs do not adequately control the pain at their maximum tolerable dose. Morphine[36,37] administered orally (maintaining patient independence), and as a slow-release tablet every 12 hours (avoiding night administration), is the drug of choice to obtain a satisfactory and prolonged control of pain. By carefully monitoring the degree and the duration of the analgesic effect of the administered morphine dosage in the first few days, it is possible to determine rapidly, with daily increases, the optimal dose and schedule of the drug with the least side-effects.

The most common undesirable effects of morphine are constipation, nausea, vomiting and somnolence. Treatment of constipation includes a colonic stimulant in conjunction with a fecal softener and rectal measures (suppositories and enemas).[38] The best drug, if tolerated, to control nausea and vomiting is haloperidol. If vomiting is due to delayed gastric emptying, gastrokinetic antiemetics such as metoclopramide or domperidone are preferable. Somnolence in most patients is an initial side-effect that disappears after several days without varying the dose of the drug. Occasionally, the analgesic effect can be potentiated by the addition of an NSAID. Respiratory depression does not represent a problem when morphine is taken orally at regular intervals and doses to control pain.[39]

The elderly patient is quite sensitive to opioid drugs.[40] Plasma clearance of morphine is reduced by 50 per cent in the elderly compared to a younger patient.[40] The pharmacokinetics of the opioid can be further altered in the elderly cancer patient by concomitant malnutrition and/or liver dysfunction and/or nephropathy. In view of the hepatic metabolism and renal secretion of opioid drugs and their metabolites, a deficit of renal and hepatic functions indicates the need for extreme caution in deciding on drug dosage. Often, hypotension occurs in hypovolemic elderly patients with cardiovascular insufficiency.[41] Moreover, opioid drugs can aggravate pre-existing cognitive dysfunctions and worsen chronic constipation, leading to fecal impaction, colonic dilatation, and obstruction.[41] Methadone is an efficacious analgesic drug similar in effect to morphine, but due to its slow elimination and long plasma half-life, the risk of overdose is high. Therefore, its use is contraindicated in elderly patients.

Other opioid drugs such as pethidine, pentazocine, hydromorphone and levorphanol do not offer advantages compared to morphine, which remains the most important drug in the control of neoplastic pain. Buprenorphine is a strong agonist–antagonist opioid drug indicated for patients with swallowing problems. It is produced as a sublingual tablet, but its usage for chronic pain is limited by a ceiling effect. It must never be administered after an agonist opioid drug as it could cause a pain relapse. Elderly patients do not tolerate buprenorphine well; it frequently provokes hallucinations, sweating and tachycardia.

Phenomena of drug tolerance or physical and psychological dependence are not relevant in cancer patients receiving opioid drugs orally to control pain.[42,43]

Neuropathic pain may require adjuvant medication in addition to the three levels of analgesic treatment.[43–45] Table 10.3 lists adjuvant medication for cancer pain according to the WHO analgesic ladder, as modified by Zimmerman et al.[28] Neuropathic pain secondary to polyneuropathy induced by chemotherapy, plexopathy or post-herpetic neuralgia may respond well to antidepressant drugs such as imipramine or amitriptyline. In elderly patients, amitriptyline is too toxic, but dothiepin is a useful alternative.

Combined therapy of opioid and antidepressant drugs is associated with an increased risk of anticholinergic effects in the elderly patient. In excruciating neuropathic pain, anticonvulsant drugs (carbamazepine) are indicated.[46]

When pain is due to nerve or spinal cord compression, corticosteroids, via their anti-inflammatory effect and by reducing the tumor mass, are often helpful in reducing the pain.[47]

Calcitonin and diphosphonates can produce satisfactory pain relief for patients with osteolysis caused by bone metastasis.

In elderly cancer patients with different kinds of pain, adjuvant drugs, chosen according to the pathogenesis of the pain, can be used, with individual dosage, in association with analgesics according to the WHO three-step ladder. Using the WHO recommendations, it is possible to obtain satisfactory pain relief in most patients with cancer pain.[48]

When it is not feasible to administer analgesics orally due to repeated vomiting, dysphagia and subacute intestinal obstruction, alternative methods for drug

Table 10.3   Adjuvant medication for cancer pain according to the WHO analgesic ladder

Adjuvant drugs	Symptoms	Examples
Antidepressants	Neuropathic pain Depression	Impramine Amtriptyline Doxepine
Anticonvulsants	Shooting or excruciating neuropathic pain	Carbamazepine Clonazepan
Corticosteroids	Nerve compression Intracranial pressure	Dexamethasone Prednisolone
Calcitonin Biphosphonates	Bone pain	
Myotonolytics	Spasm of skeletal muscle	Baclofen Tizanidine
Neuroleptics	Agitation Emesis	Chlorpromazine Haloperidol Levomepromazine
Laxatives	Constipation	

delivery are subcutaneous administration by means of a pump[49,50] or mechanical implanted devices for continuous intravenous or subcutaneous drug infusion.[51] More recently a transdermal patch containing fentanyl, a potent opioid analgesic, has been developed. This provides continuous controlled systemic delivery of fentanyl through intact skin over 72 hours. With its avoidance of the oral route and ability to space out doses every 3 days, this kind of therapy may have other benefits in terms of convenience and reduced disturbance of family carers' routines. However, the amount of fentanyl systemically available may be greater in elderly patients, compared to young adults, by up to 20 per cent, due to prolonged half-life and reduced clearance. Elderly patients should be observed carefully for signs of fentanyl toxicity, and the dose reduced if necessary.

Group III therapy

Analgesic therapy can be effectively administered via the spinal route through a peridural or subarachnoid catheter when oral or parenteral administration of opioid drugs produces insufficient analgesia or excessive side-effects.[52] Theoretically, the presence of opioid receptors was demonstrated in the gelatinous substance of the spinal dorsal horn.[53] Two or three daily intrathecal or epidural injections of microdoses of opioids will produce prolonged and excellent analgesia and typical side-effects of oral or parenteral morphine are seen less frequently. However, in elderly patients, urinary retention is common with this form of therapy and often requires bladder catheterization.

Intracerebroventricular injection of opioid drugs is also advocated.[54] Because of its invasive nature, this method, although efficacious, even with small doses of opioids, must be reserved for those cases in which the spinal route did not result in sufficient analgesia. In patients with a relatively long life expectancy, opioid drugs can be administered in the subarachnoid or intraventricular spaces via a totally subcutaneously implanted infusion pump.[55] These systems minimize the necessity for continued assistance and cooperation of patients when home-care treatment is feasible.

Nerve blocks constitute, in selected cases, a useful and necessary treatment to control neoplastic pain. Substances employed are principally local anesthetics and neurolytic agents, whereas corticosteroids and α-antagonists are less effective. Local anesthetics, due to their brief duration of action (e.g. bupivacaine 0.5 per cent; 4–12 hours duration) have a diagnostic role before proceeding to a neurolytic block. However, a series of sympathetic nerve blocks with local anesthetics can be very useful in ischemic pain[56] or in sympathetic reflex dystrophy.[57]

When a local anesthetic block (diagnostic block) has been found to be effective in controlling pain, a neurolytic agent can be injected to induce a longer lasting effect. A neurolytic block with alcohol or phenol is applied at the level of the peripheral somatic nerve (e.g. intercostal nerve) where the painful territory depends on one or two nerves. Neurolysis of several nerves is not well-tolerated by patients. In addition, alcoholic blocks can produce neuritis in some patients, with pain more severe than the pre-existing one. Neurolytic block of the celiac nerve utilizing different techniques is effective in controlling oncologic pain in the upper abdominal organs.[58–62] Subarachnoid neurolytic blocks, once frequently advocated, are now almost exclusively used in saddle pain from tumor infiltrating the perineal area, because of the risk of motor neurological lesions. As this type of block may cause bladder and bowel dysfunction in 40–50 per cent of cases, it is reserved for those patients with urinary and colonic deviations. Neurolytic blocks of cranial nerves (e.g. one or more branches of the trigeminal nerve or Gasser's ganglion) have been recently replaced by radiofrequency thermorhizotomy, a more selective and precise method than alcohol or phenol blocks.

Neurosurgical procedures to control neoplastic pain, either by conventional or stereotaxic techniques and with their innate operative and age-related risks (e.g. spinal posterior rhizotomy, trigeminal rhizotomy, dorsal route entry zone (DREZ) lesion, anterolateral cordotomy) must be considered as last resort therapy reserved for those patients in a relatively good general condition who have not responded to any of the aforementioned treatments.[63–65] Cervical percutaneous cordotomy represents one of the most effective analgesic techniques for neoplastic pain.[66,67] This operation is indicated for monolateral nociceptor pain and when performed by experts, it is possible to obtain immediate analgesia in 75–90 per cent of cases, which persists for many months. However, the procedure is associated with many complications, including hemiparesis, asthenia, urinary and sexual dysfunctions, respiratory insufficiency (especially in bilateral cordotomy) and dysesthesia, and therefore must be offered only to those cases who do not respond to usual analgesic treatments.[66]

Neurostimulation techniques, (e.g. transepidermal nerve, peripheral nerve, dorsal cord) are indicated for non-oncologic pain that often coexists in elderly patients with cancer pain. There are no secure data on the efficacy of these techniques in oncological pain. Finally, due to the complex emotional disturbances arising from chronic pain and from the awareness of the gravity of the illness, elderly patients with pain may benefit from aggressive use of psychological interventions, such as active psychological and psychosocial support, progressive muscular relaxation training, biofeedback, hypnosis, and psychotherapies.[68]

NUTRITIONAL SUPPORT FOR ELDERLY CANCER PATIENTS

General concepts

Due to physiological reduction of the muscular mass and reduced physical activity, the elderly patient has less energy demands, compared to the younger patient. Nevertheless, elderly patients often present clinical signs of malnutrition secondary to an inadequate food intake, either quantitatively or qualitatively. Factors responsible for this situation include alteration of the senses of smell and taste, disturbances of mastication and sometimes digestion and absorption, and economical, social and psychological reasons (purchase of foods rich in carbohydrates and fats but poor in proteins due to the lesser cost, inability to cook, depression due to solitude) that contribute to inadequate diet.[14] These factors, associated with a progressive reduction of calorific–protein reserves secondary to the physiological modifications of aging,[69] promote a clinical state of malnutrition that can be markedly potentiated by cancer therapies.

Cancer, *per se*, is often a cause of anorexia, early satiety and taste modifications.[70,71] Neoplasms of the digestive tract, in particular, can alter the patient's ability to ingest, digest, absorb and metabolize nutrients.[14] Metabolic alterations induced by cancer often result in a progressive loss of protein and development of cachexia.[72,73]

Antitumor therapies markedly contribute to deterioration of the nutritional status. Physiological modifications of body constituents and the additional effects of chemotherapy, such as nausea, vomiting, diarrhea, constipation, abdominal pain, mucositis and mucosal lesions, exert a strong adverse effect on elderly patients. Radiotherapy to any part of the gastrointestinal tract or adjacent organs can produce nutritional sequelae.[74] The sense of smell and taste, and mucosal trophism, already frequently affected in the elderly patient, are worsened by radiotherapy and consequences of radiotherapy such as enteritis, mucosal ulcers, difficulty in swallowing and decreased saliva secretion, contribute to further reduction of food consumption.[75] Oncological surgery, depending on its site and severity (e.g. head, neck, GI tract, pancreas, liver) may increase and prolong the difficulties in food ingestion, digestion and/or assimilation and in addition, increases the metabolic activity in response to post-operative stress and tissue repair. Thus, global reductions in energy and protein intake and increased energy expenditure secondary to metabolic activity of the neoplasm and related anticancer therapies create a negative balance, resulting in protein–calorific malnutrition.

Malnutrition and cancer have a negative influence on the immune system causing impaired T- and B-cell function.[76,77] This interference in immune function results in an increased frequency and severity of infection, which can be lethal in elderly cancer patients.

Finally, weight loss in cancer patients is regarded as an adverse prognostic factor, negatively affecting survival.[78] Nutritional support in elderly cancer patients is therefore aimed at reversing the host tissue wasting associated with aging and advanced malignancies, and at improving the clinical course and therapeutic outcome. Oral, enteral and parenteral methods have been used for these purposes.

Evaluation of malnutrition

It is important to evaluate the nutritional status of the patient to establish the presence of clinical or subclinical malnutrition that will require a precise nutritional therapy program, often of the artificial type, and to monitor the changes in nutritional status subsequent to treatment. This evaluation is obtained by anamnesic data (dietary habits, clinical history), anthropometric data (body weight, arm, arm muscle, and thigh circumferences, skinfold thickness), physical examination (clinical signs of malnutrition) and biochemical tests (creatinine/height ratio, serum albumin and pre-albumin, serum transferrin, retinol-binding protein).

De Wys *et al.*,[78] analyzing the data of 3047 cancer patients, observed a weight loss in the last 6 months, prior to antineoplastic therapy, in from 16 to 67 per cent of the patients according to type of tumor. Patients with gastric or pancreatic cancer had the highest incidence of malnutrition, and highly malignant lymphomas, colon, prostate and lung carcinomas were also associated with significant weight loss. Head, neck and esophageal neoplasms often provoked malnutrition due to dysphagia. A weight loss of 10 per cent of the body weight cannot be tolerated by an elderly patient undergoing anticancer therapy. Taking into consideration the high risk of reduction of oral intake during anticancer therapy, concomitant nutritional supplementation prior to or concurrent with cancer therapy is warranted at even lower levels of weight loss.

The best method for defining calorific needs is indirect calorimetry. When this method is not available, the Harris–Benedict formula can be used to calculate the basal energy expenditure. However, a calorific regimen of 35–40 kcal/kg per day is sufficient in most patients.[79,80] These values must be increased in the presence of sepsis or during antitumor treatment. The quota of nitrogen should be proportional to the prescribed energetic amount in a ratio kcal/g of nitrogen of 130/1.

The water needs, all too often disregarded, are particularly important in the elderly patient in whom the physiological mechanisms that help to maintain hydration are less efficient. Water needs are calculated according to body surface (1200 ml/m^2 per day) and the balance between water intake and output per day.

Certain clinical parameters such as thirst, cutaneous and mucous membrane dryness, presence or absence of edema, and systemic blood pressure, are helpful determinants of the state of hydration. A guideline for the daily basic water requirement is generally 30 ml/kg of body weight or 1 ml/kcal. Water needs increase significantly in the presence of fever, vomiting, diarrhea or fistulas. Under these circumstances, particular attention must also be paid to the increased and specific needs for mineral salts and trace elements.

Finally, an evaluation of vitamin requirements is necessary to avoid deficiency states, often pre-existing in the elderly cancer patient, and to prevent hypervitaminosis caused by an excessive proportion of lipid-soluble vitamins in certain preparations.[81]

Methods of alimentation

The various means used to correct nutritional deficits in elderly cancer patients are oral nutrition, enteral nutrition via a nasogastric or nasoenteral tube or via percutaneous endoscopic gastrostomy or jejunostomy and parenteral nutrition, either partial or total.

Oral

Oral feeding is the optimum route, the most physiological, and the preferred method of the patient. In order to utilize this mode of nutrition efficiently and for as long as possible, physicians and nurses must evaluate regularly all local and systemic factors that can interfere with an adequate oral intake in elderly patients.

Examination of the mouth may reveal evidence of an inadequate dentition, signs of gingivitis, stomatitis or alterations of mucosal integrity, the presence of a fungal infection or painful, ulcerating lesions and decreased saliva secretion. These conditions can be primary or secondary to anticancer treatments. Dental care prior to chemotherapy and fluoride trays designed by the dentist to protect teeth and mucosae from the effects of radiotherapy are useful measures to improve oral intake. Routine mouthwashes of the oral cavity with baking soda and water or, if indicated, with antifungal solutions, help to promote healing of oral cavity lesions. The use of alcohol-based substances or standard commercial mouthwashes can damage the oral mucosae and therefore are not advisable. Topical anesthetics and artificial saliva may relieve pain and the xerostomia that often impedes oral intake.

A diet consisting of a wide range of appetizing foods will help to overcome the alterations in the sense of smell and taste due to tumor or food aversions acquired during anticancer therapies. In the case of refusal of first beef and pork and then poultry and fish, eggs and milk can be substituted as sources of protein. Liquid or semiliquid foods that are not heavily flavored and do not require excessive mastication are often preferred by the elderly patient. Fresh fruits, vegetables and milk shakes often appeal to patients with taste alterations and the use of different flavors and mild seasoning improves the taste of foods. Elderly patients often have very precise food preferences and it is therefore essential to involve them in planning their oral diet.

Anorexia is often followed by early satiety. Six to seven small meals are better tolerated by patients compared to three major daily meals. Milk is a complete food that even in a dry form can be added to other food. Lactose-free milk preparations are available for people with lactose intolerance. Liquid formula diets of neutral taste but rich in proteins and calories can be mixed to habitual diets to increase the protein–calorific intake. Therefore, the availability of products of artificial concentrates of different flavors and composition, delivered in small, frequent volumes, is able to satisfy the quantitative and qualitative nutritional requirements and taste needs of the elderly patient.

Enteral

When oral feeding becomes impossible due to severe dysphagia or upper GI obstruction, artificial enteral nutrition must be resorted to, but only if intestinal function is maintained. The use of very flexible, thin, soft nasogastric or duodenal tubes (or sounds) makes the treatment possible for many weeks with few or no signs of local irritation.[82] Many artificial nutritional solutions can be administered by enteral therapy. Natural hake diets or combined artificial diets are more viscous and necessitate larger caliber sounds. Correct management of the sound is necessary to prevent obstruction (adequate solubility and fluidity of the food mixture, frequent washes, pump usage) and misplacement (ascultation, X-ray control). Accidental removal of the nasogastric tube due to coughing or vomiting is a frequent occurrence and therefore its use is contraindicated in patients with excessive cough or undergoing highly emetogenic chemotherapy. If artificial nutrition must last more than 4–5 weeks and if the nasogastric tube is not tolerated or contraindicated for the above mentioned reasons, or because of the presence of pharyngeal or esophageal stenosis, percutaneous endoscopic gastrostomy (PEG) is indicated.[83] Different preparations of complete, balanced artificial solutions containing proteins (milk, soya protein, casein), maltodextrin, fat, mineral salts, trace elements and vitamins are available for hospital and home nutrition via PEG.[84] Jejunostomy is the route of choice for long-term artificial enteral nutrition or for patients with gastric (pyloric) and duodenal stenosis.

Diet formulas with oligopeptides, amino acids, oligosaccharides, medium-chain triglycerides, and essential fatty acids are particularly indicated in elderly cancer patients with a malabsorption syndrome. During enteral feeding, meta-bolic side-effects are few and very infrequent. In contrast, the appearance of gastroenteric disturbances such as diarrhea, vomiting, abdominal distention and pain are frequent symptoms in the initial phases of therapy and can be overcome by decreasing the infusion rate, reducing the solutions' osmolarity and the usage of pumps. Constipation often develops in elderly patients after long periods of treatment and can be prevented or improved with fiber-containing solutions.

Parenteral

Parenteral nutrition is indicated when nutritional demands can no longer be maintained by the enteral route or if enteral nutrition is contraindicated (intest-inal occlusion, high-jet fistulas, vomiting, uncontrollable diarrhea, complex abdominal surgery, severe malnutrition). Major attention in the use of total parenteral nutrition (TPN) in elderly cancer patients is required due to the limitations imposed by the aging process. Elderly patients subjected to TPN have a reduced tolerance of lipids compared to younger patients.[85] In addition, the presence of chronic pathologies affects the administration of precise parenteral solutions. The commercial solutions for parenteral nutrition vary according to type and concentration, and their preparation in one bag allows the correct balance between macro- and micronutrients and minimizes the risk of contamination by infectious or chemical agents. Administration of the parenteral solution by an infusion pump at a predetermined rate reduces the incidence of metabolic complications such as hyperosmolarity and hyperglycemia.

Central venous catheterization, required because of the high osmolarity of the infused solutions, is responsible for an increased risk of venous thrombosis and catheter-related sepsis in elderly cancer patients. Soft material catheters, such as polyurethane and silicone, reduce the incidence of thrombosis. Sepsis can be minimized by subcutaneous tunneling of the venous catheter and adequate, sterile medication and care of the cutaneous entry-site and the hub of the catheter.[86] Insertion of the catheter via the subclavian approach (subclavian vein to the superior vena cava), in contrast to the jugular vein approach, offers many advantages with regard to patient compliance and nursing management. If brief (4–7 days) TPN is required, central venous catheterization can be per-formed via a peripheral vein, but this approach is associated with a higher risk of thrombosis and phlebitis due to the greater contact of the catheter with the vascular system. The use of totally implanted systems, characterized by a sub-cutaneous port attached to the catheter, is helpful in organizing nocturnal and domiciliary discontinuous therapy in compliant patients.

The major complications associated with parenteral nutrition can be avoided by careful choice of nutritional substrates including water, strict monitoring of the patient by means of clinical and biochemical analysis, and correct manage-ment of the infusion system.

In conclusion, malnutrition is an unfavorable prognostic factor when evaluat-ing neoplastic disease and is capable of worsening the quality of the life of the patient. Elderly cancer patients, compared to younger patients, are at higher risk of developing malnutrition and, therefore, the maintenance of adequate nutrition and the eventual recovery from nutritional deficit are fundamental objectives in the correct clinical management of the elderly cancer patient. The results of numerous controlled clinical trials have demonstrated that TPN used in patients independent of their nutritional state did not modify survival rates and chemotherapy or radiotherapy tolerance,[87,88] whereas in markedly malnourished cancer patients, peri-operative TPN reduced the incidence of post-surgical complications[89] and was capable of improving that nutritional state during chemotherapy.[90]

We believe that artificial nutrition is generally indicated in elderly cancer patients with malnutrition, those at risk of developing malnutrition secondary to anticancer therapies or those presenting with prolonged GI tract effects caused by antineoplastic therapies. However, qualitative and quantitative limitations must be imposed in the nutritional support of patients no longer responsive to specific oncological treatments or in terminally ill patients.

REFERENCES

1. Rowe JW, Bradley EC. The elderly cancer patient: Pathophysiological considerations. In: Yanci KR ed. *Perspectives on prevention and treatment of cancer in the elderly.* New York: Raven Press, 1983: 33–41.
2. Masoro ES. Metabolism. In: Finch CE, Scheider EL eds. *Handbook of the biology of aging,* 2nd edn. New York: Van Nostrand Reinhold, 1985: 540–63.
3. Balducci L, Phillips DM, Wallace C *et al.* Cancer chemotherapy in the elderly. *American Family Physician* 1987; **35**: 133–43.
4. Howard Ruben J. Pharmacokinetics considerations of chemotherapy administration in the elderly. In: Welch-McCaffrey D ed. *Nursing considerations in geriatric oncology.* Columbus, OH: Adria Laboratories, 1986: 9–22.
5. Kohn R. Aging and age-related diseases: normal processes. In: Johnson HA ed. *Relation between normal aging and disease.* New York: Raven Press, 1985: 1–44.
6. Lipschts DA, Udupa KB. Age and the hematopoietic system. *Journal of the American Geriatrics Society* 1986; **34**: 448–545.
7. Gurevitch A. Dermatologic disorders. In: Steinberg F ed. *Care of the geriatric patient,* 6th edn. St Louis: Mosby, 1983: 199–215.
8. Davison W. Adverse drug reactions in the elderly: general consideration. In: Butler RN, Bearn AG eds. *The aging process: therapeutic implications.* New York: Raven Press, 1984: 101–11.
9. Palumberg S, Hirsjari E. Mortality in geriatric surgery. *Gerontology* 1979; **25**: 103–12.
10. Begg CB, Cohen L, Ellerton J. Are the elderly predisposed to toxicity from cancer chemotherapy? *Cancer Clinical Trials* 1980; **3**: 369–74.
11. Begg CB, Carbone PP. Clinical trials and drugs toxicity in the elderly. *Cancer* 1983; **52**: 1986–92.
12. Lipschitz DA, Goldestein S, Reis R *et al.* Cancer in the elderly: Basic science and clinical aspects. *Annals of Internal Medicine* 1985; **102**: 218–28.
13. Brady LW, Marko AM. Radiation therapy in the elderly patient. In: Vaeth JM, Meyer J eds. *Frontiers in radiation therapy and oncology,* vol. 20, *Cancer and the elderly.* Basel: Karger, 1986: 80–92.
14. Hardy C, Wallance C, Khansur T *et al.* Nutrition, cancer and aging: an annotated review. II. Cancer, cachexia and aging. *Journal of the American Geriatrics Society* 1986; **34**: 219–88.
15. Kehlet H. The modifying effect of general and regional anesthesia on the endocrine-metabolic response to surgery. *Regional Anaesthesie* 1982; **7**: 538.

16. Pflug AE, Halter JB, Tolas AG. Plasma catecholamine levels during anesthesia and surgical stress. *Regional Anaesthesie* 1982; **7**: 549.
17. Bonica JJ, Benedetti C. Post operative pain. In: Condon RE, De Cosse JJ eds. *Surgical care: a physiologic approach to clinical management.* Philadelphia: Lea & Febiger, 1980: 394–414.
18. Bonica JJ. *The management of pain: cancer pain,* vol. 1. Philadelphia: Lea & Febiger, 1990: 409–68.
19. Bond MR. Psycological and emotional aspects of cancer pain. In: Bonica JJ, Ventafridda V eds. *Advances in pain research and therapy,* vol. 2. New York: Raven Press, 1979: 81–8.
20. Harkins SW, Chapman CR. Detection and decision factors in pain perception in young and elderly men. *Pain* 1976; **2**: 253.
21. Woodrow KM. Pain tolerance: Differences according to age, sex, and race. *Psychosomatic Medicine* 1972; **34**: 545–8.
22. Crook J, Rideout E, Browne G. The prevalence of pain complaints in a general population. *Pain* 1984; **18**: 299.
23. Harkins SW, Nowlin JB. Personality factors and chronic pain complaint in community dwelling elderly persons. Presented at the 93rd Annual Convention of the American Psychological Association, Los Angeles, 23–27 August 1985.
24. Moss MS, Lawton MP, Glicksman A. The role of pain in the last year of life of elderly persons. *Gerontologist* 1986; **26**: 165A.
25. Foley KM. Pain syndromes in patients with cancer. In: Bonica JJ, Ventafridda V eds. *Advances in pain research and therapy,* vol. 2. New York: Raven Press, 1979: 58–78.
26. Twycross RG, Fairfields S. Pain in far-advanced cancer. *Pain* 1982; **14**: 303.
27. Zimmerman M. Cancer pain: pathogenesis, therapy, and assesment. In: Senn HJ, Glaus A eds. *Supportive care in cancer patients,* vol. II, *Recent results in cancer research.* Berlin: Springer-Verlag, 1991: 8–221.
28. Zimmerman M, Handwerker HO, Schmerz G. *Konzepte und arztliches Handeln.* Berlin: Springer-Verlag, 1984.
29. Devor M. Central changes mediating neuropathic pain. In: Dubner R, Gebhart GF, Bond MR eds. *Proceedings of the 5th World Congress on Pain.* Amsterdam: Elsevier, *Pain research and clinical management* vol 3. 1988: 114–28.
30. Arner S, Meyerson B. Lack of analgesic effect of opioids on neuropathic and idiopathic form of pain. *Pain* 1988; **33**: 11–22.
31. Bonica JJ, Benedetti C. Management of cancer pain. In: Moossa AR, Robson MC, Schimpff SG eds. *Comprehensive textbook of oncology.* Baltimore: Williams & Wilkins, 1986: 443–77.
32. Bonadonna G, Molinari R. Role and limits of anticancer drugs in the treatment of advanced cancer pain. In: Bonica JJ, Ventafridda V eds. *Advances in pain research and therapy,* vol. 2. New York: Raven Press, 1979: 131–44.
33. Gurtler R, Quadt C. Die chemo- und hormonotherapie bei Krebsschmerzen. In: Tontscher G ed. Berlin: Akademie-Verlag, 1988: 60–74.
34. WHO. *Cancer pain relief.* Geneva: World Health Organization, 1986.
35. Nuki G, Gurley L. Nonsteroidal analgesic antiinflammatory drugs in the elderly. In: Butler RN, Bearn AG eds. *The aging process: therapeutic implications.* New York: Raven Press, 1984: 207–28.
36. Twycross RG. Opioid analgesics in cancer pain: current practice and controversies. *Cancer Surveys* 1988; **7**: 29–53.
37. Ventafridda V. Use of systemic analgesic drugs in cancer pain. *Advanced Pain Research Therapy* 1984; **7**: 557–74.
38. Twycross RG, Lack SA. *Control of alimentary symptoms in far-advanced cancer.* Edinburgh: Churchill Livingstone, 1986.
39. Regnards CFS, Badger C. Opioids, sleep and time of death. *Palliative Medicine* 1987; **1**: 107–10.

40. Kaiko RF. Narcotics in the elderly. *Medical Clinics of North America* 1982; **66**: 1079–89.
41. Sloan RW. Drug therapy in old age. In: *Practical geriatric and therapeutics*. Oradel NJ: Medical Economics Books. 1986: 82–106.
42. Walsh TD. Oral morphine in chronic cancer pain. *Pain* 1984; **18**: 1.
43. Kanner RF, Foley KM. Patterns of narcotic drugs use in a cancer pain clinic. *Annals of the New York Academy of Sciences* 1981; **362**: 161.
44. Foley KM. The treatment of cancer pain. *New England Journal of Medicine* 1985; **313**: 84–95.
45. Foley KM. Adjuvant analgesic drugs in cancer pain management. In: Aronoff GM ed. *Evaluation and treatment of chronic pain*. Baltimore: Urban & Schwarzenberg, 1985: 425–34.
46. Swerdlow M. Anticonvulsant drugs and chronic pain. *Clinical Neuropharmacology* 1984; **7**: 51–82.
47. Twycross RG, Lack SA. *Symptoms control in far-advanced cancer: pain relief.* London: Pitman, 1983.
48. Ventafridda V, Tamburini M, Caraceni H *et al.* A validation study of the WHO method for cancer pain relief. *Cancer* 1987; **59**: 850.
49. Dickson RJ, Russel PSB. Continuous subcutaneous analgesics for terminal care at home. *Lancet* 1982: 165.
50. Campbell CF, Mason JB, Weiler JM. Continuous subcutaneous infusion of morphine for the pain of the terminal malignancy. *Annals of Internal Medicine* 1983; **98**: 51–2.
51. Dennis GC, De Witty R. Management of intractable pain in cancer patients by implantable morphine infusion systems. *Journal of the National Medical Association* 1987; **79**: 939–44.
52. Payne R. Role of epidural and intrathecal narcotics and peptides in the management of cancer pain. *Medical Clinics of North America* 1987; **71**: 313–37.
53. Pert CB, Snyder SH. Opiate receptor: demonstration in nervous tissue. *Science* 1973; **179**: 1011.
54. Lenzi A, Galli G, Gandfini M. Intraventricular morphine in paraneoplastic painful syndrome of the cervico facial region: experience in thirty-eight cases. *Neurosurgery* 1985; **17**(1): 6–11.
55. Coombs DW, Maurer LH, Sauders RL *et al.* Outcomes and complication of continuous intraspinal narcotic analgesia for cancer pain control. *Journal of Clinical Oncology* 1984; **12**: 1414–20.
56. Zenz M, Van den Berg B, Van der Berg E. Plethysmorgraphische untersuchungen zur sympathikusblockade und periduraler morphin-analgesie. *Anasthesist* 1981; **30**(10): 70–3.
57. Gerbershagen H. Blocks with local anaesthetics in the treatment of cancer pain. In: Bonica JJ, Ventafridda V eds. *Advances in pain research and therapy*, vol. 2. New York: Raven Press, 1979: 3–11.
58. Moore DC, Bush WH, Burnett LL. Celiac plexus block: a roentgenographic, anatomic study of technique and spread of solution in patients and corpses. *Anaesthesia and Analgesia* 1981; **60**: 369–79.
59. Boas RA. The sympathetic nervous system and pain relief. *Monographs in Anesthesiology* 1983; **13**: 215–37.
60. Singler RC. An improved technique for alcohol neurolysis of the celiac plexus. *Anesthesiology* 1982; **56**: 137–41.
61. Ischia S, Luzzani A, Ischia A *et al.* A new approach to the neurolytic block of the coeliac plexus: the transaortic technique. *Pain* 1983; **16**: 333–41.
62. Montero Matala A, Vidal Lopez F, Inarja Martinez L. The percutaneous anterior approach to the celiac plexus using CT guidance. *Pain* 1988; **34**: 285–8.
63. Papo I. Spinal posterior rhizotomy and commisural myelotomy in the treatment of

cancer pain. In: Bonica JJ, Ventafridda V eds. *Advances in pain research and therapy*, vol. 2. New York: Raven Press, 1979: 439–47.

64. Looser JD. Role of neurosurgery in visceral and perineal pain. In: Bonica JJ, Ventafridda V eds. *Advances in pain research and therapy*, vol. 2. New York: Raven Press, 1979: 607–14.

65. White JC, Sweet WH. *Pain and the neurosurgeon; a 40 year experience*. Springfield, IL: Charles C Thomas, 1969.

66. Ventafridda V, De Conno F, Fochi C. Cervical percutaneous cordotomy. In: Bonica JJ, Ventafridda V, Pagni CA eds. *Advances in pain research and therapy*, vol. 4. New York: Raven Press, 1982: 185–98.

67. Lipton S. Percutaneous cordotomy. In: Wall PD, Mezack R eds. *Textbook of pain*. Edinburgh: Churchill Livingstone, 1984: 632–8.

68. Holland JC, Massie MJ. Psychiatric symptoms in cancer pain patients and management of psychiatric symptoms. In: Foley KM ed. *Management of cancer pain*. New York: Memorial Sloan–Kettering Cancer Center, 1985: 217–31.

69. Chernoff R, Lipschitz DA. Nutrition and aging. In: Shils Me, Young VR eds. *Modern nutrition in health and disease*. Philadelphia: Lea & Febiger, 1988: 982–1000.

70. De Wys WD. Anorexia in cancer patients. *Cancer Research* 1977: **7**: 2354–8.

71. Bernistein IL. Etiology of anorexia in cancer. *Cancer* 1986; **58**: 1881–6.

72. Torti FM, Dieckman B, Beutler B *et al.* A macrophage factor inhibits adipocyte gene expression: an *in vivo* model of cachexia. *Science* 1985; **229**: 867–9.

73. Fong Y, Moldawe LL, Marano M *et al.* Cachetin/TNF or IL-1 induced cachexia with redistribution of body proteins. *American Journal of Physiology* 1989; **256**: R659–65.

74. Donaldson SS. Nutritional consequences of radiotherapy. *Cancer Research* 1983; **37**: 2407–13.

75. Bistrian BR. Some practical and theoretic concepts in the nutritional assessment of the cancer patient. *Cancer* 1986; **58**: 183–6.

76. Fernandes G. Nutritional factors: modulating effects on immune function and aging. *Pharmacological Research* 1984; **36**: 1235–95.

77. Good RA, West A, Day NK *et al.* Effects of undernutrition on host cells and organ functions. *Cancer Research* 1982; **42**: 7375–465.

78. De Wys WD, Begg D, Lavin PT *et al.* Prognostic effect of weight loss prior chemotherapy in cancer patients. *American Journal of Medicine* 1980; **69**: 491–7.

79. Copeland EM, Daly JM, Dudrick SJ. Nutrition as an adjunct to cancer treatment in the adult. *Cancer Research* 1977; **37**: 2451–6.

80. Bozzetti F. La nutrizione del paziente neoplastico. In: Bonadonna G, Robustelli della Cuna G eds. *Manuale di Oncologia Medica*. Milano: Masson, 1983: 877–93.

81. Garry PJ, Goodwin JJ, Hunt WC *et al.* Nutritional status in the healthy elderly population: dietary and supplemental intake. *American Journal of Clinical Nutrition* 1982; **36**: 319–31.

82. Richter G, Dehnert J. Enteral tube feeding in clinical oncology. *Infusions Therapie* 1990; **17**(6): 291–9.

83. Gauderes MWL, Ponsky FL, Iznat RF Jr. Gastrostomy without laparotomy: a percutaneous endoscopic technique. *Journal of Pediatric Surgery* 1980; **15**: 872–5.

84. Dempsey DT, Mullen JL. Macronutrient requirements in the malnourished cancer patients. How much of what and why? *Cancer* 1985; **55**: 290–4.

85. Chernoff R, Lipschitz DA. Total parenteral nutrition: consideration in the elderly. In: Rrombeau JL, Caldwell MD eds. *Clinical nutrition: parenteral nutrition*, vol. 2. Philadelphia: Saunders, 1986: 648–53.

86. De Cicco M, Panarello G, Chiaradia V *et al.* Source and route of microbial colonization of parenteral nutrition catheters. *Lancet* 1989; **2**: 1255–61.

87. McGeer AJ, Detsty AS, O'Rourke K. Parenteral nutrition in cancer patients undergoing chemotherapy: a meta analysis. *Nutrition* 1990; **6**: 233–40.
88. Klein S, Simes J, Blackburn GL. Total parenteral nutrition and cancer clinical trials. *Cancer* 1986; **58**: 1378–86.
89. The Veterans Affairs Total Parenteral Nutrition Cooperative Study Group. Perioperative total parenteral nutrition in surgical patients. *New England Journal of Medicine.* 1991; **325**: 525–32.
90. De Cicco M, Panarello G, Fantin D *et al.* Parenteral nutrition in cancer patients receiving chemotherapy: effects on toxicity and nutritional status. *Journal of Parenteral and Enteral Nutrition* 1993; **17**: 513–18.

Specific supportive problems

CHAPTER ELEVEN

Interventional radiology in the management of malignant disease

STEVEN J BIRCH, DAVID S TARVER AND RICHARD D THOMAS

INTRODUCTION

Radiologists have, for many decades, used the percutaneous puncture of blood vessels, the biliary ducts and the upper urinary tract as a means of introducing radiopaque contrast agents as an adjunct to diagnosis. It is only within the last 20 years, however, that these techniques have been adapted to provide minimally invasive forms of treatment.

The proliferation of new imaging modalities and their increasing sophistication has greatly facilitated the introduction of these new forms of therapy and by providing anatomical information in exquisite and immediate detail made possible the safe and effective techniques of percutaneous biopsy.

The field of interventional radiology is expanding rapidly with a consequent increase in the clinical involvement of diagnostic radiologists in patient care. The following is a brief review of some areas where new interventional techniques have been shown to provide help in the management of malignant disease.

MALIGNANT BILIARY OBSTRUCTION

Obstructive jaundice is a common complication of malignant disease whether arising primarily in the pancreas or biliary system or as a consequence of extrinsic compression of the bile ducts by metastatic nodal enlargement. The presence of biliary obstruction is associated with several specific consequences, such as:

- Renal failure
- Sepsis (local or remote)
- Gastrointestinal bleeding
- Impaired wound healing
- Pruritus.

The potentially serious nature of these complications argues for the relief of obstruction, where possible, at an early stage. Radical surgery offers some hope of cure in patients with localized bile duct carcinomas, ampullary carcinomas and very occasionally early pancreatic ductal carcinomas. Unfortunately, in the majority of cases, the tumour type, its extent and the medical condition of the patient preclude attempts at surgical cure and therapy must be aimed at palliation.

Thirty-day mortality rates of between 5 per cent and 33 per cent[1,2] for palliative surgery have provided the stimulus for the development of non-operative biliary drainage techniques. External biliary drainage via percutaneously placed trans-hepatic catheters failed to reduce subsequent operative mortality and led to the introduction of trans-hepatic techniques for the insertion of internal biliary stents. These techniques were, themselves, not without complication whether used pre-operatively or as palliation. The endoscopic insertion of biliary stents has now been shown to be less dangerous than percutaneous methods with a technical success rate around 85 per cent and a procedure-related mortality of less than 5 per cent.[3]

Problems do, however, occur with endoscopic stenting. Invasion of the duodenum by tumour may preclude cannulation of the bile ducts and long irregular strictures can prevent the passage of guidewires. Furthermore, tumours in the liver hilum obstructing several ducts require multiple stents to drain the whole liver and thereby reduce the risk of cholangitis in residually obstructed segments. The cannulation at endoscopy of these multiple ducts may be difficult or impossible.

These technical difficulties may be largely overcome by a combined percutaneous and endoscopic procedure. A small percutaneous catheter is used to cross the obstructing lesion from above and a long guidewire passed into the duodenum where it is snared by the endoscopist and subsequently used for the stent insertion via the endoscope. This manoeuvre raises the overall technical success rate of stent placement to almost 100 per cent.[4]

The percutaneous insertion of stents may now be reserved for those patients in whom endoscopic visualization of the duodenum is not feasible, usually as a result of previous surgery.

A number of problems are associated with biliary stents. Many will become clogged by biliary sludge after a few months and failure through stent migration and tumour overgrowth are well-recognized. Replacement is usually possible endoscopically but this requires further hospital admission.

Patency is related to both the material from which the stent is made and its internal diameter.[5] Simple polyurethane stents, both cheap and simple to introduce, are generally satisfactory in patients whose life expectancy is short, but in those where longer term drainage will be required expandable metal stents show considerable promise. These devices may be inserted both percutaneously and endoscopically but attain a final diameter of 1 cm. A recent study showed occlusion to have occurred in only 3 of 47 patients and in each of these cases the cause of occlusion was tumour ingrowth rather than biliary sludge.[6]

In conclusion, whilst radical surgery offers the only hope of cure in malignant obstructive jaundice, palliative surgery carries significant risks. In the majority of patients relief of symptoms can be achieved safely and effectively with stents inserted endoscopically, percutaneously or by a combination of both.

THERAPEUTIC EMBOLIZATION IN MALIGNANT DISEASE

Therapeutic embolization is a radiological procedure in which insoluble solid particles or immissible fluid particles are introduced into a selected part of the circulation. The particles travel with the blood flow until the branching vessels become too small to allow further passage, causing the embolic material to become lodged. The procedure has two main objectives: (1) to cause vascular occlusion – occlusive embolization; and (2) to deliver a therapeutic agent to a specific location – chemoembolization. Therapeutic embolization can be of great value in the management of malignant disease. Occlusive embolization and chemoembolization will be discussed separately, although in practice, both techniques are frequently used together.

Occlusive embolization

Malignant tumours, like normal tissue, are dependent on an adequate blood supply for survival and growth. Interruption of the blood supply can cause tumour necrosis with reduction of tumour bulk and retardation of tumour growth. The situations in which embolization might be considered are:

- uncontrolled pain, which can be relieved by reduction of tumour bulk;
- uncontrolled haemorrhage from a tumour;
- pre-operative reduction of tumour vascularity to facilitate surgery and reduce surgical blood loss;
- distressing systemic effects due to the elaboration by a tumour of biologically active substances (e.g. ectopic hormones);
- in an attempt to stimulate an immune response to a tumour by causing ischaemic damage.

Materials and methods

A variety of embolic materials are in use and can be classified into absorbable and non-absorbable categories for temporary and permanent occlusion respectively. In management of malignant disease the latter is usually appropriate. The following are examples of materials in use:

- Polyvinyl alcohol particle
- Isobutyl 2-cyanoacrylate (tissue glue)
- Steel coils, with barbs or wool tufts
- Silastic spheres
- Silicone rubber
- Detachable balloons.

Materials such as steel coils or detachable balloons occlude the larger vessels supplying a tumour. Particulate materials are designed to flow into the tumour and lodge in the capillary bed causing occlusion. The size of particles will therefore determine the performance of an embolic material. Particle size in the order of 10^{-6} m is generally appropriate. The occlusive effect of embolic material is enhanced by a subsequent foreign body reaction in the capillary bed.

Enhanced occlusive effect is achieved if the introduction of particulate material is followed by occlusion of the supplying vessel (e.g. by a steel coil).[7] If large vessel occlusion alone is used the tumour will regain some blood supply by development of collateral channels. If a tumour receives blood from more than one major vessel, all or both must be embolized individually.

Occlusive embolization is immediately preceded by a detailed angiographic study of the tumour and the surrounding structures. All embolic materials are introduced through standard angiographic catheters manipulated into an artery supplying the tumour. Catheterization involves a needle puncture at the groin under local anaesthesia. Manipulation of the catheter tip into the required vessel is facilitated by guidewires and the use of preshaped catheters. Injection of intravenous contrast medium under fluoroscopic observation demonstrates the location of the catheter tip during manipulation. Once the catheter tip is firmly in place particulate material is introduced suspended in contrast medium. Injection is continued under constant fluoroscopy until the distal capillary bed is completely obliterated and forward blood flow ceases.

Complications

Embolization in skilled hands is a safe procedure which causes the minimum of discomfort to the patient. However, there may be side-effects and complications:

1. Tumour necrosis commonly causes a post-embolization syndrome over the following few days. This consists of nausea, vomiting, ileus, pain and fever. Management is symptomatic.
2. A potential hazard is misdirection of embolic material into normal tissue. This is avoided by ensuring that the catheter tip is well-located in the required vessel and will not slip out into another vessel during injection of embolic material. Good angiography will ensure that there are no branch vessels to normal tissue distal to the injection point. A third mode of misdirection of particles is by reflux back along the catheterized vessel. This is more likely towards the end of the procedure when forward flow in the vessel becomes sluggish. Injection of particulate material should therefore be cautious and in small aliquots (1–2 ml) under fluoroscopic observation. Forward flow can be enhanced by papaverine to reduce reflex vascular spasm.
3. Hazards of radiation exposure. This is a potential complication of all radiological procedures but is unlikely to be significant in the management of malignant disease.

Examples of the use of occlusive embolization

A tumour of almost any anatomical location can be considered for arterial embolization provided essential healthy organs are not put at risk. However, the technique is most commonly used for tumours of the liver, kidney and pelvis.

Hepatic neoplasm   Primary or secondary malignancy of the liver is eminently suitable for embolization therapy. There is a wealth of experience over 30 years with the technique. The liver has a dual blood supply from the hepatic artery (30 per cent) and portal vein (70 per cent). However, hepatic neoplasms receive blood almost exclusively from the hepatic artery. Hepatic arterial embolization can therefore render neoplastic tissue ischaemic without critically reducing the supply to normal tissue. However, it must be determined beforehand that sufficient functioning liver tissue remains (at least 10 per cent of normal) and that the portal vein is patent. A combination of capillary embolization with small particles such as polyvinyl alcohol and proximal large vessel occlusion (e.g. with a steel coil) delays the development of collateral vessels and is therefore more effective even than open arterial ligation.[7,8] The technique controls pain and prolongs life expectancy in hepatocellular carcinoma.[8] In the rare neuroendocrine tumours (e.g. carcinoid, some pancreatic tumours) in which hepatic metastases elaborate the biologically active proteins, hepatic arterial embolization can control the levels of such protein and alleviate distressing systemic symptoms.[9,10]

Renal neoplasms   Renal artery embolization can control pain and haematuria associated with renal carcinoma. The technique has been used pre-operatively to facilitate surgery and reduce pre-operative blood loss. However, a recent survey of urologists suggests that this is now rarely considered necessary and not often requested in this situation.[11] The kidney is an ideal organ for embolization as the renal artery is readily accessible to the radiologist and the contralateral kidney can maintain adequate renal function. The presence of a functioning contralateral kidney must be confirmed beforehand. Reflux of embolic material across to the contralteral renal artery is a potential hazard which demands careful technique.

Bladder and uterine malignancy   Malignant tumours of the pelvis are characterized by local invasion of the pelvic wall causing considerable pain. Palliation can be achieved by tumour embolization. Blood supply to these tumours is from both internal iliac arteries. Tumour ischaemia is achieved by simultaneous embolization of both internal iliac arteries usually via bilateral femoral artery punctures.

Chemoembolization

Chemoembolization is a technique for infusing chemotherapeutic agents directly into an artery supplying a tumour. Drugs are either injected with or carried on particulate embolic material which lodges in the tumour capillary bed. The efficacy of cytotoxic drugs is directly proportional to the concentration in malignant cells with a steep dose–response curve. Chemoembolization can produce far greater local concentrations than systemic infusion or a direct arterial infusion. Lower total doses combined with high drug extraction by the tumour result in low systemic levels. High efficacy can therefore be achieved with low toxicity.

Indications

The vast majority of the experience with this technique is in the management of primary and secondary liver malignancy. The following are indications for the use of this technique:

1. A primary treatment modality in patients unfit for surgery.[12]
2. Presurgical reduction of tumour size, particularly if the tumour is large and close to the inferior vena cava.
3. Following surgery to control any residual tumour that could not be excised.

Materials and methods

Chemoembolic material is administered using the same techniques as occlusive embolization. The drug vehicle can be of a matrix (e.g. microsphere) or vesicle (e.g. microcapsules) variety. In the former, the drug is bound to the particle. In the latter, the drug is contained within the particle. The particles are designed to be reabsorbed within 7–10 days to match the kinetics of the cytotoxic drug.

Drugs most commonly used in this technique are 5-fluorouracil, 5-fluorode-oxyuridine, mitomycin C, Adriamycin and cisplatin.

Chemoembolization can be repeated at intervals depending on response to treatment providing the arterial bed remains accessible. The procedure is commonly followed by occlusive embolization. The combination is more effective than either technique used alone.[13] The combination increases contact time of the drug with the tumour and renders malignant tissue ischaemic. Chemotherapy will also attack tissue at the periphery of a tumour which tends to be most active yet less likely than deeper tissue to be rendered adequately ischaemic by vascular occlusion. If a tumour has more than one major supplying artery (e.g. a right hepatic artery from the superior mesenteric artery as well as the proper hepatic artery from the coeliac axis) it is necessary to occlude all but one vessel prior to chemoembolization of the remaining vessel.

Research is currently in progress concerning the local injection of radiopharmaceuticals (^{131}I) carried on particles of Lipiodol (a radiopaque oil) in primary or secondary liver malignancy.[14,15] The radiation dose from a radioactive source is inversely proportional to the fourth power of the distance from the source and directly proportional to the length of exposure. This technique combines intimate contact with prolonged exposure whilst minimizing exposure to healthy tissue. The radiopacity of Lipiodol also permits the size of tumour masses to be readily measured on computerized tomography in order to assess response to treatment. Encouraging results are reported using this technique.

MALIGNANT RENAL OBSTRUCTION

The interventional techniques used in renal obstruction are similar in many ways to those used in malignant obstructive jaundice. Renal obstruction occurs commonly in malignant disease, either as a direct result of urinary tract malignancy, or due to extrinsic compression of the ureters by nodal and other retroperitoneal masses or fibrosis. The presence of bilateral renal obstruction is associated with specific consequences:

- Hyperkalaemia
- Sepsis

- Uraemia
- Pruritus

and usually requires early relief.

Percutaneous nephrostomy (PCN)

PCN is the cornerstone of uroradiological interventional procedures.[16,17] It is a quick, safe and effective means of draining the upper urinary tract. It is successful in almost all cases, though minimally dilated systems are an inevitable source of some failures (about 1 per cent). Pelvic kidneys may prove impossible to access, but malrotation and horseshoe kidneys rarely present problems. Transplanted kidneys, lying superficially, are usually easily drained. The indications, contraindications and complications are listed in Table 11.1.

Method

PCN may be performed under fluoroscopic or ultrasonic guidance. If fluoroscopy is to be used, then renal function must be sufficient to allow concentration of contrast media. A bolus of intravenous contrast is given prior to the procedure and the excretory urogram produced by the kidneys acts as a target for the puncture needle. If ultrasound is used to observe the target calyx, then intra-

Table 11.1   Percutaneous nephrostomy: indications, contraindications and complications

---

Indications
Relief of obstruction
Drainage of pyonephrosis
To divert urinary flow
To facilitate:
    ureteric stent placement/exchange/extraction
    ureteric dilatation
    ureteric embolization
    nephroscopy & in face transitional cell carcinoma removal
    stone removal/dissolution

Contraindications
Coagulation disorders
Relative contraindications:
    terminal stage malignancy
    pelvic kidney

Complications
Sepsis
    local
    systemic
Haemorrhage (usually venous)
Arteriovenous fistula
Urine leakage
Puncture of bowel/gall bladder/pleura

---

venous contrast is not required. In the absence of function in the kidney to be drained, ultrasound guidance is essential.

PCN is performed under local anaesthetic, some patients also requiring intravenous sedation and analgesia. The patient lies in a prone oblique position and a puncture site midway between the 12th rib and the iliac crest, just medial to the posterior axillary line, is selected. The aim is to enter the collecting system via a lower pole calyx. This diminishes the chance of puncturing the main renal vessels, and enables the renal parenchyma to grip the catheter whereas puncture of the renal pelvis without passing through parenchyma results both in less 'grip' and more frequent urinoma formation. A fine-bore needle is placed in the calyx and through it a guidewire is introduced into the ureter. The needle is then removed leaving the wire in place and, after dilating a tract, a catheter is manoeuvred over the guidewire into the renal pelvis. The catheter used is usually a 7F pigtail. The tip of a pigtail catheter is hidden within a loop and causes less damage to the urothelium than a catheter with an unprotected tip. The pigtail loop also renders the catheter partially self-retaining. Some catheters now have a tie to fix the loop, and while these catheters are more difficult to remove accidentally, if this does occur the damage to the renal parenchyma is more substantial. To remove these catheters they must be straightened over a wire. Patients with a fixed-loop catheter therefore require an extra radiological procedure.

Minor complications arise in 10 per cent of patients in whom PCN is undertaken, while in 4 per cent major complications occur, though even in these cases the mortality rate is very low. The risk of septicaemia is such that prophylactic intravenous antibiotics should be given prior to PCN in cases where urinary tract infection is suspected. Haemorrhage is usually mild, lasts less than 24 hours and only very infrequently requires transfusion. Arteriovenous fistula development is rare (1 per cent), and these lesions are amenable to selective embolization.

Percutaneous resection of transitional cell tumour

Percutaneous resection using a sheath and resectoscope has been used instead of nephrectomy.[18] Only low-grade well-differentiated tumours should be treated in this manner, and the puncture must be as atraumatic as possible to limit the chance of tumour dissemination. The track is sterilized with an indium wire and a temporary draining nephrostomy tube is left in place. The indications, contraindications and complications of percutaneous resection of a transitional cell tumour are listed in Table 11.2.

Balloon dilatation of ureteric strictures

Balloon dilatation is a well-recognized and effective way of treating non-malignant ureteric strictures.[19,20] Alone, it is not successful in relieving ureteric obstruction in malignant disease, but in these cases it can be used to facilitate long-term stent placement.

A wire is introduced into the ureter either antegradely via a PCN, or occasionally retrogradely via a cystoscope. A balloon is placed over the wire, straddling the stricture, and then dilated to 4–8 mm diameter. A stent is placed across the dilated stricture for 4–6 weeks and drainage is secured via a nephros-

Table 11.2 Percutaneous resection of transitional cell
tumour: indications, contraindications and complications

Indications
Focal low-grade in face transitional cell carcinoma

Contraindications
Extensive tumour
High-grade in face transitional cell carcinoma
Contraindications to PCN

Complications
Seeding of the tumour
Complications of PCN

Table 11.3 Balloon dilatation
of ureteric strictures: indications,
contraindications and complications

Indications
Benign strictures:
   post-operative
   accidental ligation
Malignant strictures:
   to facilitate stent placement
Radiation strictures:
   to facilitate stent placement

Contraindications
As for PCN

Complications
Ruptured ureter
Complications of PCN

tomy for the first week. After stent removal, ureteric patency is confirmed by a
nephrostogram before renal access is lost. The success of the procedure varies
with the duration of the stricture and is significantly decreased if the stricture has
been present for more than 3 months (90 per cent success before 3 months, only
25 per cent if longer). It is therefore important that post-operative stricture
formation should be recognized and treated at an early stage. Unfortunately
strictures due to radiotherapy respond poorly, the majority recurring within 12
months. The indications, contraindications and complications of balloon dilatation are listed in Table 11.3.

Ureteric stents

Ureteric stents may be a temporary measure (e.g. following ureteric dilatation)
or a therapeutic measure.[21] Traditionally urologists have used the perurethral
approach but the limitations of working through the cystoscope in bladder and
prostatic malignancy renders many of these patients more suitable to PCN and
antegrade placement. There are two types of percutaneous stent – external and

Table 11.4   Ureteric stents: indications,
contraindications and complications

Indications
Relieve obstruction

Contraindications
Severe bladder disease
Contraindications of PCN

Complications
Stent:
   obstruction
   fracture – replacement required
   migration
Ascending sepsis
Ureteric reflux
Complications of PCN

---

internal. The former has an externally protruding segment of catheter which is
occluded. Urine enters the catheter via sideholes in the renal pelvis and flows
down through the stent into the bladder. The stent can be irrigated through the
external component, which also allows access for percutaneous exchange when
necessary. Internal, 'double-J', stents are sited with a pigtail in each of the renal
pelvis and the bladder. They are less intrusive on the patient's lifestyle but
cannot be irrigated. Exchange is necessary at intervals to avoid obstruction, stent
fracture or migration.

In 85 per cent of patients in whom cystectomy and conduit formation has
been required, fluoroscopically controlled transconduit retrograde catheterization and stenting can be used instead of the more invasive PCN and antegrade
placement.

In those patients in whom the bladder is also severely diseased, long-term
PCN drainage should be provided, rather than ureteric stenting. The indications,
contraindications and complications of ureteric stents are listed in Table 11.4.

Transrenal ureteric occlusion

Transrenal ureteric occlusion is a palliative technique.[22] It can be used to stop
urine leakage (in patients with fistulae due to malignant disease or irradiation),
or, in combination with long-term PCN drainage, to relieve severely painful
micturition due to malignant disease. Coils, tissue adhesive (butyl-2-cyanoacryl-
ate), balloons (detachable or non-detachable) or nylon plugs are placed in the
ureter via an antegradely placed catheter. Alternatively, electrocautery may be
used to occlude the ureter, and an extralumenal approach via the retroperitoneum
leading to ureteric clamping has also been described. Permanent drainage is
secured via a PCN. Experience remains limited and presently the preferred
technique is to use detachable balloons in combination with PCN drainage.
Ureteric occlusion should only be considered in patients with a short life
expectancy and distressing symptoms. The indications, contraindications and
complications of transrenal ureteric occlusion are listed in Table 11.5.

Table 11.5 Transrenal ureteric
occlusion: indications, contraindications
and complications

Indications
Leakage from fistula:
  malignant
  radiation-induced
Painful micturition in malignancy

Contraindications
Long life expectancy
Contraindications to PCN

Complications
Complications of PCN

Prostatic balloon dilatation and stenting

This is another area being explored. Using the techniques practised in the ureter, stenoses of the prostatic urethra are now being treated. Although both of these procedures are now available, the role of balloon dilatation is uncertain and experience with prostatic stenting is limited. Encouraging results are, however, being seen with obstructive symptoms. It is likely that this field will expand during the next few years.

REFERENCES

1. Pitt HA, Cameron JL, Postier RG *et al*. Factors affecting mortality in biliary tract surgery. *American Journal of Surgery* 1981; **141**: 66–71.
2. Blumgart LH, Hadjis N, Benjamin IS *et al*. Surgical approaches to cholangiocarcinoma at confluence of hepatic ducts. *Lancet* 1984; **i**: 66–70.
3. Dowsett JF, Williams SJ, Hatfield ARW *et al*. Endoscopic management of low biliary obstruction due to unresectable primary pancreaticobiliary malignancy – a review of 463 consecutive cases. *Gastroenterology* 1989; **96**: A129.
4. Robertson DAF, Hackin, CN, Birch SJ *et al*. Experience with a combined percutaneous and endoscopic approach to stent insertion in malignant obstructive jaundice. *Lancet* 1987; **ii**: 1449–52.
5. Hacking CN. Percutaneous techniques for the relief of jaundice. In: Johnson CD, Imrie CW eds. *Pancreatic disease: Progress and prospects*. Berlin: Springer-Verlag, 1991: 29–43.
6. Adam A, Chetty N, Roddie M *et al*. Self-expandable stainless steel endoprostheses for the treatment of malignant bile duct obstruction. *American Journal of Radiology* 1991; **156**: 321–5.
7. Chuang VP, Soo CS, Wallace S. Ivalon embolization in abdominal neoplasms. *American Journal of Roentgenology* 1981; **136**: 729–33.
8. Cloux ME, Lee RGL, Duszlak EJ *et al*. Peripheral hepatic artery embolization for primary and secondary hepatic neoplasms. *Radiology* 1983; **147**: 407–11.
9. Tarver DS, Birch SJ. Life-threatening hypercalcaemia secondary to pancreatic tumour secreting parathyroid hormone-related protein – successful control by hepatic artery embolization. *Clinical Radiology* 1992; **3**: 204–5.
10. Odurny A, Birch SJ. Hepatic arterial embolisation in patients with metastatic carcinoid tumours. *Clinical Radiology* 1985; **36**: 597–602.

11. Lanigan D, Jurriaans E, Hammonds JC, Wells IP, Choa RG. The current status of emobilization in renal cell carcinoma – a survey of local and national practice. *Clinical Radiology* 1992; **3**: 176–8.
12. Ohnishi K, Tsuchiya S, Nakayama T *et al.* Arterial chemoembolisation of hepatocellular carcinoma with mitomycin C microcapsules. *Radiology* 1984; **152**: 51–5.
13. Takayasu K, Shima Y, Muramatsu Y *et al.* Hepatocellular carcinoma. Treatment with intraarterial iodized oil with and without chemotherapeutic agents. *Radiology* 1987; **162**: 345–51.
14. Bretagne JF, Raoul JL, Bourgnet P *et al.* Hepatic artery injection of I-131-labelled Lipiodol. *Radiology* 1988; **168**: 547.
15. Hind RE, Loizidou M, Perring S *et al.* Biodistribution of Lipiodol following hepatic arterial injection. *British Journal of Surgery* 1992; *79*: 952–4.
16. Banner MP. Interventional radiology in the urinary tract. *Current Imaging* 1989; **1**: 10–20.
17. Cope C. Percutaneous interventional uroradiology. Cook Incorporated, *Atlas of Interventional Radiology* 1989; **11**: 1–22.
18. Nurse ED, Woodhouse CRJ, Kellett MJ, Dearnley DP. Percutaneous removal of upper tract tumours. *World Journal of Urology* 1989; **7**: 131–4.
19. Beckmann CF, Roth RA, Bighle W III. Dilatation of beneign ureteric strictures. *Radiology* 1989; **172**: 437–41.
20. Lang EK. Transluminal dilatation of ureteropelvic junction strictures and strictures at ureteroneocystectomy sites. *Radiologic Clinics of North America* 1986; **24**: 601–14.
21. Mitty HA, Train JS, Dan SJ. Placement of ureteral stents by antegrade and retrograde techniques. *Radiologic Clinics of North America* 1986; **24**: 587–600.
22. Gunther RW, Klose K, Alken P, Bohl J. Transrenal ureteral occlusion using a detachable balloon. *Radiology* 1982; **142**: 521–3.

CHAPTER 12

Calcium and skeletal complications of cancer

ROBERT E COLEMAN————————————————————

INTRODUCTION

Bone metastases are common in advanced cancer, representing 99 per cent of malignant tumours in bone, and most clinicians will be familiar with the symptoms and problems they cause. The middle-aged woman with a past history of breast cancer who develops bone pain due to destructive metastatic involvement of the skeleton, steadily increasing disability over several years and culminating in premature death is all too common. Indeed, at any one time there are 15 000–20 000 women in the UK with bone metastases from breast cancer. Consider also that 85 per cent of men with advanced prostate cancer and 65 per cent of patients with lung cancer will develop skeletal metastases and the clinical importance of metastatic bone disease becomes obvious.

In general, the treatment of bone metastases is aimed at palliating symptoms, with cure only rarely a realistic aim (e.g. lymphoma), and dependent on the underlying disease.[1] However, the clinical course of patients with metastatic bone disease can be long, and although, the prognosis of patients with bone metastases from lung cancer is but a few months, the median survival of women with metastatic bone disease from breast cancer is 2 years,[2] while up to 20 per cent of men with advanced prostate cancer will survive 5 years.[3] In these conditions particularly, effective palliative therapy is essential to maintain a good quality and useful life.

External beam radiotherapy remains the treatment of choice for localized bone pain.[4] Rapid pain relief can usually be expected from a short course with minimal side-effects. For tumours responsive to hormonal or cytotoxic agents appropriate regimens should be prescribed and, especially in breast and prostate cancers, may produce useful control of disease. However, drug resistance almost always develops leading to progressive disease and the associated morbidity of skeletal destruction. Orthopaedic intervention may be necessary for the structural complications of bone destruction and some, although by no means all patients with bone metastases, will develop hypercalcaemia requiring specific treatment.

Underlying all the morbidity associated with skeletal metastases is the presence of an increased rate of bone resorption, mediated largely by the osteoclast.[5] Until recently, the management of osteolytic lesions and hypercalcaemia associated with malignancy has been far from ideal due to the toxicity or limited efficacy of the available therapies. In recent years, however, the bisphosphonates, agents with potent and sustained inhibitory effects on osteoclastic bone resorption, have emerged as effective treatments for hypercalcaemia[6–8] and appear extremely promising in the management of osteolysis associated with malignancy.[9–11]

NORMAL BONE METABOLISM

Shaping of the skeleton and the build-up of bone mass occurs during childhood and early adult life, while throughout adult life, within focal sites scattered throughout the skeleton, microscopic quantities of old bone are being replaced. This is an orderly process, essential for bone strength and occurring in response to mechanical stress, mediated by a complex interaction of hormones, paracrine growth factors and cytokines.[12] Bone resorption is mediated by the osteoclast, while bone formation requires the presence and function of osteoblasts.[13]

Under normal circumstances and at any one time, 80–95 per cent of the adult bone surface is in a quiescent state and covered by residing osteoblasts, while the rest is involved in various stages of the remodelling cycle. The total duration of a remodelling cycle in young adults is estimated to be around 200 days. After completion of bone formation, the lacunae created by the osteoclasts are then filled with newly deposited bone. If the osteoblasts have deposited exactly the same amount of bone as has been previously removed by the osteoclasts the remodelling cycle is in balance. In the situation of an imbalance of remodelling, a remodelling cycle will end with either a small gain in bone (positive balance) or, as is more frequently the case in malignancy, a small loss of bone (negative balance).[14]

The skeleton contains approximately 99 per cent of the total body calcium and in normal health, it is the precise hormonal regulation of the tiny extraosseus fraction which ensures homeostasis. As part of the lifestyle of bone and to facilitate bone turnover, a daily exchange of about 500 mg of calcium occurs between bone and extracellular fluid. The daily amount of calcium absorbed from the gut, primarily under the control of 1,25-dihydroxy-vitamin D, is roughly equivalent to the 150–200 mg of calcium that is excreted by the kidneys every day.

The kidney is the organ principally responsible for the acute control of calcium, and filters approximately 10 g of calcium in 24 hours.[15] A total of 98 per cent is reabsorbed, 65 per cent in the proximal tubule, 25 per cent in the ascending limb of the loop of Henle, and 10 per cent in the distal tubule. Only distal tubular reabsorption is controlled by parathyroid hormone (PTH), through an increase in adenylate cyclase activity which allows fine tuning of the renal handling of calcium. Renal calcium excretion can, if necessary, increase to about 600 mg/day. However, if the filtered load of calcium increases to more than 3–5 times normal levels, the kidney's capacity to excrete a sufficient quantity of calcium is overwhelmed.

PATHOPHYSIOLOGY AND CLINICAL FEATURES

Bone metastases

Bone metastases are especially common from carcinomas arising in the breast, prostate and lung, and these three tumours alone account for 80 per cent of patients with bone metastases.[16] These cancers, plus multiple myeloma and carcinomas of the thyroid and kidney demonstrate a phenomoneon known as osteotropism, meaning they possess an extraordinary affinity for bone. In breast cancer this correlates with positive steroid receptors,[2] and in prostate cancer with histological grade.

Irrespective of the tissue of origin of the cancer, the distribution of bone metastases is predominantly in the axial skeleton, particularly the spine, pelvis and ribs, rather than the appendicular skeleton, although lesions in the proximal femora and humeri are not uncommon. This distribution is similar to the red bone marrow in which slow blood flow possibly assists attachment of metastatic cells.

Much progress has been achieved in understanding the mechanism by which tumour cells cause invasion and destruction of bone (Fig. 12.1). Tumour cells can be seen in resorption bays on bone surfaces and may erode bone directly by the production of proteolytic enzymes. However, much more important is the indirect action of cancer cells, with the increased bone resorption and formation which occurs in metastatic bone disease resulting from the activation of normal bone cells. Numerous studies have demonstrated that malignant cells secrete many of the factors known to stimulate the proliferation and activity of osteo-clasts resulting in osteolysis.[17–19] These include transforming growth factors, prostaglandins, tumour necrosis factors and parathyroid hormone-related protein.

It is now generally accepted that osteoclast activation is the key step in the establishment and growth of all bone metastases, while recognizing that stimu-lation of osteoblastic activity occurs also. In some cancers, particularly multiple myeloma and most breast cancers, osteolysis predominates although areas of new bone formation are usually identifiable histologically even if not visible on plain radiographs. In others, osteosclerosis occurs where either new bone is laid down away from the normal resorption bays and/or condensation of new bone occurs within the infiltrated bone marrow stroma. However, increased osteolysis is also present and presumably prostate cancer cells have a dimorphic effect on bone.

It is the predominance of lysis or sclerosis which gives rise to the character-istic radiographic appearances of bone metastases. When bone resorption pre-dominates, focal bone destruction occurs and bone metastases have a lytic appearance. Conversely, in bone metastases associated with increased osteoblast activity (e.g. prostate cancer) the lesions appear sclerotic on X-ray. Even when one element predominates both processes are greatly accelerated in the sur-rounding bone.[18] This is most apparent in the appropriately termed 'mixed' lesions, seen most commonly in breast cancer, in which both lytic and sclerotic components are clearly visible.

Clinically, lytic bone metastases are much more frequent and cause most morbidity. Pathological fractures and hypercalcaemia are seen less often in

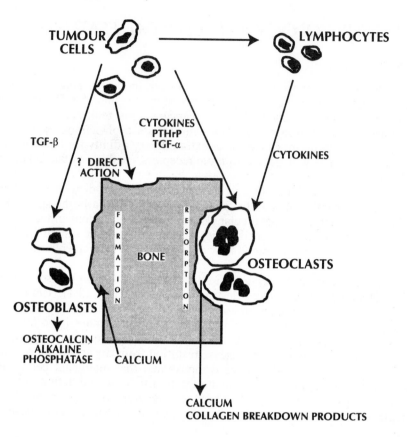

Fig. 12.1. Pathophysiology of bone metasatases. Cancer cells stimulate bone cell function through the production of locally acting paracrine factors. PTHrP, parathyroid-related protein; TGF, transforming growth factor.

patients with sclerotic lesions, while pain when present, may be caused by a minor lytic component which is difficult to demonstrate on conventional radiographs. Bone pain is not a feature of conditions such as osteopetrosis or myelofibrosis where bone sclerosis occurs but osteolysis is absent.

Hypercalcaemia of malignancy

Hypercalcaemia is probably the most common metabolic complication of malignant disease and is clinically important because of the associated morbidity. If left untreated, moderate to severe hypercalcaemia (serum calcium 3.0 mmol/l) causes a number of unpleasant side-effects related to dysfunction of the gastrointestinal tract, kidneys and central nervous system. With even greater elevations in serum calcium, renal function and conscious level deteriorate, and death ultimately ensues as the result of cardiac arrhythmias due to severe hypercalcaemia and acute renal failure.

Whilst there are many similarities between the biochemical features of humoral hypercalcaemia of malignancy and hyperparathyroidism, these dis-

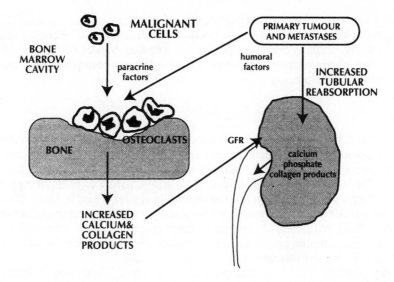

Fig. 12.2. Mechanisms of hypercalcaemia. Local osteolysis and humoral effects often coexist.

orders are seldom mistaken for one another in clinical practice. Patients with cancer-associated hypercalcaemia almost invariably have clinically advanced tumours by the time hypercalcaemia has developed; thus, the diagnosis of hypercalcaemia of malignancy is usually apparent at the bedside or with the aid of a few simple screening investigations. Regrettably however, physicians not trained in the treatment and support of cancer patients regularly mistake the symptoms of malignant hypercalcaemia for those of cancer disease and/or treatment.

Hypercalcaemia is not distributed evenly in the cancer population and is most frequent in squamous cell carcinomas of the lung, adenocarcinomas of the breast and kidney, and in certain haematological malignancies, particularly multiple myeloma and lymphoma. These differences relate in part to a diversity in the pattern of bone-metastatic involvement, but more importantly, they are due to the selective release of humoral hypercalcaemic factors by some tumours.

In most cases, hypercalcaemic cancer patients have increased osteoclastic bone resorption, either multifocally such as in the case of myeloma or metastatic breast carcinoma or systemically, stimulated by parathyroid hormone-related peptides (PTHrP)[19] and possible other tumour products. While often associated with metastatic bone disease, many instances of cancer-associated hypercalcaemia are due to the systemic release of these bone-resorbing humoral factors rather than local bone dissolution (Fig. 12.2).

Local osteolytic hypercalcaemia is attributed to excessive hydroxyapatite-calcium release by tumour metastases. Prostaglandins, growth factors which stimulate prostaglandin function, and cytokines, particularly interleukin 1 and tumour necrosis factors, appear to be involved in local osteoclast activation although the precise contribution of each factor remains to be defined.

Additional mechanisms are important in some situations.[20] The most important is impaired renal perfusion due to dehydration. Calcium is a potent diuretic causing salt and water loss and depletion of the intravascular space.[21] In myeloma, renal impairment may also result from deposition of Bence–Jones proteins. Finally, some lymphomas produce active metabolites of vitamin D which may cause hypercalcaemia through increased bone resorption and intestinal absorption of calcium.

Pain

Pain is the principal symptom of bone destruction resulting from stimulation of pain receptors in the periosteum and endosteum. Non-steroidal anti-inflammatory agents and opiates are often necessary for general relief of pain and radiotherapy for local treatment. The ideal dose and schedule of radiotherapy are not known with certainty but recent studies suggest that a single large fraction or short intensive courses of treatment are as effective as conventional fractionation for short-term pain relief.[4] However, bone regeneration is inhibited by large fractions of irradiation particularly if in excess of 800 cGy, the toxicity is greater and the need for retreatment may be more frequent.[22]

Many patients have multiple painful bony sites. Wide-field external beam irradiation can be useful or alternatively therapeutic radiopharmaceuticals such as strontium-89 are now available. Strontium-89 imitates calcium and is preferentially taken up at sites of new bone formation.[23] It has been shown to localize efficiently at the sites of prostatic bone metastases and through selective beta-particle irradiation at these sites provides pain relief in up to 80 per cent of patients. The response lasts for an average period of 6 months whilst causing only mild haematological effects.[24]

Pathological fractures

Metastatic destruction of bone reduces its load-bearing capabilities. Microfractures cause pain and rib fractures are common. Vertebral collapse frequently occurs resulting in loss of height, kyphoscoliosis and a degree of restrictive lung disease. However, it is fracture of a long bone or fracture–dislocation and epidural extension of tumour in the spine which causes most disability. Because the development of a fracture is so devastating to a cancer patient, increasing emphasis is being placed on attempts to predict metastases at risk of fracture and the use of pre-emptive surgery.

Fractures are common through lytic metastases and weight-bearing bones, the proximal femora being the most commonly affected sites. Damage to both trabecular and cortical bone is structurally important but it is the relevance of cortical destruction which is most clearly appreciated. Over the years several radiological features have been identified which may predict imminent fracture. Fracture is likely if lesions are large, predominantly lytic and erode the cortex. Prophylactic internal fixation is the treatment of choice for such lesions, followed by radiotherapy. Untreated pathological fractures rarely heal and although radiotherapy may achieve local tumour control, bony union remains unlikely. Radiotherapy inhibits chondrogenesis, a prerequisite for fracture healing, and with large areas of bone destruction there may be insufficient matrix remaining for adequate repair. Pathological fractures are not only a manifestation of terminal disease and orthopaedic surgery is usually the treatment of choice and certainly the only modality likely to restore mobility as well as relieve pain.[25]

When there is greater than a 50 per cent vertebral collapse, compression of the spinal cord becomes more likely. Invasion of the epidural space with compression of the spinal cord and nerve roots necessitates urgent corticosteroids and radiotherapy or surgical intervention to reduce permanent neurological damage. Debate persists over the relative merits of surgery and radiotherapy in this situation. However, for patients with spinal instability which causes extreme pain on movement, surgical spinal stabilization can be dramatically effective.[25]

THE BISPHOSPHONATES

Some 25 years ago the presence of inorganic pyrophosphate was discovered in plasma and urine and shown to impair the formation and aggregation of calcium phosphate crystals. Pyrophosphate is not, however, clinically useful because of its failure to act when given orally and its rapid hydrolysis when given parenterally. One exception has been dental calculus, pyrophosphate now being the main antitartar agent used worldwide in toothpastes.[26]

The search for analogues which would display similar physicochemical activity but resist the enzymatic hydrolysis and metabolism led to the discovery of the bisphosphonates. Monophosphonates and bisphosphonates have been known for some time through various industrial applications, amongst others as water softeners. The double phosphonate group on the terminal carbon atom is common to all bisphosphonates and confers a strong binding affinity for calcified bone matrix. All bisphosphonates bind to bone mineral and through effects on the surface charge on hydroxyapatite, exert a marked physicochemical effect on hydroxyapatite crystal physiology. Whilst this form of chemical interaction may account for the effect of some bisphosphonates on bone mineralization and even impair the ability of osteoclasts to 'recognize' bone mineral binding sites, direct cellular mechanisms are probably more important in explaining the effect of bisphosphonates on osteoclastic bone resorption.[26]

The degree of activity of individual bisphosphonates varies greatly from compound to compound according to the length and substitution of the aliphatic carbon backbone. Amino derivatives such as pamidronate, with an amino group at the end of the side-chain, are extremely active.[27] Studies in murine tumours have shown the bisphosphonates have neither a direct antitumour activity, nor an effect on the efficacy of conventional anticancer drugs. All effects on bone resorption, tumour growth in bone, metastasis formation and direct invasion of bone are attributable to the effects of osteoclast activity.[27]

The effect of bisphosphonates on the osteoclast is due to a number of factors, including a direct toxic effect of ingested bisphosphonate (particularly clodronate) on the resorbing osteoclast,[28] an inhibition of the differentiation of osteoclast precursors into mature osteoclasts, disruption of the chemotactic gradient between bone and osteoclasts and interference with the recognition and attachment of mature osteoclasts to the bone surface.[29]

Clinical interest results from the extremely firm binding of bisphosphonates to hydroxyapatite in bone. Consequently, they have revolutionized radionuclide bone scanning, enabling sensitive localization of bone pathology and some, through their inhibition of bone resorption, have exciting therapeutic properties. Three bisphosphonates are currently licensed for therapeutic use: etidronate (ethane-1-hydroxy-1,1-bisphosphonate; Didronel), clodronate (dichloromethane bisphosphonate; Loron, Bonefos) and pamidronate (3-amino-1-hydroxypropylidene-1,1-bisphosphonate; Aredia).

Following intravenous administration of a bisphosphonate, around 25 per cent of the injected dose is excreted by the kidney and the remainder is taken up by bone. All bisphosphonates suffer from poor bioavailability and at present only oral formulations of clodronate and etidronate are commercially available. They must be taken on an empty stomach as they bind to calcium in the diet and can cause gastrointestinal toxicities such as nausea, vomiting, indigestion and diarrhoea. Oral pamidronate is still in development but in preliminary studies, a well-tolerated enteric coated capsule has proved effective in inhibiting osteolysis despite the expected poor absorption.[30]

In general, the bisphosphonates are safe providing they are administered as a slow infusion. Rapid intravenous injection runs the risk of acute hypocalcaemia, renal failure and thrombophlebitis. Pamidronate may cause an acute-phase response following the first infusion manifested by transient fever and lymphopenia but this is rarely of clinical consequence.[27] Anecdotal reports of renal impairment following high doses of clodronate and etidronate exist but nephrotoxicity is not a clinically important problem with any of the available compounds.

MANAGEMENT OF HYPERCALCAEMIA OF MALIGNANCY

Non-bisphosphonate treatment

In recent years, the therapeutic options for controlling hypercalcaemia have increased considerably with the development of new compounds. However, an understanding of the older, more traditional therapies is helpful in order to appreciate the advantages of the bisphosphonates in the management of hypercalcaemia of malignancy. The basic principles of management involve rehydration to restore glomerular function and the use of drugs to inhibit osteoclastic bone resorption. The scientific basis for some treatments is lacking,[31] and recommendations have frequently been based on small non-randomized studies that were conducted before adequate rehydration of the patient had been achieved and confounded by concomitant anticancer therapy.

Occasionally the secretion of humoral factors by a primary tumour results in hypercalcaemia. In such cases the serum level may be corrected by surgical removal of the tumour. Typically however, the malignancy is advanced and treatment is palliative. Immobilization should be avoided where possible as this may precipitate hypercalcaemia, since the lack of weight-bearing may induce increased osteoclastic and reduced osteoblastic activity.

Absorption of calcium from the gut is usually reduced in patients with hypercalcaemia of malignancy. Cancer patients are frequently malnourished and should be encouraged to eat what they like, when they like, irrespective of the food's calcium content. The only exception where restriction of dairy products seems sensible is in the rare patient with lymphoma (usually T-cell) associated with raised levels of vitamin D metabolites.

Dehydration is an inevitable feature of symptomatic hypercalcaemia. As serum calcium levels rise, the function of the distal renal tubule becomes progressively impaired and further sodium loss occurs. The average sodium deficit is about 10 mmol/kg body weight and saline rehydration remains essential to replace this loss, restore glomerular function and increase urinary excretion of calcium.[21]

Rehydration with 3–4 l/day of 0.9 per cent normal saline over 48 hours will relieve many of the symptoms of hypercalcaemia but is rarely effective in totally controlling hypercalcaemia. Furthermore, unless effective specific treatment is available for the causative tumour or the underlying accelerated bone resorption inhibited, hypercalcaemia will usually recur. Diuretics are frequently prescribed but are usually not necessary, while thiazide diuretics actually increase tubular reabsorption of calcium and therefore should be avoided. Although loop diuretics do increase saline-induced urinary calcium excretion, large volumes of saline have to be given to prevent intravascular dehydration necessitating close haemodynamic monitoring. Although this approach may be effective it is labour-intensive, potentially hazardous and recurrence of hypercalcaemia is to be expected.

In the past the control of malignancy-associated hypercalcaemia has rested principally with the use of calcitonin and mithramycin as inhibitors of osteoclast action. Previous studies using agents such as non-steroidal anti-inflammatory agents and corticosteroids, have yielded disappointing results in cancer-associated hypercalcaemia. Corticosteroids have been widely used in the treatment of hypercalcaemia but their effects are unpredictable. Some patients, particularly those with steroid-responsive tumours, namely lymphomas, multiple myeloma and the occasional patient with breast cancer, respond well with serum calcium reaching a nadir within one week. However, in most solid tumours steroids add little to the response achieved by intravenous rehydration.[32]

Intravenous phosphate is a rapidly effective means of correcting hypercalcaemia associated with malignancy and other disorders, but its effect is transient and may be associated with serious adverse reactions such as circulatory collapse and acute renal failure. It is now reserved for refractory life-threatening hypercalcaemia where the equivalent of 1.5–3 g (50–100 mmol) of elemental phosphorous is infused over 12–24 hours. Oral phosphate can be useful, but causes gastrointestinal side-effects in 50 per cent of patients.

Calcitonin has a dual action on calcium homeostasis and in addition to its rapid inhibitory effect on bone resorption, promotes urinary calcium excretion. Despite this, calcitonin has proved disappointing with a hypocalcaemic effect which is often incomplete and transient, waning after 2–3 days of therapy despite continued administration. *In vitro* studies have suggested that inhibition of bone resorption could be sustained by concomitant administration of glucocorticoids, but clinical results have been inconsistent.[33]

Before the introduction of the bisphosphonates, mithramycin was probably the most reliably effective agent. Through a direct cytotoxic effect on the osteoclast, a single intravenous dose of 1-1.5 mg will usually lower serum calcium levels within 72 hours, but rebound hypercalcaemia typically occurs 5–10 days later.[34] Multiple doses are more effective and can control serum calcium for several weeks. However, the associated nausea and vomiting, and bone marrow, renal and hepatic toxicities usually limit the duration of repeated treatment.

Recently gallium nitrate has been shown to control hypercalcaemia and is now approved for use in the USA. The mechanism of action is poorly understood but randomized comparative studies have shown gallium nitrate to be superior to both calcitonin[35] and etidronate.[36] Gallium is nephrotoxic at high dose and has to be given in small intravenous doses over several days, features which limit its suitability for widespread use.

Bisphosphonate treatment of hypercalcaemia

The importance of accelerated osteoclastic bone resorption in the pathogenesis of cancer-associated hypercalcaemia has been stressed earlier. All three commercially available bisphosphonates are effective for the treatment of hypercalcaemia[6–8] and are now the agents of first choice in the management of this component of hypercalcaemia. The inhibitory effect of the bisphosphonates on bone resorption and their calcium-lowering effects depend on the initial plasma calcium level and the total dose used.[37–39] The decrease of plasma calcium is generally small on the first day of treatment, but becomes greater thereafter. On average, normocalcaemia occurs 3–7 days (median 4 days) after the start of treatment.

Severe hypercalcaemia requires higher doses for normalization than moderate hypercalcaemia. In patients with severe life-threatening hypercalcaemia, the rate of improvement may be suboptimal at the beginning of treatment. In such cases, combined therapy with a rapidly acting agent such as calcitonin may be preferable.[40] Transient hypocalcaemia may be encountered after intravenous bisphosphonate therapy. This is mostly asymptomatic and occurs between 2 and 14 days after treatment and lasts for a few days. This may result from the suppressed plasma levels of parathyroid hormone in these patients and disturbed calcium homeostasis. While orally administered bisphosphonates are also efficacious,[38] this mode of administration has been quickly supplanted by the intravenous route partly because nausea and vomiting are common in hypercalcaemic cancer patients, thus limiting the value of an orally administered drug, but also because of the poor intestinal absorption of the bisphosphonates.

An important point to be aware of when treating hypercalcaemia of malignancy with bisphosphonates is that these drugs are only effective against the bone-resorptive component of hypercalcaemia. The renal components of hypercalcaemia, including impairment of glomerular filtration (GFR) due to dehydration and increased renal tubular reabsorption of calcium due to sodium depletion and/or hormonal factors must be treated in their own right. For the above reasons, rehydration remains an important adjunct to bisphosphonate treatment, particularly in the initial stages of therapy when dehydration and renal impairment are prominent features.

Initial studies of intravenously administered bisphosphonates generally employed multidose regimens. More recent studies have shown, however, that single infusions of pamidronate or clodronate are equally effective in the control of hypercalcaemia of malignancy.[41–44] The efficacy of the bisphosphonates appears to be unrelated to the duration of infusion, with a 2-hour infusion of pamidronate as efficacious as infusion over 24 hours.[44]

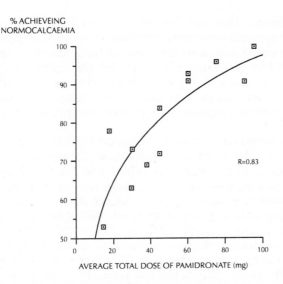

Fig. 12.3. Dose–response relationship for pamidronate in the treatment of hypercalcaemia of malignancy. The proportion of patients achieving normocalcaemia is plotted against the total dose administered. (Data obtained from ref. 27.)

Dose-ranging studies have demonstrated that a dose/efficacy relationship exists, although the clinical importance of this has been questioned. Detailed and systematic dose–response studies have only been performed with pamidronate.[37,38] In addition, review of all published studies of pamidronate for hypercalcaemia provides indirect evidence of a dose–response relationship. When the dose used in each study is plotted against the number of patients achieving normocalcaemia there is a striking relationship ($r = 0.83$; $P < 0.001$) between the total dose and the success rate, with a 90–95 per cent success rate corresponding to a dose of around 80 mg (Fig. 12.3).

The duration of normocalcaemia following a single bisphosphonate treatment has been difficult to define because of concomitant anticancer therapy. In the studies performed with pamidronate to date, recurrences of hypercalcaemia were observed 1–8 weeks (median 2–3 weeks) after treatment, their onset appearing to be relatively early after small doses.[6,41] The duration of the effect is probably dose-dependent and also related to a certain degree on the variation in skeletal uptake of the bisphosphonate. The wide variation in duration of response probably reflects also the varying rates of tumour-induced osteolysis. In a small study of patients with osteolysis from breast cancer but without hypercalcaemia, the duration of response to a single infusion of pamidronate 60 mg was investigated.[45] A remarkable variation in effect was seen with the excretion of urinary calcium suppressed to within the normal range for less than 3 weeks to more than 10 weeks.

Only a few comparative studies with other treatments have been performed. Sleeboom *et al.* compared pamidronate – given as daily 15 mg infusions over 2 hours – with volume repletion.[46] Pamidronate was clearly superior to simple volume repletion and, in parallel with control of serum calcium, also improved renal function. In a randomized study pamidronate was found to be significantly better than both mithramycin or corticosteroids and calcitonin in controlling the hypercalcaemia associated with a wide variety of malignant tumours.[47] Calcitonin/corticosteroids had the fastest effect but this was incomplete, while the duration of normocalcaemia was longest with pamidronate. Similarly, a more recent, larger study comparing pamidronate and mithramycin showed a higher proportion achieving normocalcaemia with pamidronate (88 per cent vs. 41 per cent).[48]

Three randomized comparative studies of different bisphosphonates have been performed. In the first, Ralston and co-workers showed that a single intravenous infusion of pamidronate (30 mg) was more effective in controlling hypercalcaemia than a single intravenous infusion of clodronate (600 mg) or three consecutive daily infusions of etidronate (7.5 mg/kg per day).[49] The superiority of pamidronate was reflected in a slightly more rapid onset of action, a significantly greater reduction in serum calcium levels by day 6 and a more prolonged duration of action. Normocalcaemia was achieved within 6 days in 88 per cent following pamidronate, compared with 38 per cent with clodronate and 31 per cent with etidronate. This study has been criticized for the use of a relatively low dose of clodronate by current standards but the dose of pamidronate was likewise somewhat less than current recommendations would suggest. As a result, a second randomized trial was performed which has shown the superiority of pamidronate over clodronate in patients with tumor-induced hypercalcaemia, not only in terms of success rate, but more importantly in the duration of normocalcaemia. The median duration of action of clodronate was 14 days compared with 28 days for pamidronate.[50] In a third study pamidronate was compared with etidronate. One week after starting treatment, 58 per cent of pamidronate vs. 27 per cent of etidronate recipients were normocalcaemic.[51]

Published experience of the continuing efficacy of bisphosphonates in patients with relapsing hypercalcaemia is limited. In those patients who were retreated the antihypercalcaemic effect was reported to be generally good.[52] However, the possibility of a weaker response with an increased number of treatments in advanced cancer can be a problem. In view of the long half-life of the bisphosphonates in bone, the reason for this apparent decrease in efficacy is as yet unclear. An increasing influence of tubular reabsorption of calcium, direct destruction of bone by cancer cells which is independent of osteoclast activation or further, as yet unspecified, pathogenetic factors in malignant hypercalcaemia, may all play a role here.

Finally, it should be emphasized that bisphosphonate therapy of cancer-associated hypercalcaemia is, in most cases, an essential palliative measure to relieve symptoms of hypercalcaemia. Where possible, specific antitumour therapy such as surgery, radiotherapy, chemotherapy and hormone therapy, should also be instituted as this provides the key to long-term control of the tumour itself and its associated hypercalcaemia.

TUMOUR-INDUCED OSTEOLYSIS

The dominant role of the osteoclast in tumour-induced osteolysis and the ability of bisphosphonates to block osteoclast-mediated bone destruction together form the rationale for its use in patients with bone metastases.[1] Over the past 5–10 years a number of studies have been conducted with three aims: first, the reduction of local osteolysis by the tumour, minimizing structural damage, and reducing morbidity; secondly the prevention of new metastatic lesions; and thirdly, the protection of bone from systemic mediators of resorption, either secreted by the tumour or an extension of normality as occurs in osteoporosis.

The early clinical studies with bisphosphonates for osteolysis were small and uncontrolled but nevertheless, improvements in bone pain and biochemical responses were seen. Since these preliminary reports, a number of phase II studies of intravenous pamidronate every 2–4 weeks as the sole treatment of osteolysis due to bone metastases from advanced breast cancer have been performed.[9,53–56] They have reported similar results indicating strongly that, although these studies were not placebo-controlled, real symptomatic, biochemical and radiological benefit was achieved. In summary, they show that relief of pain occurs in one half of patients and bone healing, as evidenced by sclerosis of lytic lesions, is observed in about one quarter. Selective inhibition of bone resorption occurred with a reduction in urinary calcium excretion but without inhibiting osteoblast activity. Beneficial effects have not been confined to breast cancer. In a preliminary study of pamidronate for bone metastases from hormone-resistant prostate cancer, osteoclast inhibition resulted in pain relief, stabilization of rising tumour markers and improvements in bone biochemistry.[55]

Two large randomized studies of oral bisphosphonate therapy in breast cancer have been published.[10,11] In the first, from Leiden, pamidronate was given in combination with conventional anticancer therapy.[10] One hundred and seventy women with bone metastases from breast cancer were randomized to oral pamidronate or a control group, systemic therapy being left to the discretion of the physician. Impressive results in favour of the combined treatment were seen with a statistically significant reduction in the incidence of hypercalcaemia, pathological fractures and pain and improved quality of life[58] (Table 12.1). The overall complication rate of bone involvement (per 100 patient years) was fifty-two for the treatment group and ninety-four for the control group ($P < 0.01$). However, the lack of a placebo treatment for the control group makes it impossible to exclude the possibilities, albeit unlikely, of observer bias and/or a

Table 12.1 Effect of oral pamidronate on complications of bone metastases

	Event rate per 100 patient years		
	Pamidronate	*Control*	*P value*
Hypercalcaemia	4	15	< 0.05
Fractures	10	22	< 0.01
Pain	21	46	< 0.01
Radiotherapy	22	44	< 0.01
Change in systemic treatment	36	69	< 0.01
Prophylactic surgery	3	5	NS
All complications	52	94	< 0.01

From van Holten-Verzantvoort *et al.*[10]

Table 12.2   Effect of oral clodronate on complications of bone metastases

	Number of episodes		
	Clodronate	*Placebo*	*P value*
Hypercalcaemia	28	52	< 0.01
Deaths from hypercalcaemia	7	17	< 0.05
Vertebral fractures	84	124	< 0.025
Vertebral deformity	168	252	< 0.001
All events (per 100 patient years)	219	305	< 0.001

From Paterson *et al.*[11]

placebo effect. A second, more recent placebo-controlled study with clodronate also reports an impressive reduction in the frequency of hypercalcaemia, vertebral fractures and deformities (Table 12.2).[11]

The results of double-blind randomized placebo-controlled trials of intravenous pamidronate in breast cancer patients with lytic bone metastases have recently been completed.[59,60] The results were particularly impressive in the chemotherapy trial which included 382 patients. The mean skeletal morbidity rate (number of skeletal-related events per year) was 2.1 in the pamidronate group compared to 3.3 in the placebo group ($P < 0.005$). There was a significant reduction in the proportion of patients having any skeletal-related event, in the number of non-vertebral pathological fractures, and in the proportion of patients having radiation or surgery to bone.

Three large randomized placebo-controlled trials in multiple myeloma have been published.[61,62,63] In the first trial in 350 patients with newly diagnosed myeloma, it was shown that 2.4 g of clodronate daily for 2 years resulted in a significant reduction in the proportion of patients developing progression of osteolytic bone lesions (24 per cent versus 12 per cent).[61] Subsequently, a trial in 548 patients evaluated the efficacy of 1600 mg daily of clodronate given at the time of diagnosis. The reduction in skeletal complication rate was not observed initially, but became apparent when the effect of chemotherapy wore off. At the time of disease progression, there were fewer patients with increased back pain or deterioration in performance status, and fewer new vertebral fractures.[62]

The efficacy of intravenous pamidronate was convincingly demonstrated in a double-blind, placebo-controlled trial of 392 patients with myeloma who received either 90 mg pamidronate or placebo infusions monthly in addition to their antimyeloma chemotherapy regimen. The proportion of patients developing any skeletal-related event (defined as a pathological fracture, irradiation of bone or surgery on bone, hypercalcaemia or spinal cord compression) was significantly ($P < 0.001$) smaller in the pamidronate than in the placebo-group, 24 per cent versus 41 per cent. Quality of life score, performance status, pain score, incidence of pathologic fractures and the need for radiotherapy were all favorably affected by pamidronate therapy.[63]

Several small randomized studies have also been reported. Elomaa *et al.* randomly assigned thirty-four patients with progressive bone metastases from breast cancer to receive either oral clodronate or placebo in addition to their most recent systemic therapy. Those who received oral clodronate required less analgesics, had fewer requirements for radiotherapy or episodes of hypercalcaemia, and developed fewer new bone lesions than patients receiving palcebo.[64] A study in multiple myeloma, also with clodronate, showed a reduction in pain, fewer new lytic lesions and a non-significant improvement in survival in the bisphosphonate-treated group but again, the study was not placebo-controlled.[65] Two negative randomized studies have been reported. A randomized double-blind placebo-controlled study of etidronate in fifty-seven patients with hormone-resistant prostate cancer showed no advantage for oral etidronate in terms of symptom response or analgesic requirements.[66] Similarly, a preliminary report of aminoglutethimide as endocrine treatment with or without intravenous pamidronate for bone metastases from advanced breast cancer has failed to show any influence of pamidronate on the course of bone metastases over and above that achieved with endocrine therapy alone.[67]

CONCLUSIONS

What conclusions can be drawn about the use of bisphosphonates for the treatment of tumour-induced osteolysis? The bisphosphonates, particularly pamidronate and clodronate, are clearly the treatment of choice for hypercalcaemia of malignancy. In addition, useful palliation with parenteral pamidronate for patients with advanced bone disease is a consistent finding. Somewhat surprisingly, the bone healing observed with parenteral pamidronate has yet to be reported following continuous oral therapy with any of the three currently available compounds. New more potent bisphosphonate analogues are in early clinical development and may be more effective. However, it may be that despite the obvious convenience of oral bisphosphonates, high-dose intermittent intravenous treatment is superior.

About 20 per cent of all patients with advanced breast cancer will have metastatic disease confined to the skeleton and symptoms of bone destruction. For those patients who have disease which has become resistant to endocrine treatment, bisphosphonates are a non-toxic alternative to chemotherapy. Likewise, patients with endocrine-resistant prostate cancer who commonly have disease confined to the skeleton may benefit from a similar approach.

Attention is now turning to the possibility of preventing metastatic bone disease. Osteoclast activation by malignant cells is a fundamental step in the development of all bone metastases and inhibition of osteolysis by bisphosphonates has successfully inhibited the development of bone metastases in animals.[21] In the light of these findings, clinical trials of adjuvant bisphosphonate therapy in patients at high risk of developing bone metastases are just beginning (Table 12.3). It is hoped that the results of the current trials will determine the true value of this potentially exciting new development in the management of advanced malignancy.

Table 12.3 The current role of bisphosphonates in malignancy

Hypercalcaemia	Treatment of choice
Tumour-induced osteolysis	Useful palliation as single agent & contribution to systemic therapy
Prevention of bone metastases	Trials underway
Protection of the normal skeleton	Possible role in post-oophorectomy/ cytotoxic-induced castration

REFERENCES

1. Dodwell DJ, Howell A. The systemic treatment of bone metastases. In: Rubens RD, Fogelman I eds. *Bone metastases – diagnosis and treatment.* London: Springer-Verlag, 1991: 121–42.
2. Coleman RE, Rubens RD. The clinical course of bone metastases from breast cancer. *British Journal of Cancer* 1987; **55**: 61–6.
3. Nesbit RM, Baum WC. Endocrine control of prostatic carcinoma: clinical and statistical survey of 1818 cases. *Journal of the National Cancer Institute* 1984; **68**: 507–17.
4. Price P, Hoskin PJ, Easton D *et al.* Low-dose single fraction radiotherapy in the treatment of metastatic bone pain. *Radiotherapy & Oncology* 1988; **6**: 247–55.
5. Scher HI, Yagoda A. Bone metastases: pathogenesis, treatment and rationale for use of resorption inhibitors. *American Journal of Medicine* 1987; **82** (Suppl. 2A): 6–28.
6. Body JJ, Borkowski A, Cleeren A *et al.* Treatment of malignancy-associated hypercalcaemia with intravenous aminohydroxypropylidene bisphosphonate (APD). *Journal of Clinical Oncology* 1986; **4**: 1177–83.
7. Hasling C, Charles P, Mosekilde L. Etidronate disodium for treating hypercalcaemia of malignancy: A double blind, placebo-controlled study. *European Journal of Clinical Investigation* 1988; **16**: 433–7.
8. Bonjour J-P, Philippe J, Guelpa G *et al.* Bone and renal components in hypercalcaemia of malignancy and responses to a single infusion of clodronate. *Bone* 1988; **9**: 123–30.
9. Coleman RE, Woll PJ, Miles M *et al.* 3-Amino-1,1 hydroxypropylidene bisphosphonate (APD) for the treatment of bone metastases from breast cancer. *British Journal of Cancer* 1988; **58**: 621.
10. van Holten-Verzantvoort AT, Bijvoet OLM, Cleton FJ *et al.* Reduced morbidity from skeletal metastases in breast cancer patients during long-term bisphosphonate (APD) treatment. *Lancet* 1987; **ii**: 983–5.
11. Paterson TJ, Powles TJ, Kanis JA *et al.* Clodronate decreases skeletal morbidity in patients with bone metastases from breast cancer: A double blind controlled trial. *Proceedings of the American Society for Clinical Oncology* 1992; **11**: 49.
12. Parfitt AM. Bone remodeling: relationship to the amount and structure of bone, and the pathogenesis and prevention of fractures. In: Riggs B, Melton LJ III eds. *Osteoporosis: etiology, diagnosis and management.* New York: Raven Press, 1988: 133–54.
13. Raisz LG, Rodan GA. Cellular basis for bone turnover. In: Avioli LV, Krane SM eds. *Metabolic bone disease and clinically related disorders.* Philadelphia: W.B. Saunders, 1990: 1–41.
14. Mundy GR. Bone resorption and turnover in health and disease. *Bone* 1987; **8** (Suppl. 1): S9–16.

15. Mundy GR. Calcium homeostasis – role of the gut, kidney and bone. In: *Calcium homeostasis: hypercalcaemia and hypocalcaemia.* London: Martin Dunitz, 1989: 16–27.
16. Abrams HL, Spiro R, Goldstein N. Metastases in carcinomas: analysis of 1000 autopsied cases. *Cancer* 1950; **23**: 74–85.
17. Boyce BF. Normal bone remodelling and its disruption in metastatic bone disease. In: Rubens RD, Fogelman I eds. *Bone metastases – diagnosis and treatment.* London: Springer-Verlag, 1991: 11–30.
18. Galasko CSB. Mechanisms of bone destruction in the development of skeletal metastases. *Nature* 1976; **263**: 507–8.
19. Bundred NJ, Ratcliffe WA, Walker RA *et al.* Parathyroid hormone related protein is a humoral mediator in breast cancer. *British Medical Journal* 1991; **303**: 1506–9.
20. Percival RC, Yates AJP, Gray RES *et al.* Mechanisms of malignant hypercalcaemia in carcinoma of the breast. *British Medical Journal* 1985; **291**: 776–9.
21. Hosking DJ, Cowley A, Bucknoll CA. Rehydration in the treatment of severe hypercalcaemia. *Quarterly Journal of Medicine* 1982; **200**: 473–81.
22. Shocker JD, Brady LW, Risch VR *et al.* Radiation therapy for bone metastases – The Hahnemann experience. In: Weiss L, Gilbert HA eds. *Bone metastasis.* Boston: GK Hall, 1981: 436–42.
23. Blake GM, Zivanovich MA, Blaquiere RM *et al.* Strontium-89 therapy: Measurement of absorbed dose to skeletal metastases. *Journal of Nuclear Medicine* 1988; **29**: 549–57.
24. Lewington VJ, McEwan AJ, Ackery DM *et al.* A prospective, randomised double-blind crossover study to examine the efficacy of strontium-89 in pain palliation in patients with advanced prostate cancer metastatic to bone. *European Journal of Cancer* 1991; **27**: 954–8.
25. Galasko CSB. The role of the orthopaedic surgeon in the treatment of skeletal metastases. In: Rubens RD, Fogelman I eds. *Bone metastases – diagnosis and treatment.* London: Springer-Verlag, 1991: 207–22.
26. Fleisch H. Bisphosphonates: mechanisms of action and clinical applications. In: Peck WA ed. *Bone and mineral research,* vol. 1. Amsterdam: Exerpta Medica, 1983: 319–57.
27. Fitton A, McTavish D. Pamidronate: a review of its pharmacological properties and therapeutic efficacy in resorptive bone disease. *Drugs* 1991; **41**: 289–318.
28. Flanagan AM, Chambers TJ. CL_2MDP inhibits resorption through injury of osteoclast that resorbs CL_2MDP coated bone. *Bone & Mineral* 1989; **6**: 33–43.
29. Boonenkamp PM, van der wee Pals LJA, van Wijk-van Lennep MML *et al.* Two modes of action of bisphosphonates on osteolytic resorption of mineralised bone matrix. *Bone & Mineral* 1986; **1**: 27–39.
30. Coleman RE, Dirix LY, Dodwell D *et al.* Phase I/II evaluation of effervescent and enteric coated oral pamidronate for bone metastases *European Journal of Cancer* 1991; **27**: 945–6.
31. Warrell RP. Questions about clinical trials in hypercalcaemia. *Journal of Clinical Oncology* 1988; **6**: 759–61.
32. Percival RC, Yates AJP, Gray RES *et al.* The role of glucocorticoids in the management of malignant hypercalcaemia. *British Medical Journal* 1984; **289**: 287.
33. Binstock ML, Mundy GR. Effect of calcitonin and glucocorticoids in combination on the hypercalcaemia of malignancy. *Annals of Internal Medicine* 1980; **93**: 907–10.
34. Slayton RE, Schinder BJ, Elias E *et al.* New approach to the treatment of hypercalcaemia – the short term treatment with mithramycin. *Clinical Pharmacology and Therapeutics* 1971; **12**: 833–7.
35. Warrell RP Jr, Israel R, Frisone M *et al.* Gallium nitrate for acute treatment of cancer

related hypercalcaemia A randomised double-blind comparison to calcitonin. *Annals of Internal Medicine* 1988; **108**: 669–74.

36. Warrell RP Jr, Murphy WK, Schulman P *et al.* Gallium nitrate for treatment of cancer-related hypercalcaemia: A randomised double-blind comparison to etidronate. *Proceedings of the American Society for Clinical Oncology* 1990; **9**: 65.

37. Thiébaud D, Portman L, Jaeger Ph *et al.* Oral versus intravenous APD in the treatment of hypercalcaemia of malignancy. *Bone* 1986; **7**: 247–53.

38. Body JJ, Pot M, Borkowski A *et al.* Dose-response study of aminohydroxypropylidene bisphosphonate in tumor-associated hypercalcaemia. *American Journal of Medicine* 1987; **82**: 957–63.

39. Thiébaud D, Jaeger Ph, Jacquet AF *et al.* Dose response in the treatment of hypercalcaemia of malignancy by a single infusion of the bisphosphonate AHPrBP (APD). *Journal of Clinical Oncology* 1988; **6**: 762–8.

40. Ralston SH, Alzaid AA, Gardner MD *et al.* Treatment of cancer associated hypercalcaemia with combined aminohydroxypropylidene diphosphonate and calcitonin. *British Medical Journal* 1986; **292**: 1549–50.

41. Coleman RE, Rubens RD. 3(Amino-1,1-hydroxypropylidene) bisphosphonate (APD) for hypercalcaemia of breast cancer. *British Journal of Cancer* 1987; **56**: 465–9.

42. Body JJ, Magritte A, Seraj F *et al.* Amino-hydroxypropylidene-1,1-bisphosphonate (APD) treatment for tumour-associated hypercalcaemia: a randomized comparison between a 3-daytreatment and single 24 hour infusions. *Journal of Bone Mineral and Research* 1990; **4**: 923–7.

43. Kanis JA, McCloskey EV, Paterson AHG. Use of diphosphonates in hypercalcaemia due to malignancy. *Lancet* 1990; **i**: 170–1.

44. Morton AR, Cantrill JA, Howell A. Disodium pamidronate for the management of hypercalcaemia of malignancy: comparative studies of single dose versus daily infusions and of infusion duration. In: Burckhardt P ed. *Disodium pamidronate (APD) in the treatment of malignancy related disorders.* Toronto: Hogrefe & Huber, 1989: 85–9.

45. Dodwell DJ, Coleman RE, Daley-Yates P *et al.* Intravenous pamidronate: pharmacokinetic and duration of effect studies in women with skeletal breast cancer. *Journal of Cancer Research and Clinical Oncology* 1990: 15th UICC Hamburg, abstract B3. p 401.

46. Sleeboom, HP, Bijvoet OLM, van Oosterom AT *et al.* Comparison of intravenous (3-amino-1-hydroxypropylidene)-1,1-bisphosphonate and volume repletion in tumour-induced hypercalcaemia. *Lancet* 1983; **ii**: 239–43.

47. Ralston SH, Gardner MD, Dryburgh FJ *et al.* Comparison of animohydroxypropylidene diphosphonate, mithramycin, and corticosteroids/calcitonin in treatment of cancer-associated hypercalcaemia. *Lancet* 1985; **i**: 907–10.

48. Thurlimann B, Waldburger R, Senn HJ *et al.* Mithramycin and pamidronate (APD) in symptomatic tumour-related hypercalcaemia – a comparative randomised cross-over trial. In: Bijvoet OLM, Lipton A eds. *Osteoclast inhibition in the management of malignancy related bone disorders.* Bern: Hogrefe & Huber, 1991: 27–32.

49. Ralston SH, Gallacher SJ, Patel U *et al.* Comparison of three intravenous bisphosphonates in cancer-associated hypercalcaemia. *Lancet* 1989; **ii**: 118.

50. Purohit OP, Radstone CR, Anthony C *et al.* A randomised double-blind comparison of intravenous pamidronate and clodronate in the hypercalcaemia of malignancy. *British Journal of Cancer* 1995; **72**: 1289–93.

51. Ritch P, Gulcalp R, Wiernik P *et al.* Pamidronate (APD) and etidronate disodium (EMDP) in hypercalcaemia of malignancy. In: Rubens RD ed. *The management of bone metastases and hypercalcaemia by osteoclast inhibition.* Bern: Hogrefe & Huber, 1990.

52. Thiébaud D, Jaeger P, Burckhardt P. Response to retreatment of malignant hyper-

calcaemia with the bisphosphonate AHPrBP (APD): respective role of kidney and bone. *Journal of Bone and Mineral Research* 1990; **5**: 221–6.

53. Morton AR, Cantrill JA, Pillai GV *et al.* Sclerosis of lytic bone metastases after disodium aminohydroxypropylidene bisphosphonate (APD) in patients with breast cancer. *British Medical Journal* 1988; **297**: 772–3.

54. Leyvraz S, Thiébaud D, von Fliedner V *et al.* Use of disodium bisphosphonate (APD) in the treatment of breast cancer and myeloma bone metastases In: Rubens RD ed. *The management of bone metastases and hypercalcaemia by osteoclast inhibition.* Bern: Hogrefe & Huber, 1990: 76–80.

55. Grabelsky S, Lipton A, Harvey H *et al.* Pamidronate disodium (APD) – A dose seeking study in patients with breast cancer. *Proceedings of the American Society for Clinical Oncology* 1991; **10**: 42.

56. Tyrrell CJ on behalf of the Aredia Multinational Cooperative Group. Role of pamidronate in the management of bone metastases from breast cancer: Results of a non-comparative multicenter phase II trial. *Annals of Oncology* 1994; **5** (Suppl 7): S37–S40.

57. Clarke NW, Holbrook IB, McClure J *et al.* Osteoclast inhibition by pamidronate in metastatic prostate cancer: a preliminary study. *British Journal of Cancer* 1991; **63**: 420–3.

58. van Holten-Verzantvoort AT, Zwinderman AH, Aaronson NK *et al.* The effect of supportive pamidronate treatment on aspects of quality of life with advanced breast cancer. *European Journal of Cancer* 1991: **27**: 544–9.

59. Hortobagyi GN, Porter L, Blayney D *et al.* Reduction of skeletal related complications in breast cancer patients with ostelytic bone metastases receiving chemotherapy (CT), by monthly pamidronate sodium (PAM) (Aredia^R) infusion. *Proceedings of the American Society for Clinical Oncology* 1996; **15**: 108 (Abstr. 99).

60. Theriault RL, Lipton A, Leff R *et al.* Reduction of skeletal related complications in breast cancer patients with osteloytic bone metastases receiving hormone therapy, by monthly pamidronate sodium (Aredia^R) infusion. *Proceedings of the American Society for Clinical Oncology* 1996; **15**: 122 (Abstr. 152).

61. Lahtinen R, Laakso M, Palva I *et al.* for the Finnish Leukaemia Group. Randomised, placebo-controlled multicentre trial of clodronate in multiple myeloma. *Lancet* 1992; **340**: 1049–52.

62. McCloskey EV, Maclennan ICM, Drayson M *et al.* Effect of clodronate on progression of skeletal disease in multiple myelomatosis. *European Journal of Cancer* 1995; **31**A (suppl 5): S162.

63. Berenson JR, Lichtenstein A, Porter L *et al.* for the Myeloma Aredia Study Group Efficacy of pamidronate in reducing skeletal events in patients with advanced multiple mieloma. *New England Journal of Medicine.* 1996; **334**: 488–93.

64. Elomaa I, Blomqvist C, Porrka L *et al.* Diphosphonates for osteolytic metastases. *Lancet* 1985; **i**: 1155–6.

65. Merlini G, Parrinello GA, Piccinini L *et al.* Long-term effects of parenteral dichloromethylene diphosphonate (C12MDP) on bone disease of myeloma patients treated with chemotherapy. *Haematology & Oncology* 1990; **8**: 23–30.

66. Smith JR. Palliation of painful bone metastases from prostate cancer using sodium etidronate: results of a randomized, prospective, double-blind, placebo-controlled study. *Journal of Urology* 1989; **141**: 85–7.

67. Millward MJ, Cantwell BMJ, Carmichael J *et al.* A randomised trial of the addition of disodium pamidronate (APD) to endocrine therapy for advanced breast cancer with bone metastases. *Proceedings of the American Society for Clinical Oncology* 1991; **10**: 42.

CHAPTER 13

Morphine metabolism: an evaluation of recent research and its clinical implications

CAROL L. DAVIS————————————————————————————

INTRODUCTION

The control of pain frequently plays a major part in the management of patients with cancer and the role of morphine in this respect is well-documented. This chapter will concentrate on recent advances in our understanding of morphine metabolism and an attempt will be made to put these in a clinical context.

Opium is produced from one particular species of poppy, *Papaver somniferum* (Fig. 13.1), and is obtained by lacerating the unripe seedheads of the plant and then harvesting the exuded sap. The analgesic and hypnotic properties of opium are common knowledge and artefacts connected with its use date back some 4000 years to the twenty-first century BC. It was not, however, until the early nineteenth century that a German pharmacist, Friedrich Serturner, described and isolated the principal analgesic component of opium. He called it morphium after Morpheus, the Greek god of dreams who was himself the son of Hypnos, the god of sleep. The name was later changed to morphia and then to morphine.

By the turn of the century morphine had become established in Western medicine as its actions were more predictable than those of opium. The chemical structure of morphine was established in 1926[1] but its synthesis was not achieved until 1952.[2] Of the powerful analgesics which have been synthesized from morphine, diacetylmorphine, or diamorphine, is probably most widely used. It is rapidly metabolized to two major metabolites, monoacetylmorphine and morphine, which are both active.[3] Diamorphine has several physicochemical properties which it does not share with morphine and which have generated considerable controversy over the years.[4] The difference in analgesic potency between morphine and diamorphine is now recognized to be considerably less than previously thought.[5] A discussion of diamorphine, however, is not within the scope of this chapter.

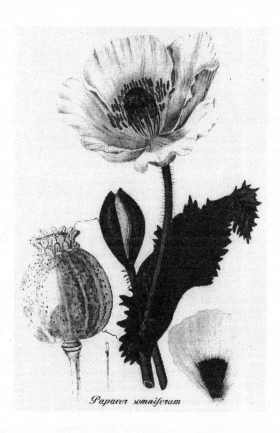

Fig. 13.1. Opium poppy, *Papaver somniferum* 1836. (By courtesy of the Herbarium and Library Royal Botanic Gardens, Kew.)

MORPHINE METABOLISM

As long ago as 1890 Ashdown reported the isolation of glucuronic acid from human urine after the administration of morphine.[6] It was not until the 1940s and 1950s that research confirmed that this substance was a metabolite of morphine and that it was a morphine conjugate, morphine 3-glucuronide (M 3-G).[7,8] At about the same time Thompson and Gross isolated a further glucuronide metabolite, a diglucuronide, from the urine of dogs.[9] These compounds were thought to be the sole glucuronide metabolites of morphine and so most subsequent laboratory and clinical research concentrated on them. In 1968 Yoshimura and co-workers demonstrated the existence of another morphine monoglucuronide, morphine 6-glucuronide (M 6-G)[10] and described the synthesis of this compound. They used a thin-layer chromatographic technique for its detection and went on to report that after the administration of morphine, M 6-G was found in both the urine and bile of rabbits[11] and in the urine of humans.[12] Radioimmunoassay techniques were then developed and were widely employed throughout the 1970s and early 1980s.

Using thin-layer chromatography and radioimmunoassay only very small quantities of M 6-G could be detected in human urine after morphine administration[13] and so M 6-G was thought to be of little relevance in humans. After perfecting a high performance liquid chromatography (HPLC) technique, whch proved to be both sensitive and more specific than the assays previously employed, Svensson *et al.* were able to demonstrate that M 6-G was produced in greater quantities in humans than had been previously recognized.[14,15] Subsequently, cross-reactivity was demonstrated between the morphine and M 6-G antibodies that had been employed in the previous radioimmunoassays.[16] More recently, this problem has been overcome by development of a differential radioimmunoassay technique.

Wahlstrom *et al.* recently demonstrated that glucuronidation of the active laevo-rotatory (−) enantiomer of morphine in humans results in the preferential production of M 3-G whilst considerably more M 6-G is produced after glucuronidaton of the dextro-rotatory enantiomer.[17] The reverse is true in rats and, in addition, the amount of M 6-G produced differs markedly between different species[18]. The extrapolation of metabolic data derived from animals to humans should, therefore, be avoided. Glucuronidation in the 3- position is mediated by uridine pyrophosphoglucuronyl transferase (UDGPT) whilst that at the 6- position is probably catalysed by a different enzyme. M 6-G and to a lesser extent M 3-G have been found to be more lipophilic than other glucuronides which are usually highly polar compounds and unable to cross the blood–brain barrier. The two morphine monoglucuronides have been shown to exist in conformational equilibria between extended, more hydrophilic, and folded, more lipophilic, forms[19].

The predominant site of morphine metabolism is the liver[19] although other sites including the intestinal wall[20,21] the kidneys[22] and the brain[17] are also involved. In patients with normal liver function, extrahepatic glucuronidation accounts for less than 10 per cent of the total clearance of morphine but the percentage may rise in patients with impaired liver function.[23] The potential clinical significance of this will be discussed later.

In addition to M 3-G and M 6-G which account for approximately 75 per cent and 15 per cent, respectively, of the total metabolites of morphine (Fig. 13.2), many other metabolites are known to be formed after morphine administration. These include morphine 3,6-diglucuronide, morphine 3-ethereal sulphate, morphine 6-ethereal sulphate, codeine, normorphine and normorphine glucuronides.[24] The analgesic property of codeine is well-known and may well be shared by some of these other compounds but they are formed in such small amounts that it is unlikely that they contribute to the analgesic action of morphine. Recent work, therefore, has concentrated on the monoglucuronide metabolites of morphine.

The analgesic efficacy of morphine after single-dose oral administration is low compared to that achieved after parenteral administration. After repeated oral doses, however, the analgesic effect is enhanced and it has been postulated that this could be due to the fact that after repeated doses active metabolites account for much of the analgesic activity.[25] Evidence has been put forward to support the existence of an enterohepatic circulation of morphine in dogs[26] and if this

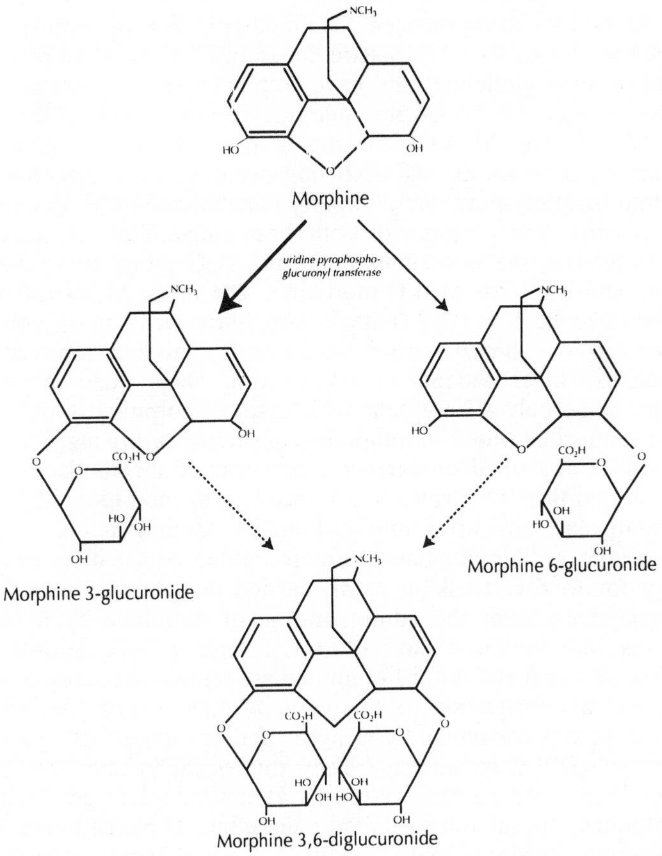

Fig. 13.2 Glucuronidation of morphine.

exists in humans then it may have clinical significance. After the administration of oral morphine a double peak in plasma morphine levels has been reported[27] and high concentrations of M 6-G have been found in bile.[28] Other groups have not been able to confirm these findings, and so this issue remains unresolved. It appears that the relationship between the pharmacokinetics and pharmacodynamics of morphine is even more complicated than hitherto thought.

PHARMACOKINETICS OF MORPHINE

Many investigators have reported the pharmacokinetics of morphine administered by various routes but clinical interpretation of their results is difficult. Different sampling methods and non-specific assay techinques have been employed and up to tenfold differences in basic pharmacokinetic parameters have been demonstrated. Hoskin reviewed fifty-seven published studies and found considerable disparity in the method of sample collection.[29] After studying the influence of various factors on plasma and serum levels of morphine,

M 3-G and M 6-G he recommended the standardization of sample collection using plasma samples collected in plastic heparinized tubes. Most recent studies have adhered to these guidelines and have employed specific assays.

In 1983 Sawe et al. confirmed the quantitative importance of the morphine metabolites M 3-G and M 6-G[30] in four cancer patients on doses of oral morphine varying between 80 and 2520 mg per day. They demonstrated that after oral administration morphine is rapidly metabolized to M 3-G and M 6-G and that the plasma concentrations of both these metabolites far exceed that of the parent compound, the mean molar plasma AUC ratios being 34:1 for M 3-G:morphine and 3.9:1 for M 6-G:morphine. The mean M 3-G:M 6-G AUC ratio was found to be 9:1. The same investigators went on to compare the pharmacokinetics of morphine after single-dose oral and intravenous (IV) administration to cancer patients in severe pain. They found the mean oral bioavailability to be only 47 per cent which, since morphine is well-absorbed from the gastrointestinal tract,[31,32] might be considered surprising. This apparent anomaly could be explained by extensive presystemic metabolism and indeed Sawe demonstrated that the mean urinary recovery of morphine, M 3-G and M 6-G was virtually the same after both oral and IV administration.

Using a specific radioimmunoassay for morphine and a differential radio-immunoassay for M 6-G Hosking et al. carried out pharmacokinetic studies on normal volunteers after the administration of morphine by a number of routes[33]. In this study the mean plasma M 6-G:morphine AUC ratios were found to be 2.0. 10.9, 11.1 and 10.5 after IV, immediate-release oral, slow-release oral and slow buccal administration respectively. Another major pharmacokinetic study of morphine was conducted by Osborne and co-workers using a modification of Svensson's HPLC technique.[34] They studied the behaviour of morphine and its metabolites in ten normal volunteers after single-dose administration of IV, oral, sublingual, buccal and sustained release buccal preparations,[35] and the peak plasma concentrations (Cmax) of both M 3-G and M 6-G exceeded that of the parent compound after all routes of administration. The mean ratios of plasma AUC for M 6-G:morphine were shown to be 1.4:1 after IV and 8.6:1 after oral administration; these results mirror those of both Hosking and Sawe and confirm the importance of first-pass metabolism in the liver after oral administration. Furthermore, they raise the possibility that the analgesic efficacy of morphine might be mediated through different mechanisms after different routes of administration.

The pharmacokinetics of sustained-release oral preparations of morphine have been investigated in several single-dose studies and the mean Cmax has been found to occur between 2 and 2.4 hours after administration.[36–38] Despite the fact that, in patients with advanced cancer, the relative bioavailability of controlled-release morphine has been shown to be less than after immediate-release morphine,[36,39] there is substantial clinical evidence that these preparations share the same analgesic efficacy and toxicity profile.[40] It is now accepted practice that once a patient has been stabilized on a 4-hourly regime of immediate-release morphine, a controlled-release preparation can be substituted so that the drug only needs to be given 12 hourly. The total daily dose remains the same;[5] there is evidence that a loading dose of the sustained-release preparation is not required.[41]

Drug administration by the buccal and sublingual routes rather than the oral route not only results in faster absorption and a more rapid achievement of therapeutic levels, but also avoids first-pass metabolism. When Osborne *et al.* studied the pharmacokinetics of an immediate-release buccal preparation of morphine[35] they found the M 6-G:morphine AUC ratio to be 5.1. This value is approximately midway between the ratios achieved after administration by the oral and IV routes and so it seems likely that when a buccal dose of morphine is given, a significant proportion is swallowed and absorbed into the portal circulation.

Somewhat surprisingly, both Hoskin and Osborne found the bioavailability and the M 6-G:morphine plasma AUC ratio of a slow-release buccal preparation of morphine to be very similar to that of immediate-release oral morphine.[35,36] Whilst several studies have shown that the time that peak plasma morphine concentration is achieved (*T*max) is between 5 and 8 hours after administration of a slow-release buccal tablet,[33,35,42] a much shorter *T*max has been described by two other groups of investigators.[43,44] This dichotomy is probably accounted for by differences in drug formulation although inter-individual differences such as the length of time that the tablet remains in the buccal sulcus may also be important. Apart from one study in which a cross-reacting radioimmunoassay was employed,[45] the sole published report of the pharmacokinetics of sublingual morphine is again by Osborne *et al.*,[35] who found the main pharmacokinetic parameters to be very similar to those achieved after administration of immediate-release buccal morphine. These studies were performed on normal volunteers and require confirmation in a clinical setting.

The few studies of the pharmacokinetics of morphine after rectal administration have produced variable results and in none of them was the plasma M 6-G concentration assayed.[45–48] In contrast, the pharmacokinetics of IV, intramuscular[26,49] (IM) and subcutaneous (SC) morphine have been widely studied. Over the last decade it has become accepted that in cancer patients with opiate-requiring pain in whom oral administration is, for whatever reason, impossible, the preferred route of opiate administration is SC.[5] Moreover whilst adequate analgesia can be provided by regular SC injections, the method of choice is continuous SC infusion.[50–52] Although the pharmacokinetics of both bolus SC injections and continuous SC infusions have been studied,[26,53] very few investigators have compared the pharmacokinetics after administration by other routes. Brunk and Delle described the pharmacokinetics after single doses of morphine given by bolus SC, IM and IV injections[32] and found a very similar plasma half-life in each case. Their finding that higher serum morphine concentrations were achieved between 15 minutes and 3 hours after SC and IM than after IV administration may well have been due to the use of a morphine assay which, in retrospect, cross-reacted with the morphine glucuronides. A comparison of the efficacy of morphine administered by continuous SC infusion and by continuous IV infusion in patients with postoperative pain, found no significant difference in either the requirement for breakthrough analgesia or the serum morphine levels achieved.[54]

Systemically administered opioid drugs achieve their analgesic action through interaction with opioid receptors in the central nervous system and in the small proportion of those patients in whom toxicity is considerable and, sometimes, dose-limiting the continuous administration of low-dose spinal opioids provides a useful therapeutic alternative. Of the spinal routes available, the intrathecal route is enjoying increasing popularity.[55,56] Usually only small numbers of patients at any one centre are treated in this way and there is, therefore, a dearth of clinical and pharmacokinetic data. Studies to date have demonstrated that profound analgesia can be produced with small doses of morphine[57,58] and it is hoped that the increasing use of spinal opiods, particularly in patients with postoperative pain, will generate further research in this area.

In summary, pharmacokinetic studies employing specific assays have already yielded clinically useful results but undoubtedly need to be extended. Most have been carried out in normal subjects after administration of only a single dose and so these results should not be extrapolated to patients in chronic pain. There is a need for further investigation of the pharmacokinetics of morphine using assays specific for both morphine and its major metabolites. Most importantly, the clinical relevance of such data is limited unless the relationship between the pharmacokinetics and the pharmacodynamics of morphine can be established.

PHARMACODYNAMIC ASPECTS

Pharmacodynamic studies seek to establish a link between the biochemical and physiological effects of drugs and their mechanisms of action. The clinical effects of morphine are both well-recognized and well-documented[59] and studies have been conducted with the aim of establishing a relationship between plasma morphine concentration and analgesia, miosis and respiratory depression. Whilst the latter are easily measured objectively, analgesia is difficult to quantify even within an individual patient whilst inter-patient comparison is even harder. For these reasons the speed of onset of analgesia and its duration have been more widely studied than the quality of pain relief. The rate of onset of analgesia has been found to be 15 minutes, 1.4 hours and over 2 hours after morphine administration by the intravenous,[60] intramuscular[61] and epidural[62] routes respectively. Several studies have tried to define the relationship between duration and degree of analgesia and plasma morphine concentration but most have failed to demonstrate any correlation[63–67] between the two. Hanks *et al.* however, found a correlation between adequacy of pain relief and plasma morphine concentration after the administration of oral sustained release morphine[68] and Nordberg *et al.* described a relationship between the duration of analgesia and both peak levels and the AUC of morphine in the CSF.[69] Interestingly the same investigators found no correlation between plasma and CSF concentrations after intramuscular morphine[63] and questioned the validity of studies which have assessed morphine levels in plasma rather than in CSF. The contribution of M 6-G to the clinical effects of morphine has not yet been assessed.

ANIMAL STUDIES OF MORPHINE MONOGLUCURONIDES

Both M 6-G and M 3-G have been synthesized[16] but of the two compounds only the former has been shown to have analgesic activity. After M 6-G was administered subcutaneously to mice, the analgesic potency was found to be four times greater than that of morphine,[70] whilst after intracerebral administration the analgesic potency ratio of M 6-G:morphine has been found to be at least 45:1[70] and, in one study, as much as 200:1.[71] Furthermore, the duration of analgesia after M 6-G administration was significantly greater than that following administration of morphine.[72]

M 3-G had been thought to be of no clinical significance but there is now evidence that it can antagonize the analgesic effects of morphine.[73] Moreover, Gong *et al.* has recently described, in rats, antagonism of the antinociceptive effects of intrathecal and intracerebral M 6-G by M 3-G.[74] Although these findings have not been substantiated by other workers[75] they suggest that M 3-G may not be as inert as previously thought and add a further twist to the tale.

ANALGESIC EFFICACY OF MORPHINE MONOGLUCURONIDES IN HUMANS

There have been, to date, no reported studies of the administration of M 3-G to humans although the analgesic efficacy of M 6-G was first reported in 1988. Osborne *et al.* conducted a phase I-type study in opiate-naive cancer patients with pain and demonstrated minimal toxicity with appreciable analgesic activity, lasting between 2 and 18 hours, in 17/19 assessable patients.[76] Surprisingly, they found no correlation between the dose of M 6-G, which ranged from 0.5 to 4 mg/70 kg, and either the degree or the duration of analgesia and this requires further investigation. A further study investigated the analgesic and respiratory depressant effects of IV morphine and M 6-G in normal volunteers;[77] experimental pain was induced by limb ischaemia and using this model the analgesic potency ratio of M 6-G:morphine was found to be 3:1. The other results of this study are discussed later.

At present the only other report of the analgesic efficacy of M 6-G is a single-blind comparison of the effects of intrathecal morphine and M 6-G in three patients.[78] In this study M 6-G was shown to have only twice the analgesic potency of morphine and this is considerably lower than that demonstrated in animals after administration by the same route.[70,72]

PHARMACOKINETICS OF MORPHINE 6-GLUCURONIDE

Several studies have assessed the pharmacokinetic profile of intravenous M 6-G in both patients[79] and normal volunteers.[80] M 6-G has been shown to have a smaller volume of distribution and a lower clearance than morphine but a similar elimination half-life. Morphine has not been detected after the administration of M 6-G. In a comparative study the half-life of M 6-G was found to be similar whether it was administered by the intravenous or the subcutaneous route.[81] After oral administration the bioavailability of M 6-G is only 8 per cent (RJ Osborne, personal communication).

Further pharmacokinetic studies are needed in order that accurate and appropriate dosing schedules can be devised and then employed in a more detailed assessment of the clinical potential of this compound.

TOXICITY OF MORPHINE 6-GLUCURONIDE IN ANIMALS AND HUMANS

In Osborne's open study of M 6-G in cancer patients with pain[76] none of the twenty patients studied experienced any nausea, dysphoric symptoms, sedation of significant cardiorespiratory effects. These preliminary observations have been supported by the results of randomized, crossover studies of morphine and M 6-G in normal subjects but not, as yet, in patients. Thompson *et al.* found that nine out of ten subjects complained of nausea after receiving 10 mg/70 kg morphine intravenously whilst only one did so after receiving three different doses of M 6-G, namely 1, 3.3 and 5 mg/70 kg.[77] Hanna *et al.* have found broadly similar findings at similar dose levels although a dose of 60 mg/kg, which is equivalent to 4.2 mg/70 kg, did cause nausea in two out of five subjects.[80] In view of these observations, albeit in very small numbers, it is somewhat surprising that M 6-G has been shown to have greater emetic potential than morphine in the ferret, the most commonly used animal model of emesis.[82] It has, however, been demonstrated that in the ferret, in contrast to humans, less than 1 per cent of an administered dose of morphine is metabolized to M 6-G[18] and this finding serves to emphasize, yet again, the interspecies variations that exist in morphine metabolism.

Intravenous M 6-G has been shown to cause significantly less respiratory depression, as measured by changes in transcutaneous carbon dioxide concentration and expired carbon dioxide concentration, than equi-analgesic doses of morphine in normal volunteers.[77] Respiratory depression is, however, seen when high plasma concentrations of M 6-G are achieved[83,84] and M 6-G, in doses up to 60 mg/kg, has been shown to reduce the ventilatory response to inhaled carbon dioxide but to a lesser extent than morphine.[85] Conversely, in a series of experiments in awake dogs, Pelligrino *et al.* found that intraventricular administration of M 6-G caused dose-dependent ventilatory depression[86] and when compared to morphine, M 6-G was 5–10 times more potent as a ventilatory depressant. In animals the LD_{50} of M 6-G has been shown to be less than that of morphine, the ratio being 0.8:1.[70] If, however, the differences in analgesic potency are also taken into consideration then it becomes apparent that in animals, as well as in humans, equi-analgesic doses of M 6-G are considerably less toxic than the parent compound.

MORPHINE ADMINISTRATION IN RENAL FAILURE

The exaggerated and prolonged toxicity seen after morphine administration to patients suffering from renal failure is both well-documented[87,88] and a common clinical problem. Pharmacokinetic studies employing radioimmunoassay techniques[89] suggested that these effects were due to accumulation of morphine and demonstrated that both the clinical and the pharmacologic effects could be reversed by renal transplantation.[90] With the use of more specific analytical techniques it has become evident that it is accumulation of the metabolites and not persistence of the parent compound that is the cause of toxicity in these patients. This was first described by Osborne *et al.* who also demonstrated that respiratory depression persisted for several days after morphine treatment was discontinued and was associated with high plasma levels of both M 3-G and M 6-G. Subsequently, the same group of workers demonstrated that a short period of peritoneal dialysis did not significantly alter either the pharmacokinetic parameters or the clinical effects. Peritoneal dialysis would thus seem an inappropriate intervention in the treatment of patients with morphine intoxication due to renal insufficiency. In contrast, renal transplantation resulted in a rapid decline in plasma glucuronide levels as soon as the transplanted kidney started to work (RJ Osborne, personal communication).

In the only other report of the effects of dialysis on morphine pharmacokinetics Bion *et al.* showed that a 3–5 hour period of haemodialysis resulted in a 48 per cent mean fall in plasma morphine concentration.[91] The method of sample analysis employed did not distinguish between morphine and its glucuronide metabolites but nonetheless this study clearly demonstrated that haemodialysis is an efficient way of reversing the pharmacologic and clinical effects of morphine intoxication in patients with renal failure.

In clinical and normal volunteer studies M 6-G appears to be less toxic than equi-analgesic doses of morphine. However, the evidence that the morphine monoglucuronides and not the parent compound accumulate in renal failure make it likely that the toxicity seen after morphine administration to patients with impaired renal function is due to the very high concentration of metabolites achieved. These studies highlight the need for extreme care in the use of morphine in patients with significant renal impairment but, at present, there are no recommendations for dose adjustment in such patients and it is to be hoped that future research will address this issue.

OPIOID RECEPTORS

If morphine and M 6-G were found to have different opioid receptor binding affinities then the clinical differences between the two compounds might be explained.

Despite the fact that the existence of an opioid receptor was first postulated as long ago as 1953[92] controversy remains over both the classification of opioid receptors and their function. In 1976 Martin *et al.* reported the results of receptor binding studies in animals[93] and described three distinct opioid receptors, mu, kappa and sigma. The discovery of the endogenous opioids in 1975[96] generated further interest in opioid receptors and subsequently two further receptors, the delta and epsilon receptors, were characterized.[94,95] Since then many different receptor models have been proposed.

Over a decade ago Pasternak and his colleagues postulated the existence of a common opioid receptor, the mu_1 receptor, with a high binding affinity for both morphine and delta agonists and of another receptor, which they named mu_2, which possessed a lower affinity for these compounds.[97] They demonstrated that the ratio of mu_1:mu_2 receptors was 3:7. Both they and other researchers went on to suggest that activation of the low-affinity mu_2 receptor modulated much of the toxicity of morphine, particularly respiratory depression and gastrointestinal toxicity.[96–100] It was shown that M 6-G has a fourfold lower affinity for this receptor than morphine, but although supraspinal analgesia is primarily mediated by the mu_1 receptor,[93,102,103] no substantive difference has been demonstrated in the binding of morphine and M 6-G at the mu_1 receptor.[71,101]

There is thus some evidence, at a receptor level, to explain the differences in toxicity between M 6-G and morphine but the apparent increased analgesic potency of M 6-G remains unexplained. Further evaluation of the interactions between morphine, M 6-G and opioid receptors at a molecular level along with increased understanding of the ways in which opioid receptor binding initiates or inhibits a phsyiological response might shed light on this matter.

MORPHINE ADMINISTRATION AND HEPATIC DYSFUNCTION

Little is known about the effects of impaired hepatic function on morphine metabolism in humans. Evidence has been put forward that morphine disposition is unchanged in patients with moderate to severe cirrhosis, relative to normal subjects,[104] but in retrospect none of the six cirrhotic patients in this study had gross abnormality of liver function. In contrast other studies have shown that liver dysfunction influences the metabolism and pharmacokinetics of morphine. Whilst in patients with normal liver function, extrahepatic glucuronidation accounts for less than 10 per cent of the total clearance of morphine, the percentage has been shown to be as high as 30 per cent in patients with impaired liver function.[23] Mazoit *et al.* found a longer terminal half-life, reduced clearance and a significantly increased AUC in cirrhotic patients.[105] Both a marked reduction in morphine clearance and a prolongation of terminal elimination half-life have been demonstrated in rats with artificially induced liver dysfunction.[106]

There appears little doubt that liver dysfunction can affect morphine metabolism and that this must be of clinical significance but there are insufficient data available on which to base changes in clinical practice. The treatment of such patients therefore remains largely empirical.

AGE-RELATED CONSIDERATIONS

It is well-recognized that there are age-related variations in the pharmacokinetics of a variety of drugs but literature on this aspect of opiate pharmacokinetics is sparse.

Morphine pharmacokinetics and pharmacodynamics in children could be influenced by many factors including reduced protein binding,[107] increased volume of distribution[108] and greater permeability of the blood–brain barrier.[109] Furthermore, the capacity for renal elimination of drugs matures rapidly and is equivalent to that in adults from 6 months of age. Hepatic enzyme systems mature even more quickly and drugs with a high rate of first-pass metabolism in the liver are metabolized more quickly in children than in adults.[110] Some of these factors would increase morphine metabolism and clearance in children whilst others would militate against this and the situation is complicated still further by the fact that at least one of the metabolites possesses analgesic activity. The pharmacodynamic studies which have addressed this issue have shown considerable variation in morphine requirements in children of different ages.[111,112]

In the adult the clinical finding of a relationship between age and duration of analgesia after the administration of intramuscular morphine[113] has been substantiated by a pharmacokinetic study conducted perioperatively in middle-aged and elderly patients. This confirmed significantly greater clearance of morphine in the younger patients, aged between 36 and 55, than in the older group, aged between 65 and 83.[114]

Current practice reflects the paucity of pharmacokinetic studies in both children and the elderly. There is no firm consensus of opinion on either the optimum starting dose or the most appropriate dosing intervals for either immediate-release or slow-release morphine in children of different age groups. Likewise increasing age in the adult is not usually a consideration in the choice of the most appropriate opiate regime.

CONCLUSION

Although the rational prescription of any drug does not rely solely on a comprehensive understanding of its pharmacokinetics and metabolism these aspects are nonetheless important and may influence patient management. In particular, a knowledge of the pharmacokinetics of morphine in different clinical settings can lead to the identification of patient populations in which particular caution should be exercised. The inconsistent results of the early morphine pharmacokinetic studies led to considerable confusion but the more recent application of specific analytical techniques has allowed its administration to be based on sound pharmacokinetic principles. Further research, however, must be aimed at more thoroughly elucidating the effects of both impaired renal and hepatic function and of age on the pharmacokinetics of both morphine and M 6-G so that a rationale can be determined for the prescription of morphine in these groups.

Preliminary reports that the morphine metabolite, M 6-G, has greater analgesic potency but less toxicity than the parent compound are exciting but should be considered in the light of the fact that morphine, when properly employed, is an excellent strong analgesic and that its toxicity is rarely dose-limiting. There are, nevertheless, some clinical situations such as parturition and myocardial ischaemia when a less toxic drug may be indicated. Furthermore, if in chronic dosing studies M 6-G proves to be less constipating than morphine then it might deserve a place in analgesic practice although its limited oral bioavailability would limit its use in the treatment of chronic pain. This difficulty could be circumvented either by engineering other substituted morphine analogues with greater lipid solubility or by the utilization of other routes such as buccal administration. Until the results of current clinical and laboratory trials aimed at a more thorough evaluation of the therapeutic potential of M 6-G are available the use of this compound must remain experimental.

In 1870 William Rhind, a surgeon, when describing narcotic plants wrote that opium 'requires much skill and managment in its exhibition'.[115] This still holds true for all the opiate drugs.

REFERENCES

1. Van Duin CF, Robinson R, Smith JC. The morphine group. Part III. The constitution of neopine. *Journal of the Chemistry Society* 1926; 903–12.
2. Gates M, Tschudi G. The synthesis of morphine. *Journal of the American Chemistry Society* 1952; **74**: 1109–10.
3. Lockridge O, Mottershaw-Jackson N, Eckerson HW, Ladu BN. Hydrolysis of diacetylmorphine (heroin) by human serum cholinesterase. *Journal of Pharmacology and Experimental Therapeutics* 1980; **215**: 1–8.
4. Twycross RG. Choice of strong analgesic in terminal care: diamorphine or morphine? *Pain* 1977: **3**: 93–104.
5. Regnard CFB, Tempest S. Pain. In: *A guide to symptom relief in advanced cancer*, 3rd Ed. Manchester: Haigh Ltd. 1992: 5–22.
6. Ashdown HH. Report on certain substances found in the urine which reduce the oxide of copper upon boiling in the presence of an alkali. *British Medical Journal* 1890; **i**: 169–72.
7. Oberst FW. Free and bound morphine in the urine of morphine addicts. *Journal of Pharmacology* 1940: **69**: 240–51.
8. Woods LA. Distribution and fate of morphine in non-tolerant and tolerant dogs and rats. *Journal of Pharmacology and Experimental Therapeutics* 1954: **112**: 158–75.
9. Thompson V, Gross EG. Excretion of combined morphine in the tolerant and non-tolerant dog. *Journal of Pharmacology* 1941: **72**: 138-45.
10. Yoshimura H, Oguri K, Taukamoto H. Metabolism of drugs. LX. The synthesis of codeine and morphine glucuronides. *Chemical Pharmacology Bulletin* 1968: **16**: 2114–19.
11. Yoshimura H, Oguri K, Taukamoto H. Metabolism of drugs. LXII. Isolation and identification of morphine glucuronides in urine and bile of rabbits. *Biochemical Pharmacology* 1969: **18**: 279–286.
12. Oguri K, Ida S, Yoshimura H, Tsukamoto H. Metabolism of drugs. LXIX. Studies on the urinary metabolites of morphine in several mammalian species. *Chemical Pharmacology Bulletin* 1970: **18**: 2414-19.
13. Boerner U, Abbott S, Roe RL. The metabolism of morphine and heroin in man. *Drug Metabolism Review* 1975; **4**: 39–73.
14. Svensson J-O, Rane A, Sawe J, Sjoquist F. Determination of morphine, morphine-3-glucuronide and (tentatively) morphine-6-glucuronide in plasma and urine using ion-pair high-performance liquid chromatography. *Journal of Chromatography* 1982; **230**: 427–32.
15. Svensson J-O. Determination of morphine, morphine-6-glucuronide and normorphine in plasma and urine with high-performance liquid chromatography and electrochemical detection. *Journal of Chromatography* 1986; **375**: 174–8.
16. Aherne GW, Littlejohn P. Morphine-6-glucuronide, an important factor in interpreting morphine radioimmunoassays. *Lancet* 1985; **ii**: 210–11.
17. Whalstrom A, Pacifici GM, Lindstom B, Hammar L, Rane A, Human liver morphine UDP-glucuronyl-transferase enantio-selectivity and inhibition by opioid congeners and oxazepam. *British Journal of Pharmacology* 1988; **94**: 864–70.
18. Kuo CK, Hanioka N, Hoshikawa Y, Oguri K, Yoshimura H. Species difference of site-selective glucuronidation of morphine. *Journal of Pharmacobiology and Dynamics* 1991; **14**; 187–93.
19 Carrupt P-A, Testa B, Belchalany A, Taylor NE, Descas P, Perrissoud D. Morphine-

6-glucuronide and morphine-3-glucuronide as molecular chameleons with unexpected lipophilicity. *Journal of Medical Chemistry* 1991; **34**: 1272–5.

20. Koster AS, Frankhuijzen-Sierevogel AC, Noordhoek J. Distribution of glucuronidation capacity (1-naphthol and morphine) along the rat intestine. *Biochemical Pharmacology* 1985; **34**: 3527–32.

21. Pacifici GM, Bencini C, Rane A. Presystemic glucuronidation of morphine in humans and rhesus monkeys: subcellular distribution of the UDP glucuronyl-transferase in the liver and intestine. *Xenobiotica* 1986; **16**: 123–8.

22. Schali C, Rach-Ramel F. Transport and metabolism of [^{3}H] morphine in isolated, non-perfused proximal tubular segmets of the rabbit kidney. *Journal of Pharmacology and Experimental Therapeutics*. 1982; **223**: 811–15.

23. Crotty B, Watson KJ, Desmond PV *et al*. Hepatic extraction of morphine is impaired in cirrhosis. *European Journal of Clinical Pharmacology* 1989; **36**: 501–6.

24. Yeh SY. Urinary excretion of morphine and its metabolites in morphine-dependent subjects. *Journal of Pharmacology and Experimental Therapeutics* 1975; **192**: 201–10.

25. Hanks GW, Hoskin PJ, Aherne GW, Turner P, Poulain P. Explanation for potency of repeated oral doses of morphine? *Lancet* 1987; **ii**: 723–5.

26. Walsh CT, Levine RR. Studies of the enterohepatic circulation of morphine in the rat. *Journal of Pharmacology and Experimental Therapeutics* 1975; **195**: 303–10.

27. Hoskin PJ, Hanks GW. Morphine: pharmacokinetics and clinical practice. *British Journal of Cancer* 1990; **62**: 705–7.

28. Hanks GW, Wand PJ. Enterohepatic circulation of opioid drugs. Is it clinically relevant in the treatment of cancer patients? *Clinical Pharmacokinetics* 1989; **17**: 65–8.

29. Hoskin PJ, Alsayad-Omar O, Hanks GW, Johnston A, Turner P. The influence of blood sample preparation on measured levels of morphine and its major metabolites. *Annals of Clinical Biochemistry* 1989; **26**: 182–4.

30. Sawe J, Dahlstrom B, Rane A. Steady-state kinetics and analgesic effect of oral morphine in cancer patients. *European Journal of Clinical Pharmacology* 1983; **24**: 537–42.

31. Sawe J, Svensson JO, Rane A. Morphine metabolites in cancer patients on increasing oral doses – no evidence for autoinduction or dose-dependence. *British Journal of Clinical Pharmacology* 1983; **16**: 85–93.

32. Brunk SF, Delle M. Morphine metabolism in man. *Clinical Pharmacology and Therapeutics* 1974; **16**: 51–7.

33. Hoskin PJ, Hanks GW, Aherne GW, Chapman D, Littlejohn O, Filshie J. The bioavailability and pharmacokinetics of morphine after intravenous, oral and buccal administration in healthy volunteers. *British Journal of Clinical Pharmacology* 1989; **27**: 499-505.

34. Joel SP, Osborne RJ, Slevin ML. An improved method for the simultaneous determination of morphine and its principal glucuronide metabolites. *Journal of Chromatography* 1988; **430**: 394–9.

35. Osborne RJ, Joel SP, Trew D, Slevin ML. Morphine and metabolite behaviour after different routes of morphine administration; demonstration of the importance of the active metabolite morphine 6-glucuronide. *Clinical Pharmacology and Therapeutics* 1990; **47**: 12-19.

36. Khojasteh A, Evans W, Reynolds RD, Thomas G, Savarese JJ. Controlled-release oral morphine sulphate in the treatment of cancer pain with pharmacokinetic correlation. *Journal of Clinical Oncology* 1987; **5**: 956–61.

37. Leslie ST, Rhodes A, Black FM. Controlled release morphine sulphate tablets – a study in normal volunteers. *British Journal of Clinical Pharmacology* 1980; **9**: 531–4.

38. Pinnock CA, Derbyshire DR, AChola KJ, Smith G. Absorption of controlled release

morphine sulphate in the immediate post-operative period. *British Journal of Anaesthesia* 1986; **58**: 868–71.

39. Poulain P, Hoskin PJ, Hanks GW *et al*. Relative bioavailability of controlled release morphine tablets (MST Continus) in cancer patients. *British Journal of Anaesthesia* 1988; **61** 569–74.

40. Hanks GW. Controlled-release morphine (MST Contin) in advanced cancer. The European experience. *Cancer* 1989; **63**(suppl. 11): 2378–82.

41. Hoskin PJ, Poulain P, Hanks GW. Controlled-release morphine in cancer pain. Is a loading dose required when the formulation is changed? *Anaesthesia* 1989; **44**: 897–901.

42. Manara AR, Shelley MP, Quinn KG, Park GR. Pharmacokinetics of morphine following administration by the buccal route. *British Journal of Anaesthetics* 1989; **62**: 498–502.

43. Bell MDD, Mishra P, Weldon BD, Murray GR, Calvey TN, Williams NE. Buccal morphine – a new route for analgesia? *Lancet* 1985; **i**: 71–73.

44. Fisher AP, Vine P, Whitlock J, Hanna M. Buccal morphine premedication. A double-blind comparison with intramuscular morphine. *Anaesthesia* 1986; **41**: 1104–11.

45. Pannuti F, Rossi AP, Iafelice G *et al*. Control of chronic pain in very advanced cancer patients with morphine hydrocloride administered by oral, rectal and sublingual routes. Clinical report and preliminary results on morphine pharmacokinetics. *Pharmacology Research Committee* 1982; **14**: 2845–9.

46. Jonsson T, Christensen CB, Jordeling H, Frolund F. The bioavailability of rectally administered morphine. *Pharmacological Toxicology* 1988; **62**: 203–5.

47. Ellison NM, Lewis GO. Plasma concentrations following single doses of morphine sulphate in oral solution and rectal suppository. *Clinical Pharmacology* 1984; **3**: 614–16.

48. Hojsted J, Rubeck-Petersen K, Rask H, Bigler D, Broen E, Christensen C. Comparative bioavailability of a morphine suppository given rectally and in a colostomy. *European Journal of Clinical Pharmacology* 1990; **39**: 49–50.

49. Stanski DR, Greenblatt DJ, Lowenstein E. Kinetics of intravenous and intramuscular morphine. *Clinical Pharmacology and Therapeutics* 1978; **24**: 52–9.

50. Miser AW, Davis DM, Hughes CS, Mulne AF, Miser JS. Continuous subcutaneous infusion of morphine in children with cancer. *American Journal of Diseases in Children* 1983; **137**: 383–5.

51. Campbell, CF, Mason JB, Weiler JM. Continuous subcutaneous infusion of morphine for pain of terminal malignancy. *Annals of Internal Medicine* 1983; **98**: 51–2.

52. Bruera E, Brenneis C, Michaud M *et al*. Use of the subcutaneous route for the administration of narcotics in patients with cancer pain. *Cancer* 1988; **62**: 407–11.

53. Nahata MC, Miser AW, Miser JS, Reuning RH. Analgesic plasma concentrations of morphine in children with terminal malignancy receiving a continuous subcutaneous infusion of morphine sulfate to control severe pain. *Pain* 1984; **18**: 109–14.

54. Waldmann CS, Eason JR, Rambohul E, Hanson GC. Serum morphine levels. A comparison between continuous subcutaneous infusion and intravenous infusion in post-operative patients. *Anaesthesia* 1984; **39**: 768–71.

55. Sjoberg M, Applegren L, Einarsson S *et al*. Long term intrathecal morphine and bupivacaine in 'refractory' cancer pain. Results from the first series of 52 patients. *Acta Anaesthesia Scandanavia* 1991; **35**: 30–43.

56. Crul BJP, Delhass EM. Technical complications during longterm subarachnoid or epidural administration of morphine in terminally ill patients: a review of 140 cases. *Regional Anaesthesia* 1991; **16**: 209–13.

57. Yaksh TL. Spinal opiate analgesia: characteristics and principles of action. *Pain* 1981; **11**: 293–346.

58. Coombs DW, Saunders RL, Gaylor MS *et al*. Relief of continuous chronic pain by

intraspinal narcotics infusion via an implanted reservoir. *Journal of the American Medical Association* 1983; **250**: 2336–9.

59. Jaffe JH, Martin WR. Opioid analgesics and antagonists. In: Goodman Gilman A, Goodman LS, Rall TW, Murad F eds. *Goodman and Gilman's the pharmacological basis of therapeutics*. New York: Macmillan, 1985: 491–532.

60. Gourlay GK, Cherry DA, Cousins MJ. A comparative study of the efficacy and pharmacokinetics of oral methadone and morphine in the treatment of severe pain in patients with cancer. *Pain* 1986; **25**: 297–312.

61. Grabinski PY, Kaiko RF, Rogers AG, Houde RW. Plasma levels and analgesia following deltoid and gluteal injections of methadone and morphine. *Journal of Clinical Pharmacology* 1983; **23**: 48–55.

62. Kaiko RF, Wallenstein, SL, Rogers AG, Grabinski PY, Houde RW. Analgesic and mood effects of heroin and morphine in cancer patients with post-operative pain. *New England Journal of Medicine* 1981; **304**: 1501–5.

63. Nordberg G, Borg L, Hedner T, Mellstrand T. CSF and plasma pharmacokinetics of intramuscular morphine. *European Journal of Clinical Pharmacology* 1985; **27**: 677–81.

64. Rigg JRA. Ventilatory effects and plasma concentration of morphine in man. *British Journal of Anaesthesia* 1978; **50**: 759–65.

65. Samuelson H, Nordberg G, Hedner T, Lindquist J. CSF and plasma morphine concentrations in cancer patients during chronic epidural morphine therapy and its relation to pain relief. *Pain* 1987; **30**: 303–10.

66. Sawe J, Dahlstrom B, Rane A. Steady-state kinetics and analgesic effect of oral morphine in cancer patients. *European Journal of Clinical Pharmacology* 1983; **24**: 537–42.

67. Vater M, Smith G, Aherne GW, Aitkenhead AR. Pharmacokinetics and analgesic effect of slow-release oral morphine sulphate in volunteers. *British Journal of Anaesthesia* 1984; **56**: 821–7.

68. Hanks GW, Rose NM, Aherne GW, Piall EM, Fairfield S, Trueman T. Controlled-release morphine tablets. A double-blind trial in dental surgery patients. *British Journal of Anaesthesia* 1980; **53**: 1259–63.

69. Nordberg G, Mellstrand T, Borg L, Hedner T. Extradural morphine: influence of adrenaline admixture. *British Journal of Anaesthesia* 1986; **58**: 598–604.

70. Shimomura K, Kamata O, Ukei S, Ida S, Oguri K, Yoshimura H, Tsukamoto H. Analgesic effects of morphine glucuronides. *Tohuko Journal of Experimental Medicine* 1971; **105**: 45–52.

71. Abbott FV, Palmour RM. Morphine-6-glucuronide: analgesic effects and receptor binding profile in rats. *Life Sciences* 1988; **43**: 1685–95.

72. Paul D, Standifer KM, Intrurrisi CE. Pharmacological characterisation of morphine-6 beta-glucuronide, a very potent morphine metabolite. *Journal of Pharmacology and Experimental Therapeutics* 1989; **251**: 477–83.

73. Smith MT, Watt JA, Cramond TM. Morphine-3-glucuronide, a potent antagonist of morphine analgesia. *Life Sciences* 1990; **47**: 579–85.

74. Gong Q-L, Hedner J, Bjorkman R, Hedner T. Morphine-3-glucuronide may functionally antagonize morphine-6-glucuronide induced antinociception and ventilatory depression in the rat. *Pain* 1992; **48**: 249–55.

75. Suzuki N, Kalso E, Rosenberg P. Effect of simultaneous administration of morphine-3-glucuronide on the antinociception induced by intrathecal morphine-6-glucuronide. *The Scandinavian Association for the Study of Pain* 1992, abstract.

76. Osborne R, Thompson P, Joel S, Trew D, Patel N, Slevin ML. The analgesic activity of morphine-6-glucuronide. *British Journal of Clinical Pharmacology* 1992; **34**: 130–8.

77. Thompson PI, John L, Wedzicha J, Slevin ML. Comparison of the respiratory

depression induced by morphine and its active metabolite, morphine-6-glucuronide. *British Journal of Cancer* 1990; **62**: 484.

78. Hanna MH, Peat SJ, Woodham M, Knibb AA, Fung C. Analgesic efficacy and CSF pharmacokinetics of intrathecal morphine-6-glucuronide: a comparison with morphine. *British Journal of Anaesthesia* 1990; **64**: 547–50.

79. Osborne R, Joel S, Trew D, Slevin M. Analgesic activity or morphine-6-glucuronide. *Lancet* 1988; **i**: 828.

80. Hanna MH, Peat SJ, Knibb AA, Fung C. Disposition of morphine-6-glucuronide and morphine in healthy volunteers. *British Journal of Anaesthesia* 1991; **66**: 103–7.

81. Hanna MH, Zilkha TR, Peat SJ, D'Costa F, Fung C. Morphine-6-glucuronide. Pharmacokinetics after subcutaneous administration. *Proceedings of European Conference on Pain* 1991: abstract 57.

82. Thompson PI, Bingham S, Andrews PLR, Patel N, Joel SP, Slevin ML. Morphine 6-glucuronide: a metabolite of morphine with greater emetic potency than morphine in the ferret. *British Journal of Pharmacology* 1992; **106**: 3–8.

83. Hasselstrom J, Berg U, Lofgren A, Sawe J. Longlasting respiratory depression induced by morphine-6-glucuronide? *British Journal of Clinical Pharmacology* 1989; **27**: 515–18.

84. Osborne RJ, Joel SP, Slevin ML. Morphine intoxication in renal failure: the role of morphine-6-glucuronide. *British Medical Journal* 1986; **292**: 1548–9.

85. Peat SJ, Hanna MH, Woodham M, Knibb AA, Ponte J. Morphine-6-glucuronide: effects on ventilation in normal volunteers. *Pain* 1991; **45**: 101–4.

86. Pelligrino DA, Riegler FX, Albrecht RF. Ventilatory effects of fourth cerebroventricular infusions of morphine-6- or morphine-3-glucuronide in the awake dog. *Anesthesiology* 1989; **71**: 936–40.

87. Don HF, Dieppa RA, Taylor P. Narcotic analgesics in anuric patients. *Anesthesiology* 1975; **42**: 745–7.

88. Michie C, Chapman JR, Sear J, Moore RA. Opioid metabolism and the kidney. *Lancet* 1985; **i**: 586.

89. Moore RA, Sear J, Baldwin D *et al.* Morphine kinetics during and after renal transplantation. *Clinical Pharmacology and Therapeutics* 1984; **35**: 641–5.

90. Sear J, Moore A, Hunniset A *et al.* Morphine kinetics and kidney transplantation: morphine removal is influenced by renal ischaemia. *Anaesthesia and Analgesia* 1985; **64**: 1065–70.

91. Bion JF, Logan BK, Newman PM *et al.* Sedation in intensive care: morphine and renal function. *Intensive Care Medicine* 1986; **12**: 359–65.

92. Beckett AH, Casey AF. Synthetic analgesics: stereochemical considerations. *Journal of Pharmacy and Pharmacology* 1953; **6**: 986–99.

93. Martin WR, Eades CG, Thompson JA, Huppler RE, Gilbert PE. The effects of morphine- and nalorphine-like drugs in the nondependent and morphine-dependent chronic spinal dog. *Journal of Pharmacology and Experimental Therapeutics* 1976; **197**: 517–32.

94. Lord JAH, Waterfield AA, Hughes J, Kosterlitz HW. Endogenous opioid peptides: multiple agonists and receptors. *Nature* 1977; **267**: 495–9.

95. Schulz R, Fease E, Wuster M, Herz A. Selective receptors for B-endorphin on the rat vas deferens. *Life Sciences* 1979; **24**: 843–50.

96. Hughes J. Isolation of an endogenous compound from the brain with pharmacological properties similar to morphine. *Brain Research* 1975; **88**: 295–308.

97. Wolozin BJ, Pasternak GW. Classification of multiple morphine and enkephalin binding sites in the central nervous system. *Proceedings of the National Academy of Sciences, USA* 1981; **78**: 6181–5.

98. Pasternak GW, Wood PJ. Minireview: Multiple mu opiate receptors. *Life Sciences* 1986; **38**: 1889–98.

99. Ling GS, Spiegel K, Nishimura SL, Pasternak GW. Dissociation of morphine's

analgesic and respiratory depressant actions. *European Journal of Pharmacology* 1983; **86**: 487–8.

100. Ling GS, Spiegel K, Lockhart SH, Pasternak GW. Separation of opioid analgesia from respiratory depression: evidence for different receptor mechanisms. *Journal of Pharmacology and Experimental Therapeutics* 1985; **232**: 149–55.

101. Hucks D, Thompson PI, McLoughlin L *et al*. Explanation at the opioid receptor level for differing toxicity of morphine and morphine 6-glucuronide. *British Journal of Cancer* 1992; **65**: 122–6.

102. Frederickson RCA, Smithwick EL, Shuman R, Bemis KG. Metkephamid, a systemically active analog of methionine enkephalin with potent opioid δ-receptor activity. *Science* 1981; **211**: 603–5.

103. Yaksh TL. *In vivo* studies on opiate receptor systems mediating antinociception. I. Mu and delta receptor profiles in the primate. *Journal of Pharmacology and Experimental Therapeutics* 1983; **226**: 303–16.

104. Patwardhan RV, Johnson RF, Hoyumpa A *et al*. Normal metabolism of morphine in cirrhosis. *Gastroenterology* 1981; **81**: 1006–11.

105. Mazoit JX, Sandouk P, Zetlaoui P, Scherrman JM. Pharmacokinetics of unchanged morphine in normal and cirrhotic subjects. *Anesthesia and Analgesia* 1987; **66**: 293–8.

106. Knodell RG, Farleigh RM, Steele NM, Bond JH. Effects of liver congestion on hepatic drug metabolism in the rat. *Journal of Pharmacology and Experimental Therapeutics* 1982; **221**: 52–7.

107. Reed MD, Besunder JB. Developmental pharmacology: otogenic basis of drug disposition. *Pediatric Clinics of North America* 1989; **36**: 1053–74.

108. Koehntop DE, Rodman JH, Brundage DM, Hegland MG, Buckley JJ. Pharmacokinetics of fentanyl in neonates. *Anesthesia and Analgesia* 1986; **65**: 227–32.

109. Way WL, Costley EC, Way EL. Respiratory sensitivity of the newborn infant to heperidine and morphine. *Clinical Pharmacology and Therapeutics* 1965; **6**: 444–61.

110. Kelly H. Pharmacotherapy of paediatric lung disease: differences between children and adults. *Clinical Chest Medicine* 1987; **8**: 681–94.

111. Mickell JJ, Pedigo SA, Lucking SE, Albert. Age-related differences in the use of morphine, diazepam and pancuronium for mechanically ventilated children. *Developmental Pharmacology and Therapeutics* 1990; **14**: 20–8.

112. Burne R, Hunt A. Use of opiates in terminally ill children. *Palliative Care* 1987; **1**: 27–30.

113. Kaiko RF. Age and morphine analgesia in cancer patients with post-operative pain. *Clinical Pharmacology and Therapeutics* 1980; **28**: 528–33.

114. Sear JW, Hand CW, Moore RA. Studies on morphine disposition: plasma concentrations of morphine and its metabolites in anesthetized middle aged and elderly surgical patients. *Journal of Clinical Anaesthetics* 1989; **1**: 164–9.

115. Rhind W. *History of the vegetable kingdom*. London: Blackie & Son, 1870: 546–8.

CHAPTER 14

Haemostatic abnormalities in patients with cancer

STUART ROATH AND JOHN L. FRANCIS————————————

INTRODUCTION

Patients with malignancies, whether haematological or solid tumours, can be at increased risk of bleeding, clotting or both. This may be due to the disease itself or to complications associated with treatment. Management of such problems with appropriate support for the patient is essential to allow treatment to continue, to prevent or avoid complications of treatment or simply to reduce morbidity in the patient who has established disease, whether it is treatable or not. It should also be emphasized that a high proportion of patients with malignant disease have subclinical abnormalities of haemostasis.

HAEMOSTATIC ABNORMALITIES IN THE CANCER PATIENT

Acquired disorders of haemostasis in patients with cancer can be classified in the same way as those associated with non-malignant states and are usually due to problems with the vasculature, thrombocytopenia or thrombocytopathies, coagulation factor deficiencies and defects, and fibrinolytic abnormalities.

Vessel wall defects

Vasculitis due, for example, to endotoxins or immune complexes may cause bleeding in cancer patients with acquired infections, especially in septicaemia with encapsulated organisms.[1] Vasculitis causing purpura due to paraproteins is well described and amyloid itself, either in association with paraproteinaemia, or occasionally with other tumours, can also give rise to purpura. Occasionally the paraprotein may be deposited at critical temperatures, as in cryoglobulinaemia[2] or pyroglobulinaemia. Wäldenstrom's macroglobulinaemia may often be associated with both hyperviscosity and purpura.[3] Problems with circulatory stasis and associated purpuric bleeding may be caused by large molecular weight proteins such as IgM (and less commonly IgA or IgG), or when considerably increased populations of leucocytes are seen in some myeloid malignancies (acute leukaemias and chronic myelogenous leukaemia).[4]

Platelet abnormalities

Thrombocytopenia

Bleeding due to abnormally low platelet numbers is probably the commonest cause of bleeding associated with malignancies.[5] As a rule, patients are at risk of bleeding spontaneously if their platelet counts are less that $25 \times 10^9/l$ (normal values vary from laboratory to laboratory but $150–400 \times 10^9/l$ is a typical normal laboratory range). Individuals with platelet counts between 25 and 50 $\times 10^9$ are at risk of bleeding if stressed, for example by surgery or dental extraction. Patients with platelet counts of over 50×10^9 will probably escape haemorrhage unless the situation is compounded by a defect in the coagulation pathway, extreme stress such as prolonged surgery, cardiopulmonary bypass, hypotension, infection or a platelet function defect, for example induced by drugs such as aspirin.

Thrombocytopenia is often taken to be an indicator of disseminated intravascular coagulation (DIC) but, as discussed below, in patients with cancer, may also occur as a result of malignant infiltration of the bone marrow, immune complications, or as a side-effect of radiotherapy or chemotherapy. The incidence of thrombocytopenia in patients with disseminated malignancy may be as high as 38 per cent but is probably much lower (5–10 per cent) in patients with lesser tumour burdens. In patients with cancer complicated by DIC, over 90 per cent of cases will be thrombocytopenic. Thrombocytopenia may be due either to failure of platelet production, the commonest cause, or reduced platelet survival in the circulation due to either antibody-mediated removal or consumption in clotting.[6]

Failure of platelet production

Megakaryocyte numbers in the bone marrow may be diminished due to aplastic or hypoplastic states, clonal diversion of megakaryocyte production, occupancy of bone marrow by non-haemic tissue or bone marrow fibrosis (which may be associated with any of the above).

Bone marrow aplasia or hypoplasia can occur *de novo*, although its major importance in malignancies is that it may be associated with aggressive anti-tumour treatment. Most of the alkylating agents are myelosuppressive and can give rise to thrombocytopenia. This is usually in combination with neutropenia; because other side-effects limit the use of some alkylating agents, they are not regarded as highly bone marrow damaging. However, deliberate marrow ablation with increased doses will be invariably cytotoxic. Paradoxically, in situations where the marrow is occupied, for example, by low-grade lymphoma, the use of such agents may be accompanied by an increase in circulating platelets, presumably because of the preferential antitumour effect.

Antimetabolites interfering with DNA synthesis usually are cycle-active and may be temporarily myelosuppressive and cause thrombocytopenia. (They are also immunosuppressive and occasionally can be used in the treatment of immune thrombocytopenias.) Many other drugs such as anthracyclines and

Table 14.1 Drugs used in malignancies that may be
associated with thrombocytopenia

Primary bone marrow suppression (anticancer drugs)
Alkylating agents
Antimetabolites
Procarbazine
Quinolones
Anthracyclines
Cytarabine
Actinomycin D ⎫
Vinca alkaloids ⎬ less suppressive
Asparaginase ⎪
Cisplatin ⎭
Radiotherapy and bone/marrow-seeking isotopes

Non-anticancer agents
Massive blood transfusion
Chloramphenicol
Thiazides
Oestrogens and tamoxifen
Allopurinol
Hydantoin

---

antimitotics (e.g. the vinca alkaloids) can cause myelosuppression and thrombocytopenia. Bleomycin seems occasionally to have a rather specific action on both platelet destruction and production. Corticosteriods are traditionally platelet-sparing and may even raise the platelet count if there is an immunological element to its suppression. Some hormones may have a mild depressant effect on platelet production. Since it is not practicable to remove the offending drug, the normal method of management of thrombocytopenia due to myelosuppression is to replace the platelets. Table 14.1 lists some of the drugs associated with thrombocytopenia.

Other causes of aplastic or hypoplastic states include radiotherapy – total bone marrow aplasia is deliberately induced when sufficient radiotherapy is given as the conditioning treatment for bone marrow transplantation. Platelet support is obviously needed in this situation.

Clonal diversion of megakaryocyte production presumably occurs where there are stem cell disorders – some primitive leukaemias – where failure to form a megakaryocytic lineage may occur.

Occupancy of the bone marrow by lymphoma or cancer is a common cause of failure of platelet production which, either for mechanical reasons or due, for example, to disturbance of cytokine control, causes failure of megakaryocyte differentiation.

Bone marrow fibrosis due to marrow damage following chemotherapy or radiotherapy may result in production of fewer and sometimes more poorly functioning platelets than normal. Extramedullary haemopoiesis may be associated with marrow fibrosis; this may compensate for the failure of bone marrow production. In such situations platelets are often misshapen, oversized, and may be functionally incompetent.

Peripheral blood loss or destruction

In some situations, the bone marrow may produce adequate numbers of platelets but thrombocytopenia may occur because of peripheral blood loss or destruction. One of the causes for this is the consumption of platelets in coagulopathies and this will be described later. Another group of disorders associated with thrombocytopenia – the immune thrombocytopenias – may be isoimmune or autoimmune.

Isoimmune thrombocytopenia is relatively straightforward as it is due to alloantibodies, often following sensitization to antigenic platelets (which may have been given with otherwise properly typed blood transfusions) or because of previous pregnancies. It is interesting that the antiplatelet A1 isoantibody which is the one commonly involved may destroy autologous PLA1-negative platelets! In such conditions the only management is to ensure that PLA1-negative platelets are used when such support is needed.

Autoimmune thrombocytopenia has been well-documented in lymphoproliferative neoplasms – chronic lymphatic leukaemia and lymphomas – and also in Hodgkin's disease. There are also case reports from various cancers but these are less frequent. The disorder may be suspected when severe thrombocytopenia is noted in the absence of bone marrow depression due to disease or drugs and may be confirmed by the presence of free or platelet-associated platelet antibodies in about 80 per cent of all cases.

Drug-induced thrombocytopenia may be associated with a number of drugs, some of which produce bone marrow suppression or suppress megakaryocyte production. There are also a few agents that damage platelets; some are associated with the formation of platelet antibodies where the platelet may be secondarily involved in an immunological reaction and many others are reported to have been associated with thrombocytopenia where the mechanism is not understood.

Bone marrow transplantaion

Following ablative therapy, recovery of platelets to normal numbers may be prolonged by many months or even years. This may be immune[7] but since it can occur in autologous transplantation, other mechanisms must also operate.

Hypersplenism

'Hyperfunction' of the spleen, often but not invariably associated with splenomegaly, can be associated with low platelet counts. The nature of the splenic pathology may be irrelevant. Splenic platelet pooling and destruction are obvious mechanisms but do not account for all cases.

Viral infections

Viral infections may be associated with malignancies and may be reponsible for coagulation abnormalities, especially but not exclusively thrombocytopenia. CMV, HIV-1 viruses, parvoviruses and hepatitis viruses have all been implicated. In HIV-1 infections, 3–8 per cent are said to be thrombocytopenic[8] as are

30–45 per cent of AIDS patients.[9] Anticardiolipid antibodies have also been detected[10] with correspondingly abnormal coagulation profiles (e.g. prolonged INRs or APTTs).

Thrombocytopathies

Patients with cancer may bleed because of defective platelet function associated with normal, slightly reduced or even elevated platelet counts.[6] Such acquired defects of platelet function are either due to drugs such as aspirin or other non-steroidal anti-inflammatory medications, or alternatively, associated with myelo-proliferative disorders where adequate or raised numbers of platelets are produced whose adhesion, contraction or aggregation is inadequate.[11] Patients with an excessive number of platelets (more than $700 \times 10^9/l$) may be at particular risk from bleeding, clotting or both.[6] Retinal or cerebral haemorrhages seem to be particular hazards in such patients.

Commonly used platelet function screening tests include the template bleeding time[12] and the tourniquet (Hess) test. Although these tests may often be abnormal in patients with malignant disease, they generally add little to the diagnosis of a haemostatic defect, and may cause unnecessary bruising and bleeding in those patients with acute DIC. Shortened bleeding times are also observed in cancer patients. In one series, almost half the patients with disseminated malignancy had bleeding times below the lower limit of normal, and this has been taken as evidence of hypercoagulability.[13]

The identification of platelet function defects in patients with malignant disease is made difficult by the frequent use of interfering drugs in such individuals and the presence of thrombocytopenia. The latter is probably the more important cause of haemorrhagic problems in cancer patients,[14] although various platelet function defects may occur. These have included reduced platelet adhesion, impaired aggregation to adenosine diphosphate (ADP) and poor clot retraction, deficiency of platelet factor 3 and spontaneous *in vitro* platelet aggregation.[6] Increased platelet aggregation to ADP and adrenaline has also been reported.[13,15]

The pathogenesis of platelet function defects remains relatively unclear. Defects may arise as a result of partial stimulation of the platelets, directly or indirectly, by malignant tissue, or by exposure to activated clotting factors. The abnormal plasma proteins found in individuals with malignant paraprotein-aemias 'coat' the platelets and interfere with adhesion and aggregation. Patients with myeloproliferative disorders frequently exhibit platelet function defects that often result from an acquired defect of platelet prostaglandin metabolism.[11] A variety of other functional defects in these syndromes have been reported, including abnormal glucose metabolism, defective coagulant activity, low serotonin levels, abnormalities of platelet membrane glycoproteins and receptors and abnormal calcium ion homeostasis. Patients with myeloproliferative disorders may also have an increased platelet affinity for fibrinogen, possibly due to reduced glycosylation of the adhesive receptors, glycoproteins IIb and IIIa, which may account for the thrombotic diathesis of these individuals.[16]

When platelets take part in haemostasis they undergo a process known as 'degranulation' in which the contents of their intracellular granules are released into the surrounding plasma. The subsequent detection of some of these platelet proteins [particularly β-thromboglobulin (β-TG) and platelet factor 4] is a sensitive indication of *in vivo* platelet activation. Plasma β-TG levels are elevated in a high proportion (>80 per cent) of patients with a variety of malignancies.[17] Levels are reduced by chemotherapy, independently of the platelet count, and β-TG levels may therefore be a useful indication of the tumour burden and response to treatment. It should be noted that β-TG levels may be raised in cancer patients even in the absence of thrombocytopenia and other coagulation abnormalities.[18] Patients with myeloproliferative disorders have significantly raised levels of plasma β-TG, even after correction for the increased platelet count.[19] Plasma levels of thrombospondin, a large adhesive glycoprotein present in platelets, which is thought to play a role in promoting metastasis,[20] are increased in various types of cancer.[21]

Thrombocytosis

The incidence of thrombocytosis in untreated patients with cancer is higher than that of thrombocytopenia, but equally variable. Interpretation of published data is made more difficult by variations in the upper normal limit used by different workers ranging from 350 to 500 $\times$ 10^9/l. Although some workers have put the incidence as high as 57 per cent,[22] others have reported thrombocytosis in only 10–18 per cent of patients.[13,23] In one large study, 36 per cent of patients had platelet counts over 350 $\times$ 10^9/l and it was noteworthy that the platelet counts increased in the months before death.[24] Such an increase in platelet count cannot be managed or prevented by warfarin therapy. Despite variations in published reports, it is evident that thrombocytosis is common in patients with malignant disease and it appears that it may be a valuable indicator of malignancy in patients in whom the diagnosis is uncertain. Thrombocytosis may also be an independent indicator of poor prognosis in patients with cervical cancer.[25]

Deficiencies and defects of the coagulation factors

Screening tests of blood coagulation

The most commonly used tests to screen the blood coagulation mechanism are the prothrombin time (PT), the activated partial thromboplastin time (APTT) and the thrombin clotting time (TCT). The PT measures the combined efficiency of the extrinsic clotting pathway (Factors II, V, VII and X), while the APTT assesses the intrinsic system (Factors II, V, VII, IX, X, XI and XII). The TCT is only sensitive to factors affecting the conversion of fibrinogen to fibrin (fibrinogen concentration, abnormal forms of fibrinogen and inhibitors such as heparin degradation products).

Prolongation of the PT in patients with DIC may be due to markedly decreased (< 1.0 g/l) fibrinogen levels, the presence of high levels of fibrin(ogen) degradation products (FDP) or reduction in the plasma levels of Factors II, V, VII and X. Of the clotting factors, Factor V is readily degraded by plasmin during acute DIC and is therefore the most likely factor to be significantly reduced. Nevertheless, not all individuals with a prolonged PT have a decrease in Factor V concentration. In patients with a broad spectrum of malignant disease the PT is prolonged in approximately 14 per cent of cases,[15,26,27] but this will be much higher (about 40 per cent) in cases with established DIC.[23]

As with PT, APTT may also be prolonged by severe fibrinogen deficiency, elevation of FDP and degradation of Factor V. Depletion of Factor VIII, the other major plasmin-sensitive coagulation factor, as well as reductions in Factors IX and XI, may also contribute to a prolonged APTT. The incidence of a prolonged APTT is more difficult to establish, possibly because of the much greater range and sensitivity of commercially available APTT reagents. However, it is probably less than 10 per cent in unselected patients, although as expected, it will be much higher in those individuals with diagnosed DIC.[15,23,26]

Shortened APTTs may also occur, although the frequency of this finding appears to be lower. The presence of DIC makes little difference to the incidence of a shortened APTT.[23] The cause of a shortened APTT and/or PT is less obvious than the reasons for prolongation, but may be related to the presence of activated clotting factors or rapidly clottable early degradation products of fibrin.

Prolongation of the TCT in patients with cancer is rather more common and may be profoundly influenced by the combination of hypofibrinogenaemia and the presence of fibrin degradation products in subjects with DIC;[15,26,27] 55 per cent of patients with DIC and malignancy showed a prolonged TCT.[23] The TCT is prolonged by low fibrinogen concentrations (<1.0 g/l), but it is not generally appreciated that increased plasma fibrinogen levels (>4.5 g/l) will also give rise to a prolonged clotting time. As detailed below, raised fibrinogen levels are a common finding in patients with malignant disease and this is undoubtedly a major factor in the prolongation of the TCT in such patients.

Overall, routine screening tests of coagulation are of only limited value in detecting subclinical levels of intravascular clotting activation.[28] Typically, 50 per cent of patients without overt DIC have normal screening test results.[23] Although these tests may be more useful in the detection of acute DIC, for reasons detailed below, falling levels of fibrinogen and/or AT III, together with elevation of FDP (see later) have greater diagnostic value.[23]

Fibrinogen levels

Abnormalities in the plasma fibrinogen concentration, normally 1.5–4.0 g/l, are relatively common in patients with malignant disease. Low fibrinogen levels (hypofibrinogenaemia), however, are surprisingly uncommon, and are found in less than 5 per cent of unselected patients.[15,22,24] In individuals with DIC the incidence will be higher. Raised fibrinogen levels (hyperfibrinogenaemia), on the other hand, are much more common, and are found in 50–80 per cent of patients studied.[15,22,24] If patients with evidence of DIC are specifically excluded, over 80 per cent of patients may show hyperfibrinogenaemia. In patients with DIC however, less than 10 per cent have an increased fibrinogen level. It should be emphasized that as most cancer patients have elevated fibrinogen concentrations before the onset of DIC, a normal fibrinogen level cannot be used to exclude DIC in such patients. In this respect the use of serial estimations to detect falling levels is more useful. Like the platelet count, fibrinogen levels in cancer patients increase in the months before death.[24] An increase in the plasma cryofibrinogen level has also been observed.

Fibrinogen survival

The plasma half-life of fibrinogen is approximately 4–6 days. A decrease in this value reflects increased consumption of fibrinogen which is widely thought to result from intravascular coagulation. There is now general agreement that decreased plasma fibrinogen survival is a common feature of malignant disease.[29] In general, fibrinogen levels below about 2 g/l are associated with plasma fibrinogen survival times of less than one day. As such levels may still be within the normal physiological range; this further emphasizes the importance of serial fibrinogen assays in the diagnosis of DIC in cancer patients.

Dysfibrinogenaemia

Dysfibrinogenaemia may be defined as a qualitative defect of plasma fibrinogen which may occur in both congenital and acquired forms.[30] Acquired dysfibrinogenaemia is manifested by an impairment of fibrin polymerization and is rare in the majority of malignant diseases. It does, however, occur commonly in patients with hepatocellular carcinoma, but is much less common in patients with carcinoma of other sites which have metastasized to the liver.[31]

The presence of dysfibrinogenaemia has been considered to be a useful biological marker of primary hepatocellular carcinoma,[32] although this abnormality is often the result of underlying liver cirrhosis and is not specific for hepatoma. Since the abnormal fibrinogen may disappear following successful chemotherapy and clinical improvement and reappear prior to relapse and death, it may be a useful indicator of disease activity.[33]

Molecular markers of clotting activation

When thrombin acts on fibrinogen, the first stage in the formation of fibrin is the release of small peptides from the ends of the A(α10) and B(β11)-chains. These peptides are termed fibrinopeptides A and B respectively and their presence in increased amounts in the plasma is a sensitive indicator of *in vivo* coagulation activation. Plasma levels of fibrinopeptide A (FpA) have been extensively studied in patients and are elevated in a high proportion of patients with malignant disease. Thus, 95 per cent of those with 'active' disease have an increase in plasma FpA, while levels are normal in most patients in remission and in those without mestastases.[34] Like platelets and fibrinogen levels, FpA tends to increase as disease becomes terminal but may also be increased in localized malignancy.[35] Persistently raised FpA levels suggest treatment failure and a poor prognosis. Serial FpA measurements may therefore be a useful indicator of tumour progression or response to treatment.[36]

Other markers of clotting activation include prothrombin F1.2, a fragment which is released from prothrombin during its activation by Factor Xa and thrombin–antithrombin (TAT) complex which is formed when intravascularly generated thrombin is bound by its natural inhibitor, antithrombin III. As might be expected, plasma levels of these markers are elevated in a high proportion of cancer patients.[37] TAT has also been shown to be elevated in patients with acute promyelocytic leukaemia and acute non-lymphocytic leukaemias.[38] For reasons which remain unclear, AT III levels in such patients are frequently normal, despite other evidence of intravascular coagulation.[39]

Factor XIII deficiency

Moderate Factor XIII deficiency may occur in patients with solid tumours as well as various haematological malignancies.[13] Indeed, Factor XIII depletion is one of the most common haemostatic defects associated with leukaemias and lymphomas, although this does not necessarily herald the onset of DIC. Since only about 1–2 per cent of the normal plasma Factor XIII level is sufficient for normal clot formation, it is unlikely that this causes bleeding *per se*.[40] Nevertheless, in combination with other abnormalities, for example thrombocytopenia or other ill-defined defects of fibrin stabilization, moderate Factor XIII deficiency may contribute to poor wound healing or a haemorrhagic diathesis in these patients.

Antithrombin III (AT III)

AT III is the major physiological inhibitor of the activated clotting factors. A reduction in AT III is associated with an increased tendency towards intravascular coagulation and acquired deficiency may result from decreased synthesis or increased consumption. Increased AT III consumption due to complex formation with thrombin and other activated serine proteinases, is an early indicator of DIC, and AT III levels may provide valuable information about the course of intravascular clotting. Falling AT III levels suggest that intravascular coagulation is ongoing, while cessation of AT III consumption may indicate that treatment has successfully curbed the process.[5]

Miscellaneous coagulation defects

Patients with malignant disease may develop abnormalities of most components of the blood coagulation pathway. For example, deficiencies of the vitamin K-dependent clotting factors (II, VII, IX and X) may also arise, particularly in patients with hepatic metastases.[13] These defects would result in prolongation of the PT and APTT even in the absence of DIC. Cancer patients may also develop circulating anticoagulants, although the relationship of these to the clinical haemostatic defect is largely unknown. Some of these, especially those found in association with lung cancer or transitional cell carcinoma, have a heparin-like action.[5,41] Fibrin degradation products interfere with platelet function and fibrin formation and thus also act as circulating anticoagulants. Increased levels of clotting factors are also common in patients with malignant neoplasms[15] and patients with chronic myeloid leukaemia may have an abnormal multimeric composition of plasma von Willebrand factor (vWf).[42]

Fibrinolytic defects

Intravascular activation of the blood coagulation pathway in cancer patients is virtually inseparable from activation of fibrinolysis. Thus, evidence of fibrinolytic activation is frequently observed in patients with malignant disease.[43] This is usually manifested by a combination of depletion (consumption) of fibrinolytic proteins (plasminogen) and inhibitors (α10-antiplasmin and β-macroglobulin), and an increase in the major products of fibrinolysis (circulating plasmin and fibrin(ogen) degradation products).

Euglobulin clot lysis time

The euglobulin clot lysis time (ECLT) is the most widely used global assessment of plasma fibrinolytic activity. Shortened lysis times, indicating increased fibrinolytic activity, may be observed in around 10 per cent of patients with malignant disease, a proportion which is not significantly affected by the presence of DIC.[22]

Plasminogen levels

Plasminogen levels are decreased in many patients with cancer whose disease is complicated by DIC, but are also low in around 25 per cent of individuals without evidence of acute intravascular coagulation.[23] Plasminogen levels are usually normal in patients with prostatic cancer but increase during oestrogen therapy.[44]

Plasminogen activator activity

Increased levels of urokinase-type plasminogen activator (u-PA) antigen may be found in various forms of cancer and are generally higher in those with more advanced disease. This agrees with much of the available data on plasminogen activator activity in solid tumours, which suggests that u-PA may be a marker of malignant transformation and may also have some prognostic value.[45,46]

Fibrin(ogen) degradation products (FDP)

FDP are formed as a result of plasmin action on fibrinogen (fibrinogenolysis) or fibrin (fibrinolysis). The presence of FDP in plasma or urine therefore represents direct evidence of the activation of the fibrinolytic pathway. Most, if not all patients with malignancy and acute DIC have elevated FDP levels.[5,23] In the absence of overt DIC however, the incidence of raised FDP levels has been variously reported, but is certainly much lower. Levels are generally higher in patients with remote metastases compared to those with more localized disease and determination of FDP may therefore have some prognostic value in patients with malignant disease.[47] Modern techniques for the measurement of FDP allow the differentiation of degradation products derived from fibrin and fibrinogen. A preponderance of fibrinogen-derived cleavage products is indicative of primary fibrinolytic activation.

HYPERCOAGULABILITY IN CANCER

Hypercoagulability – a tendency towards thrombosis – is common in patients with malignancies and there is now considerable clinical and experimental evidence to support the concept of an association between blood coagulation and malignant disease first described in 1865 by Armand Trousseau.[48] The altera- tions in haemostasis are complex and many of the specific laboratory findings have already been discussed in this review. Generally there is an increase in clotting factor levels, evidence of increased fibrin(ogen) breakdown, thrombo- cytosis, evidence of platelet activation and decreases in coagulation inhibitors. There is therefore little doubt that coagulation is activated in many patients with cancer. The role of the tumour in this sequence of events remains poorly defined, but many patients with malignancies have life-threatening coagulation disorders and autopsy studies have shown that a significant proportion have evidence of thrombosis.[49]

Role of clotting activation in tumour pathology

The association of fibrin with intravascular tumour deposits is well-established and fibrin appears to be an integral part of tumour stroma in many animal and human malignancies.[50] Since tumours cannot grow significantly in the absence of adequate stroma, fibrin deposition appears to be an important determinant of malignant proliferation.[50] That fibrin is important in tumour growth and dissemi- nation has been well-shown, at least in animal models, by the beneficial effects of oral anticoagulants and other modalities that interfere with blood coagulability. Such studies, some of which have been undertaken in the authors' laboratory, have suggested that certain types of blood-borne tumour cells activate coagulation *in vivo* leading to the formation of tumour–platelet–fibrin complexes in the circula- tion.[51] Formation of such complexes apparently facilitates lodgement and sub- sequent extravasation of the tumour cell and may therefore be an essential step in the formation of metastases.[52] As discussed in more detail below, this process may depend on the ability of the circulating tumour cells to activate coagulation.

The apparently central role of clotting activation in the dissemination of malignant tumours has been the trigger for many studies into the efficacy of anticoagulant drugs in the treatment of cancer. Many of the more positive reports have been from uncontrolled studies, although a large Veteran's Administration (VA) Cooperative study begun in 1976 reported a significant survival advantage in patients with small cell carcinoma of the lung (SCCL) who received warfarin treatment.[53,54] Similar results were also published by the Cancer and Leukemia Group B while others have suggested that malignant melanoma also responds to oral anticoagulants. Another VA group study reported that a dipyridamole derivative had a favourable effect on survival in non-small cell lung cancer.[55] In general, however, such studies have not realized the promise of animal experiments in this regard. There may be at least two reasons for this. First, many of the patients entering such trials may have already developed metastases and thus the theoretical benefit of anticoagulation would be expected to be diminished. Secondly, many of these studies have not taken account of the way in which specific tumour types interact with the haemostatic system. Thus, immunolocalization studies have shown that some tumours, such as SCCL[56] and malignant melanoma,[57] produce tissue factor and are apparently associated with a complete thrombin-forming pathway. Others, such as breast and colorectal tumours express fibrinolytic activity and do not have significant procoagulant activity.[58] It therefore seems reasonable, if procoagulant activity is

Table 14.2 Partial classification of human tumours based on their interactions with haemostatic pathways[58]

Tumours having thrombin-forming (procoagulant) potential
Small cell carcinoma of the lung
Malignant melanoma
Renal cell carcinoma

Tumours having fibrinolytic potential
Colorectal carcinoma
Breast cancer
Non-small cell lung cancer

Tumours apparently lacking coagulation or fibrinolytic potential
Mesothelioma
Lymphoproliferative disorders

---

related to metastic potential, to confine trials of anticoagulant drugs to those tumours that have the ability to activate coagulation (Table 14.2).

Tumour-derived procoagulant activity

Many workers have focused on the mechanisms of clotting activation in malignant disease and it is now apparent that tumour cells and/or host cells may contribute to fibrin formation by expressing procoagulant activity (PCA).[59] Several types of PCA have been described. Tissue factor (TF) a normal constituent of many tissues, which is responsible for initiating coagulation following injury, may be expressed by tumour cells and tumour-associated macrophages.[60] TF apparently in complex with activated Factor VII (VIIa) has been described in breast and colon tumours and other situations associated with extravascular fibrin formation.[61,62] Another Factor X activator that appears to be specific for malignant cells, termed cancer procoagulant (CP), has also been described.[63] This procoagulant has the enzymatic characteristics of a cysteine proteinase and is distinct from tissue factor in its ability to activate Factor X directly, without a requirement for Factor VII.[64] Whether the presence of CP in plasma is related to haemostatic defects in patients with cancer remains to be proved but preliminary results suggest that it may prove to be a useful marker of malignant disease.[65] Experimental blockade of cellular procoagulant activity in animal models has been shown to reduce metastasis, emphasizing the potential pathophysiological relevance of tumour cell procoagulants in this process.[51,66]

Host cell-derived procoagulant activity

The presence of malignant tumours stimulates the production of TF by circulating blood monocytes. This appears to make a significant contribution to the hypercoagulable state as TF expression correlates well with markers of clotting activation, such as fibrinopeptide A.[67] The elaboration of TF by monocytes and macrophages is apparently part of the inflammatory response and is regulated by complex and poorly understood cooperativity between lymphocytes, platelets and various cytokines such as the interleukins and tumour necrosis factor.[68] Endothelial cells may also be involved in this process and damage to these cells, for example from tumour–host cells complexes, may provide an additional procoagulant stimulus.

Non-specific causes of clotting activation in cancer patients

As detailed above, there exists the possibility that tumour cells may activate coagulation either directly or by mediating an indirect response via monocytes and/or endothelial cells. Tumours may also evoke coagulation activation non-specifically by causing damage to host tissues or through induction of a host inflammatory response, for example due to secondary conditions such as pneumonia. Some tumours may activate coagulation through tumour necrosis or by production of mucin.[6]

Venous thromboembolism and cancer

The literature abounds with case reports which are often cited as evidence for the thrombogenicity of malignant tumours. Many of these describe a picture of multiple thrombotic attacks in alternating locations, commonly referred to as thrombophlebitis migrans sive saltans or recurrent thrombophlebitis.[69]

Post-mortem studies have revealed a high frequency of thromboembolism among cancer patients. Such studies have suggested that thrombosis complicates 15–25 per cent of most types of malignancy, although the incidence in certain types, for example cancer of body or tail of pancreas, may be double this figure.[49]

Attempts to ascribe the presence of thrombotic disease in patients with cancer directly to the presence of a malignant tumour have met with mixed results. Although there is little doubt that cancer patients have a higher than normal frequency of thrombosis, the possibility that this is due to the presence of additional risk factors has been difficult to exclude.[70]

In many of the published case reports, the thrombotic phenomena were the first clinical manifestations in patients subsequently found to have cancer. This has led to the suggestion that occult cancer should be suspected in patients presenting with otherwise unexplained venous thromboembolism.[71,72] Some support for this has been obtained from large-scale studies but the evidence is by no means conclusive.

FIBRINOLYTIC ACTIVATION BY TUMOUR CELLS

The ability of many types of malignant tumour to activate blood coagulation has been discussed above. However, it is now clear that many tumour types do not possess procoagulant activity but seem to be rich in activators of the fibrinolytic system. Two common tumours, those of breast and colon, have been particularly well-studied in this regard. Malignant breast and colon tumours both contain increased amounts of the urokinase-type plasminogen activator (u-PA).[45,73,74] Unlike the tissue-type plasminogen activator (t-PA), u-PA does not require the presence of fibrin to activate plasminogen and therefore lacks the local control that regulates t-PA activity. Interestingly, u-PA has growth factor activity which suggests a role for this proteinase outside that of fibrinolysis. In breast cancer, tumour u-PA levels have prognostic value and oestrogen receptor antagonists suppress u-PA expression.[45,74] In colon cancer, u-PA levels correlate well with the degree of tissue invasion, undifferentiated morphology and aggressive growth of cultured tumour cells. Thus, u-PA may prove to be a useful target for antimetastatic agents, either by inhibiting its synthesis or activity or by intefering with its binding to the u-PA receptor.

MANAGEMENT OF HAEMOSTATIC PROBLEMS IN MALIGNANCIES

Typically a patient will present with either venous or rarely arterial thrombosis, or with bleeding, sometimes with evidence of DIC.

Management of vascular problems

If associated with infection, clearly the underlying infection should be treated as vigorously as possible. Management of vascular purpuras due to paraproteins involves the reduction and removal of the paraproteins. Treatment of the underlying disease with alkylating agents or combination chemotherapy such as ABCM (Doxorubicin, Carmustine, Cyclophosphomide, Melphalan) or VAMP (Vincristine, Doxorubicin, Melphalan, Prednisolone) may be indicated, and the use of plasmapheresis with reduction of the pathological protein may be life-saving. Drug-induced non-thrombocytopenic purpura, another cause of vascular purpura, should always be suspected in situations where purpuric bleeding occurs in a patient with normal platelet count and coagulation profile. Removal of the offending drug is the treatment of choice.

Management of thrombocytopenia

If there is active bleeding due to thrombocytopenia then platelet transfusions are indicated. The quantity given should be enough to secure haemostasis and although it is reassuring to see incremental increases in circulating platelets, this may not be essential. All individuals with platelet counts $<10 \times 10^9/l$ will need platelet transfusions to prevent bleeding. Patients actually bleeding, or febrile, should be transfused if their platelet counts are less than $20 \times 10^9/l$. If surgery, lumbar puncture or dental extraction is contemplated, counts of $50 \times 10^9/l$ should be aimed at.[75] The source of the platelets needs to be considered. Platelet transfusions, like other biological products, carry certain risks. Transmission of infection is an important one, especially that of cytomegalovirus (CMV). All individuals due to receive platelet or blood transfusions should be sero tested for CMV and, if negative, should only receive CMV-negative products. It may also be true that disease in CMV-positive individuals may recur if they are otherwise immunosuppressed. Thus, if possible, they should also be given CMV-negative or irradiated platelets. There is also a case for filtering platelet preparations to remove leucocytes. Many platelet transfusions do contain a few viable lymphocytes and there is a possibility of graft-versus-host disease from transfused lymphocytes. More often though, effete leucocytes cause febrile reactions. In some institutions platelets are obtained from single donors in large quantities on cell separators rather than being skimmed from donated units of blood. There is an advantage in using a single, properly matched donor if the described safety measures are also observed – improving techniques in plateletpheresis can obtain the equivalent of 6–10 units in one process; this may be repeated twice weekly if a willing donor is available. After repeated transfusions alloantibodies to donor platelets may develop; typing and crossmatching as for red blood cells may then be necessary.[76]

Transfused platelets, however well typed, may also be rapidly destroyed in the circulation, especially in the presence of disease-associated immune thrombocytopenia (ITP). Although their transfusion is still by no means valueless, immunosuppressive therapy needs to be initiated to block the destructive process. The conventional treatment is with sizeable doses of steroids such as 60 mg of prednisolone daily by mouth; this dose can be reduced as soon as the platelet count returns to $100 \times 10^9/l$ or more, which it often does within a few days. Such steroid treatment may need to be persisted with until the underlying disease can be treated, when hopefully the ITP will burn out. Should the underlying disease however be indolent, such as chronic lymphatic leukaemia, then other immunosuppressive agents such as chlorambucil or azathioprine can be considered. Intravenous immunoglobulin (0.4 g/kg for 4 days) undoubtedly has a short-term, but welcome effect in rapidly raising the platelet count and its use may be repeated. In the longer term, danazol, a progesterone-like agent, has achieved spectacular results in some patients who would otherwise need persistent treatment. Such patients should be started at 800 mg/day reducing to 200 mg/day when a beneficial rise in platelet count has been established.

Management of drug-induced thrombocytopenia involves the withdrawal of the offending drug. Many patients with cancer are having many drugs concurrently so this may be much more difficult than it seems. However, candidate drugs should be withdrawn or replaced with others whenever this is possible. Immunosuppression with corticosteroids or other drugs is unlikely to be effective but platelet transfusions may be temporarily helpful if indicated.

Management of thrombocytopathies

The acquired platelet functional defects are only acutely manageable by replacement with fresh unaltered platelets. Most will be drug-associated and respond to withdrawal of the culprit such as aspirin or other non-steroidal anti-inflammatory agents.

Management of thrombocytosis

Thrombocytosis itself constitutes a risk factor as well as being a 'marker' of some aspects of malignant disease. Individuals with platelet counts of over 700 $\times 10^9/l$ are at risk of both clotting and bleeding. Such a risk is reduced only when the platelet count is reduced. Drugs like aspirin should not be given, but platelet reduction by antimetabolites such as hydroxyurea, alkylating agents like busulphan and radioisotopes such as radio-phosphorus may all be useful in reducing platelet numbers, although none acts very quickly. If the patient is felt to be at immediate risk, for example with recurrent arterial thromboses, then a quicker acting drug such as intravenous cyclophosphamide (1.5 g in a medium-sized patient, although the dose would have to be considered carefully in relation to concomitant treatment) might be suitable.

Management of venous thrombosis

Treatment of venous thrombosis in malignancy is that of immediate heparinization for the first 48 hours and warfarinization for at least 3 months. Assuming the thrombosis is in the lower limb, then rest and analgesia may be also required initially. The dose of heparin is usually regulated by the APTT level at about twice normal and warfarinization by the INR, which should be maintained between 2 and 4. Consideration should be given in any patient with an established malignancy and deep vein thrombosis (DVT) to warfarinizing that individual for the rest of their life. Certainly, a recurrence of the thrombotic event is an indication for continued anticoagulation.

Pulmonary embolus, presumably associated with DVT, is a serious and occasionally fatal complication in about 10–15 per cent of patients who suffer it. Treatment has traditionally been heparinization for 7–10 days[77] but thrombolytic agents are at least as effective in its management. Streptokinase, urokinase and newer clot-seeking agents such as recombinant tissue plasminogen activator (rTPA) may be used.[78] Endarterectomy has also been of value, especially in the treatment of pulmonary hypertension as a late complication. With all these drugs, especially streptokinase and urokinase, there is a risk of bleeding and only the recombinant drugs can be used on more than one or two occasions without risk of anaphylaxis. Any patient who has malignancy and has already had a pulmonary embolus should be maintained on anticoagulant therapy unless the malignancy is cured. Any patient with a known malignancy who is to have significant surgery and immobilization probably should have prophylactic anticoagulation.

Management of arterial thrombosis

Arterial thrombotic events are much less common, and more often associated with hyperviscosity syndromes in polycythaemias, myelomas, and leukaemias with high white cell counts. They are amenable to treatment like venous thromboses or by mechanical removal. Circulatory improvement, for example by volume replacement or isovolaemic red cell removal, may also be indicated.

Management of bleeding

The causes of bleeding in patients with malignancies have already been described, but may additionally be due to DIC. This may be due to products of the malignancy itself. For example, in promyelocytic leukaemia the abnormal myeloid granules have been identified as having procoagulant activity and triggering such a reaction.[79] As mentioned above, many tumours express increased amounts of tissue factor levels which may initiate DIC.

Tissue factor production by peripheral blood monocytes and endothelial cells may also act as a trigger for DIC and this inflammatory response may be greatly accelerated by the presence of infection.[80] The clinical condition, as well as appearing largely as a bleeding phenomenon, may include shock and peripheral circulatory failure. The management of DIC has always been difficult but the principle has been that of replenishment of consumed factors and platelets using fresh frozen plasma, coagulation factor concentrates and platelet concentrates, while attempting to deal with the underlying insult – the malignancy or infection.[81] More heroic measures such as the use of heparin or large doses of corticosteroids are probably of little value. The antiproteinase aprotinin (Trasylol[TM]) may temporarily help the process and be of use in securing effective haemostasis for some days at least.[82] It must be used in adequate doses, e.g. 2 million KIU daily. Again, this may at least provide a window during which successful antitumour or anti-infection treatment can be instituted.

Bleeding due to primary fibrinolytic syndromes is rare but does occur in malignancy, including sarcomas and sometimes with more common cancers. If such a diagnosis can be safely made then treatment with ε-aminocaproic acid may be effective. The dose is 5–10 g initially and then 1–2 hourly until haemostasis is secured. As indicated above, aprotinin infusion may also be beneficial in these cases although controlled trials of this agent in such patients are lacking.

Bleeding due to dysfibrinogenaemias, if diagnosed, can be treated with fresh frozen plasma as a source of normal fibrinogen, but rarely occurs except in primary hepatomas or sometimes with liver metastases. It is, in any case, debatable whether dysfibrinogenaemia *per se* causes bleeding.

Acquired anticoagulants are sometimes found[83] and may be directed against any coagulation factor, but are not often associated with bleeding. However, malignant paraproteins are well-documented as interfering with the action of clotting factors and in this sense are somewhat similar to inhibitors. Von Willebrand disease-like states can occasionally be seen[84] but, although this may be associated with, for example, a prolonged bleeding time, or laboratory coagulation abnormalities, there is no specific procoagulation treatment indicated.

CLOSING REMARKS

Numerous studies have documented haemostatic abnormalities in the plasma of patients with malignant disease, and defects of almost every haemostatic component have been described. It is clear that the incidence of such defects varies both with the sensitivity of the laboratory approach and the severity of the particular malignancy. Nevertheless, no single plasma clotting abnormality is specific for cancer. The actual mechanisms of intravascular clotting activation in cancer patients remain poorly defined. The greatest haemostatic problem of malignancy not associated with treatment is that of a thrombotic tendency which may threaten both the quality of life and life itself in patients who are not terminally ill with malignancies. It would seem that most patients with cancer might well have a thrombotic episode, although some of these may be subclinical. Studies of antihaemostatic therapies such as coumarin derivatives, heparin and aspirin, have suggested improvements in survival in some forms of cancer. It therefore seems that a case could be made for prophylactic anticoagulant treatment in cancer patients both under stress, such as those under-going surgery, or in the long term, especially if their disease is progressive.

REFERENCES

1. Cupps TR, Fanci AS. Vasculitis and neoplasm. *Major Problems in Internal Medicine* 1981; **21**: 116–19.
2. Winfield B. Cryoglobulinaemia. *Human Pathology* 1983; **14**: 350–4.
3. Strauss WG. Purpura hyperglobulinaemia of Waldenstrom. *New England Journal of Medicine* 1969; **260**: 857–60.
4. Roath S, Davenport P. Leucocyte numbers and quality: their effects on viscosity. *Clinical Laboratory Haematology* 1991; **13**: 255–62.
5. Bick RL. Alterations of haemostatsis associated with malignancy. Etiology, patho-physiology, diagnosis and management. *Seminars in Thrombosis and Hemostatsis* 1978; **5**: 1–26.
6. Bick RL. Alterations of hemostasis in malignancy. In: Bick RL, Bennett JM, Brynes RK, Cline M *et al.* eds. *Hematology clincial and laboratory practice.* St Louis: Mosby-Year Book, 1993: 1583–602.
7. Anasetti C, Ryska W, Sullivan KM *et al.* Graft vs host disease is associated with autoimmune-like thrombocytopenia. *Blood* 1989; **73**: 1054.
8. Abrams DI, Chinn EK, Lewis BJ *et al.* Hematologic manifestations in homosexual men with Kaposi's Syndrome. *American Journal of Clinical Pathology* 1984; **81**: 13–18.
9. Zon LI, Groopman JE. Hematologic manifestations of the human immunodeficiency virus (HIV). *Seminars in Haematology* 1988; **25**: 208–15.
10. Cohen AJ, Phillips TM, Kessler CM. Circulating coagulation inhibitors in the acquired immunodeficiency syndrome. *Annals of Internal Medicine* 1986; **104**: 175–80.
11. Adams GA, Schultz L, Goldberg L. Platelet function abnormalities in the myelo-proliferative disorders. *Scandinavian Journal of Haematology* 1974; **13**: 215–24.
12. Mielke CH. Measurement of the bleeding time. *Thrombosis and Haemostasis* 1984; **52**: 210–11.
13. Miller SP, Sanchez-Avalos J, Stefanski T, Zuckerman L. Coagulation disorders in cancer I. Clinical and laboratory studies. *Cancer* 1967; **20**: 1452–65.
14. Belt RJ, Leite C, Haas CD, Stephens RL. Incidence of hemorrhagic complications in patients with cancer. *Journal of the American Medical Association* 1978; **239**: 2571–4.
15. Davis RB, Theologides A, Kennedy BJ. Comparative studies of blood coagulation and platelet aggregation in patients with cancer and non-malignant diseases. *Annals of Internal Medicine* 1969; **71**: 69–80.
16. Clezardin P, McGregor JL, Dechavanne M, Clemetson KJ. Platelet membrane glycoprotein abnormalities in patients with myeloproliferative disorders and second-ary thrombocytosis. *British Journal of Haematology* 1991; **30**: 331–7.
17. Bidet JM, Ferriere JP, Besse G, Chollet P, Gaillard G, Plagne R. Evaluation of β-thromboglobulin levels in cancer patients: Effects of antitumor chemotherapy. *Thrombosis Research* 1980; **19**: 429–33.
18. Yahara Y, Okawa S, Onazawa Y, Motomiya T, Tanove K, Yamazaki H. Activation of platelets in cancer, especialy with reference to genesis of disseminated intra-vascular coagulation. *Thrombosis Research* 1983; **29**: 27–35.
19. Grossi A, Vannucchi A, Rafanelli D, Filimberti E, Ferrini PR. Beta thromboglobulin content in megakaryocytes of patients with myeloproliferative diseases. *Thrombosis Research* 1986; **43**: 367–74.

20. Walz DA. Thrombospondin as a mediator of cancer cell adhesion in metastasis. *Cancer Metastasis Reviews* 1992; **11**: 313–24.
21. Tuszynski GP, Smith M, Rothman VL et al. Thrombospondin levels in patients with malignancy. *Thrombosis and Haemostasis* 1992; **67**: 607–11.
22. Sun NCJ, McAfee WM, Hum GJ, Weiner JM. Hemostatic abnormalities in malignancy, a propective study of one hundred eight patients. Part 1. Coagulation studies. *American Journal of Clinical Pathology* 1979; **71**: 10–16.
23. Kies MS, Posch JJ, Giolama JP, Rubin RN. Haemostatic function in cancer patients. *Cancer* 1980; **46**: 831–7.
24. Edwards RL, Rickles FR, Moritz TE et al. Anormalities of blood coagulation tests in patients with cancer. *American Journal of Clinical Pathology* 1987; **88**: 596–602.
25. Hernandez E, Lavine M, Dunton CJ, Gracely E, Parker J. Poor prognosis associated with thrombocytosis in patients with cervical cancer. *Cancer* 1992; **69**: 2975–7.
26. Sun NCJ, Bowie EJW, Kazmier FJ, Elveback LR, Owen CA. Blood coagulation studies in patients with cancer. *Mayo Clinic Proceedings* 1974; **49**: 636–41.
27. Mitchell WH, Althaus J. Coagulation problems in patients with cancer. *Journal of Surgical Oncology* 1980; **13**: 323–7.
28. Ratnoff OD. Disseminated intravascular coagulation. In: Ratnoff OD, Forbes CD eds *Disorders of hemostasis*, 2nd edn. Philadelphia: WB Saunders, 1991: 292–326.
29. Slichter SJ, Harker LA. Haemostasis in malignancy. *Annals of the New York Academy of Sciences* 1974; **230**: 252–62.
30. Francis JL. Acquired dysfibrinogenaemia. In: Francis JL ed. *Fibrinogen, fibrin stabilization and fibrinolysis*. Chichester: Ellis Horwood, 1988: 128–56.
31. Francis JL, Armstrong DJ. Acquired dysfibrinogenaemia in liver disease. *Journal of Clinical Pathology* 1982; **35**: 667–72.
32. Barr RD, Ouna N, Simpson JG, Bagshawe AF. Dysfibrinogenaemia and hepatocellular carcinoma. *Quarterly Journal of Medicine* 1976; **180**: 647–59.
33. Ballard JO, Kelly GA, Kukrika MD, Sanders JC, Eyster ME. Acquired dysfibrinogenaemia in a haemophiliac with hepatoma. *Cancer* 1981; **48**: 686–90.
34. Peuscher FW, Cleton FJ, Armstrong L et al. Significance of plasma fibrinopeptide A (FPA) in patients with malignancy. *Journal of Laboratory and Clinical Medicine* 1980; **96**: 5–14.
35. Auger MJ, Galloway MJ, Leinster SJ, McVerry BA, Mackie MJ. Elevated fibrinopeptide A levels in patients with clinically localised breast carcinoma. *Haemostasis* 1987; **17**: 336–9.
36. Rickles FR, Edwards RL, Barb C, Cronlund M. Abnormalities of blood coagulation in patients with cancer. Fibrinopeptide A generation and tumor growth. *Cancer* 1983; **51**: 301–7.
37. Seitz R, Rappe N, Kraus M et al. Activation of coagulation and fibrinolysis in patients with lung cancer – relation to tumour stage and prognosis. *Blood Coagulation & Fibrinolysis* 1993; **4**: 249–54.
38. Asakura H, Saito M, Ito K et al. Levels of thrombin–antithrombin III complex in plasma in cases of acute promyelocytic leukaemia. *Thrombosis Research* 1988; **50**: 895–9.
39. Rubin RN, Kies MS, Posch JJ. Measurements of antithrombin III in solid tumor patients with and without hepatic metastases. *Thrombosis Research* 1980; **18**: 353–60.
40. Francis JL. *Fibrinogen, fibrin stabilization and fibrinolysis*. Chichester: Ellis Horwood, 1988.
41. Horne MK, Chao ES, Wilson OJ, Scialla SJ, Lynch MA, Kragel PJ. A heparin-like anticoagulant as part of global abnormalities of plasma glycosaminoglycans in a patient with transitional cell carcinomma. *Journal of Laboratory and Clinical Medicine* 1991; **118**: 250–60.
42. Lopez-Fernandez MF, Lopez-Berges C, Martin R, Pardo A, Ramos FJ, Batlle J.

Abnormal structue of von Willebrand factor in myeloproliferative syndrome is associated to either thrombotic or haemorrhagic diathesis. *Thrombosis and Haemostasis* 1987; **58**: 753–7.

43. Nand S, Messmore H. Hemostasis in malignancy. *American Journal of Hematology* 1990; **35**: 45–55.

44. Henriksson P, Blomback M, Bratt G, Eghag O, Eriksson A. Activators and inhibitors of coagulation and fibrinolysis in patients with prostatic cancer treated with oestrogen or orchidectomy. *Thrombosis Research* 1986; **44**: 783–91.

45. Duffy MJ. Plasminogen activators and cancer. *Blood Coagulation & Fibrinolysis* 1990; **1**: 681–7.

46. Duffy MJ, Reilly D, Nolan N, Ohiggins N, Fennelly JJ, Andreasen P. Urokinase plasminogen activator, a strong and independent prognostic marker in breast cancer. *Fibrinolysis* 1992; **6**: 55–7.

47. Carlsson S. Fibrinogen degradation products in serum from patients with cancer. *Acta Chirurgica Scandinavica* 1973; **139**: 499–502.

48. Trousseau A. Phlegmasia alba dolens. In: Anonymous, ed. *Clinique medicale de l'Hôtel de Paris*. Ballière, 1865: 654–6.

49. Thompson CM, Rodgers RL. Analysis of autopsy records of 157 cases of carcinoma of the pancreas with particular reference to the incidence of thromboembolism. *American Journal of Medical Science* 1952; **223**: 469–76.

50. Dvorak HF. Thrombosis and cancer. *Human Pathology* 1987; **18**: 275–84.

51. Amirkhosravi M, Francis JL. Procoagulant effects of the MC28 fibrosarcoma cell line in vitro and in vivo. *British Journal of Haematology* 1993; **85**: 736–44.

52. Honn KV, Tang DG, Crissman JD. Platelets and cancer metastasis – a causal relationship. *Cancer Metastasis Reviews* 1992; **11**: 325–51.

53. Zacharski LR, Henderson WG, Rickles FR *et al*. Rationale and experimental design for the VA cooperative study of anticoagulation (warfarin) in the treatment of cancer. *Cancer* 1979; **44**: 732–41.

54. Zacharski LR, Henderson WG, Rickles FR *et al*. Effect of warfarin on survival in small cell carcinoma of the lung. Verterans Administration Study No. 75. *Journal of the American Medical Association* 1981; **245**: 831–5.

55. Zacharski LR, Moritz T.E. Effect of RA-33 (mopidamole) on survival in carcinoma of the lung and colon. Final report of VA cooperative study no. 188 (abstract). *Thrombosis and Haemostasis* 1987; **58**: 508.

56. Wojtukiewicz MZ, Zacharski LR, Memoli VA *et al*. Abnormal regulation of coagulation/fibrinolysis in small cell carcinoma of the lung. *Cancer* 1990; **65**: 481–5.

57. Wojtukiewicz MZ, Zacharski LR, Memoli VA *et al*. Malignant melanoma. Interaction with coagulation and fibrinolytic pathways in situ. *American Journal of Clinical Pathology* 1990; **93**: 516–21.

58. Zacharski LR, Memoli VA, Costantini V, Wojtukiewicz MZ, Ornstein DL. Clotting factors in tumour tissue: implications for cancer therapy. *Blood Coagulation & Fibrinolysis* 1990; **1**: 71–8.

59. Francis JL. Haemostasis and cancer. *Medical Laboratory Sciences* 1989; **46**: 331–46.

60. Rao LVM. Tissue factor as a tumor procoagulant. *Cancer Metastasis Reviews* 1992; **11**: 249–66.

61. Francis JL, El-Baruni K, Roath OS, Taylor I. Factor X-activating activity in normal and malignant colorectal tissue. *Thrombosis Research* 1988; **52**: 207–17.

62. El-Baruni K, Taylor I, Roath OS, Francis JL. Factor X-activating procoagulant in normal and malignant breast tissue. *Hematological Oncology* 1990; **8**: 323–32.

63. Gordon SG, Franks JJ, Lewis B. Cancer procoagulant: A factor X-activating procoagulant from malignant tissue. *Thrombosis Research* 1975; **6**: 127–37.

64. Gordon SG, Cross BA. A factor X-activating cysteine protease from malignant tissue. *Journal of Clinical Investigation* 1981; **67**: 1665–71.

65. Gordon SG, Cross BA. An enzyme-linked immunosorbent assay for cancer procoagulant and its potential as a new tumor marker. *Cancer Research* 1990; **50**: 6229–34.
66. Mueller BM, Reisfeld RA, Edgington TS, Ruf W. Expression of tissue factor by melanoma cells promotes efficient hematogenous metastasis. *Proceedings of the National Academy of Sciences, USA* 1992; **89**: 11832–6.
67. Edwards RL, Rickles FR, Cronlund M. Abnormalities of blood coagulation in patients with cancer. Mononuclear cell tissue factor generation. *Journal of Laboratory and Clinical Investigation* 1981; **98**: 917–28.
68. Edwards RL, Rickles FR. The role of leukocytes in the activation of blood coagulation. *Seminars in Haematology* 1992; **29**: 202–12.
69. Lieberman JS, Borrero J, Urdaneta E, Wright IS. Thrombophlebitis and cancer. *Journal of the American Medical Association* 1961; **177**: 542–5.
70. Rahr HB, Sorensen JV. Venous thromboembolism and cancer. *Blood Coagulation & Fibrinolysis* 1992; **3**: 451–60.
71. Goldberg RJ, Seneff M, Gore JM *et al.* Occult malignant neoplasm in patients with deep venous thrombosis. *Archives of Internal Medicine* 1987; **147**: 251–3.
72. Monreal M, Lafoz E, Casals A *et al.* Occult cancer in patients with deep venous thrombosis. A systematic approach. *Cancer* 1991; **67**: 541–5.
73. Gelister JSK, Jass JR, Mahmoud M, Gaffney PJ, Boulos PB. Role of urokinase in colorectal neoplasia. *British Journal of Surgery* 1987; **74**: 460–3.
74. Yamashita JI, Inada K, Ogawa M. Plasminogen activators in breast cancer cells – review. *International Journal of Oncology* 1992; **1**: 683–6.
75. Slichter SJ. Principles of platelet transfusion therapy. In: Hoffman R, Benz EJ, Shattil SJ, Furie B, Cohen HJ eds. *Hematology, principles & practice*. New York: Churchill Livingstone, 1991: 1610–22.
76. Andreu G, Dewailly J, Leberre C *et al.* Preventation of HLA immunisation with leucocyte poor packed red cells and platelet concentrates obtained by filtration. *Blood* 1988; **73**: 964–9.
77. Barritt DW, Jordan SC. Anticoagulant drugs in the treatment of pulmonary embolism. *Lancet* 1960; **1**: 1309–12.
78. Tibbutt DA, Davies JN, Anderson JA *et al.* Comparison by controlled clinical trial of streptokinase and heparin in the treatment of life threatening pulmonary embolism. *British Medical Journal* 1974; **1**: 343–7.
79. Goualt-Heilman M, Chardon E, Sultan C, Josso F. The procoagulant factor of leukaemic promyelocytes. Demonstration of immunologic cross reactivity with human brain tissue factor. *British Journal of Haematology* 1975; **30**: 151–8.
80. Yang WP, Okabe H, Inoue M, Takatsuki K.; Role of leukocytes in the activation of intravascular coagulation in patients with septicemia. *American Journal of Hematology* 1991; **36**: 265–71.
81. Bick RL. Disseminated intravascular coagulation and related syndromes. In: Bennett JM, Brynes RK, Cline MJ *et al.* eds. *Hematology: clinical and laboratory practice.* St Louis: Mosby-Year Book, 1993: 1463–99.
82. Roath OS, Majer RV, Smith AG. The use of aprotinin in thrombocytopenic patients: a preliminary evaluation. *Blood Coagulation & Fibrinolysis* 1990; **1**: 235–9.
83. Kunkel LA. Acquired circulating anticoagulants in malignancy. *Seminars in Thrombosis and Hemostasis* 1992; **18**: 416–23.
84. Jakway JL. Acquired von Willebrand's disease in malignancy. *Seminars in Thrombosis and Hemostasis* 1992; **18**: 434–5.

CHAPTER 15

Metabolic abnormalities associated with cancer

THÉRÈSE LOUGHLIN

INTRODUCTION

In this chapter we explore metabolic abnormalities in patients with cancer. Some of these effects are brought about by the presence of tumour, its influence on general metabolism, its ability to usurp substrates from the diet, or change the pattern of biochemical utilization of protein, carbohydrate and fat metabolism. Additionally, the tumour may produce metabolic factors which influence appetite, satiety, and may directly or indirectly cause weight loss. Alternatively, problems associated with the cancer, for example, ascites, may cause large volumes of protein-rich fluid to be unavailable to the patient for anabolism, and cause symptoms and complications of themselves.

We also deal with tumours which have the ability to make hormones, and how those hormones may cause symptoms. We examine how such conditions are investigated, diagnosed and treated, on the basis of the known properties of the tumours and the hormones they secrete. Other tumours acquire the ability to synthesize hormones not classically associated with that tissue of origin, so-called ectopic hormone production. Finally we explore biochemical abnormalities which arise in the context of malignancy or its treatment.

NUTRITIONAL AND GASTROINTESTINAL ABNORMALITIES ASSOCIATED WITH CANCER

Weight loss in cancer patients

Weight loss is a frequent presentation in patients with cancer (Table 15.1).[1,2] While patients with breast cancer are least likely to present with this, patients with gastric or pancreatic carcinoma are very likely to complain of this symptom. The spectrum of abnormalities in patients with some degree of protein–calorific malnutrition may vary from subtle weight loss to extreme cachexia and emaciation (Table 15.2).[3]

The best index of weight loss is history. Loss of greater than 10 per cent of premorbid body weight represents significant weight loss. Principal changes are

Table 15.1   Potential causes of weight loss in patients with cancer

Mechanical obstruction
Anorexia and reduced intake
Loss of absorption
Selective use of nutrients for tumour synthesis
Depletion of vitamins and cofactors
Altered metabolic pathways
Organ system failure in association with metastatic disease
Hormonal effects
Infection
Consequences of therapy: chemotherapy
                          radiotherapy
                          biological therapy
                          drugs used for symptomatic relief

Table 15.2   Features
of patients with cancer
cachexia

General features
Severe weight loss
Anorexia
Lethargy
Muscle wasting
Loss of body fat
Oedema

Biochemical abnormalities
Low serum albumin
Low serum transferrin
Anaemia

loss of body fat and skeletal muscle. These changes may be objectively followed by measurement of skin-fold thickness and mid-arm muscle circumference. Weight loss is a negative prognostic indicator. Weight loss itself may be responsible for a proportion of cancer deaths. Certainly, patients who have suffered a degree of weight loss tolerate treatment with surgery, radiotherapy or chemotherapy less well, and are more likely to suffer complications of therapy. Outcomes following treatment are less likely to be favourable.

Mechanisms of anorexia and weight loss

Any lesion of the mouth, oropharynx or oesophagus can directly obstruct the passage of food into the stomach. The situation may be compounded by carious teeth or superinfection. Angular cheilosis or stomatitis, oral ulceration, or xerostomia arising later following radiotherapy may all worsen the situation. Early sense of satiety can follow after gastric surgery, compression from an enlarged liver or the presence of ascites.

Slowing of gastric emptying and general intestinal immobility may all be consequent on opiate therapy for analgesia. Inadequate hepatic or pancreatic function may follow after intestinal bypass procedures, or as a consequence of drug therapy, or metastatic disease; both may compound malabsorption problems. Small bowel absorptive capacity may be impaired following combination chemotherapy, or by superinfection associated with blind loops. Chronic constipation may result from metabolic aberrancies, e.g. hypercalcaemia, or may be associated with medication, and may exacerbate anorexia.

Diarrhoea eventually occurs in most patients with progressive weight loss.

Metabolic abnormalities in patients with weight loss

Theoretically, weight loss occurs either because of reduced intake or because of increased energy expenditure. Indirect calorimetry has been used to measure basal metabolic rate in patients with cancer and weight loss.[4] While a proportion of patients demonstrate increased energy expenditure, in some patients it is 'normal', while in others, it is reduced. A value of normal, however, indicates failure to recognize and adapt to the semi-starved state. It is not well understood why these semi-starved patients do not automatically downregulate basal energy expenditure. It has been postulated that energy-dependent metabolic cycles, e.g. protein turnover or glucose–lactate (Cori cycle) metabolism are increased; the evidence is conflicting where these hypotheses have been objectively examined. Some cancer patients certainly exhibit decreased tissue sensitivity to insulin, and decreased insulin incremental rises following a glucose load.[5] This may be one of the mechanisms by which calorific substrate is not readily available for metabolism. In other patients excessive catecholamine secretion has been noted, as has enhanced responsiveness to catecholamines, which could also cause a perturbation of calorific utilization.[6]

The state of cancer cachexia, which occurs frequently, is poorly understood. In any one individual, the mechanism appears to be multifactorial and resistant to systemic management.

Treatment

Anorexia and weight loss are often multifactorial, and in addressing the problem the approach must be broad based. Consideration should be given to the state of dental hygiene. Caries should be treated and problems with ill-fitting dentures should be recognized. Active oral hygiene, including the use of oral antiseptics, should be promoted. The role of pilocarpine as a salivary secretagogue is currently being evaluated. Artificial salivas (Glandosane) have a use in the treatment of dry mouth. The symptom of thirst should be formally investigated. Intolerance of sweetness may be circumvented by the use of alternative flavourings and spices. Meat intolerance can be counteracted by the substitution of poultry, eggs, cheese or pulses. Pain, infection, constipation and depression should each be considered separately, and appropriately treated.

Milk-based oral food supplements of high calorific and protein value, e.g. Build Up or Complan, are readily available, and may be used to supplement a normal diet. The oncologic dietician is the best person to instruct and monitor the patient and their family. The most attainable goal is probably maintenance of current body weight, rather than regaining lost weight. Regular follow-up and review of weight status is an important component of total care.

Pharmacological treatments (Table 15.3)

The observation that some patients treated with progestational agents as an endocrine strategy in the management of metastatic breast cancer, regardless of response, gained considerable weight, has led to studies of the efficacy of this therapy in other cancer states. It has been confirmed that patients treated with progestogens increase body cell mass, although a component of this must be fluid retention. Doses as low as 160 mg/day may be effective, although doses as high as 480–800 mg/day may be required.[7] Consideration should be given to the thrombogenic property of progestogens when this treatment is being considered.

Systemic glucocorticoids (prednisolone 5–15 mg/day) can also stimulate appetite, increased food intake and weight gain. They can also increase the sense of well-being. Their chronic use must take into consideration their severe side-effects, but as a short-term measure in terminally ill patients, they undoubtedly have a role to play.

Phenothiazines (haloperidol 1/mg) relieve nausea and anorexia in some patients, particularly those receiving combination chemotherapy.

Antidepressants, e.g. amitryptaline, also have a role to play, not just in the management of depression, but also because of their properties as serotonin antagonists. Hydrazine has been shown to inhibit gluconeogenesis and promote weight gain in patients with cancer, and may have a role to play in the management of anorexia and weight loss.

High doses of vitamin C (>1 g/day), have been shown to increase well-being and appetite over short periods of time.

Finally, the use of alcohol to promote appetite and a sense of well-being should be considered.

Nasogastric feeding, PEGs and total parenteral nutrition (TPN)

It is recognized that weight loss is an independent negative prognostic factor in many cancers. Additionally, it is known that patients who have sustained severe weight loss are more prone to the complications of either chemotherapy or radiotherapy, and are ultimately less likely to respond to either form of treatment. The advent of effective ways of treating malnutrition in the short term has prompted much investigation into the role and efficacy of these strategies in cancer patients. It has been demonstrated that the metabolism of the cancer-bearing host is not the same as compensated semi-starvation, and the response to

Table 15.3   Pharmacological manoeuvres in patients with weight loss

---

Progestational agents, e.g. medroxyprogesterone
Glucocorticoids
Phenothiazines
Antidepressants
Hydrazine sulphate
Vitamin C
Alcohol

---

nutritional supplementation would appear to be less than can be achieved in the malnourished patient with chronic benign disease. If weight gain can be achieved, fat deposition will occur rather than repletion of the vital lean body mass. The nature of this inhibition to the repletion of host body mass remains unknown, though it is clearly related to the continual growth and activity of the patient's neoplasm. It is now recognized, also, that correction of malnutrition does not improve prognosis over and above that which might be expected in the absence of weight loss. Furthermore, it does not improve tolerance to chemotherapy over and above that which can be maintained by improvement of voluntary oral intake. Nonetheless, there is undoubtedly a role for the employment of these strategies in those patients who might reasonably be expected to do well, when treated aggressively with chemotherapy or radiotherapy, in the short term.

In the presence of intraoral pathology or dysphagia, the positioning of a nasogastric tube allows access to the gastrointestinal tract without volitional swallowing. A silicone fine-bore nasogastric tube is inserted, generally with a stiffening guidewire in the centre to aid insertion. The position of the tube is checked either by auscultating for bubbling sounds in the gastric bed following the forceful injection of air or radiographically. A commercial liquid diet is generally used. These diets contain a mixture of oligo/polysaccharides, fats, minerals, vitamins and trace elements. In general, they contain 1 kcal/ml and are administered via an electric pump at the rate of 25–100 ml/h. The most common problem associated with these feeds is diarrhoea, and they may have to be introduced very cautiously, and their rate of administration increased very gradually to offset this side-effect.

If the nasogastric route is not tolerated, or if long-term enteral feeding is planned, then the feeding tube may be inserted directly into the stomach via a gastrostomy. A percutaneous endoscopic gastrostomy (PEG) can be sited without recourse to general anaesthesia.

Where the gut is not functioning, parenteral feeding has to be employed. Parenteral feeds are hypertonic and tend to cause phlebitis if infused into peripheral veins; therefore, infusion into central veins is recommended. Currently, a standard 3 l regimen is employed, containing 14 g nitrogen, generally as amino acids, and 2400 kcal. The energy source is a mixture of hyperosmolar dextrose and lipid, each contributing 50 per cent of the total energy. Because of the hyperosmolar glucose solutions, and the relative glucose intolerance seen in cachexia patients, insulin may have to be administered concurrently. The infusion also contains essential vitamins and minerals. These sterile bags are connected to a silastic catheter which has previously been tunnelled into a subclavian, external or internal jugular vein. A different lumen is used for transfusion products, antibiotics and chemotherapy. Therapy should be monitored, checking electrolyte levels, including magnesium and phosphate, glucose, and triglycerides. Ketonuria may also be used to monitor the progress of these patients. The major complications of this therapy are sepsis and thrombophlebitis.

Withdrawal of TPN should be gradual as patients are prone to develop hypoglycaemia.

ASCITES

Malignant ascites commonly results from the presence of multiple peritoneal seedlings of metastatic disease. In these patients the pathogenesis of ascites is thought to be mediated by a combination of lymphatic obstruction and the increased production of peritoneal fluid.[8] Less commonly it occurs in association with extensive liver metastases, and disruption of normal hepatic architecture. In these cases, high portal venous pressure, and reduced albumin synthesis, may also be important mechanistically. It occurs most commonly with carcinoma of the colon, pancreas, stomach, ovary or breast and is a negative prognostic sign. The median survival in all patients from the onset of ascites is 20 weeks, although the range is quite variable.

Ascites tends to be a late event in association with carcinomas of the gastro-intestinal tract, but may be an early and presenting feature in patients with carcinoma of the ovary (Table 15.4). Patients complain of abdominal distention, and associated changes in posture, nausea and early satiety, as well as respiratory compromise. Physical examination reveals a tense, distended abdomen, shifting dullness in the flanks and a fluid thrill. Plain abdominal films may show a 'ground glass appearance', while ultrasound and CT scans will confirm the presence of the fluid, and may reveal small quantities of ascitic fluid before it is clinically discernible. Diagnostic paracentesis should be undertaken. Fluid aspirated should be sent for biochemical analysis (protein concentration and LDH), microbiological analysis and cytology. Cytological analysis for malignant cells is not as sensitive a diagnostic test as might be expected, yielding confirmation of the diagnosis in approximately 50 per cent of patients. The most specific index is the ratio of serum to ascitic LDH. This figure has been shown to have a sensitivity of 80 per cent and a specificity of 100 per cent. While high levels of ascitic carcinoembryonic antigen (CEA) are associated with malignancy, this is not always the case, but may provide a useful clue.

The most critical therapeutic manoeuvre should be consideration of systemic therapy for the underlying malignancy. Since one third of carcinomas of the ovary will present with ascites, the diagnosis must be substantiated, surgery undertaken and the disease histologically staged before consideration of subse-

Table 15.4 Carcinomas in which ascites commonly occurs

Colon
Pancreas
Stomach
Ovary
Breast (less commonly)
Treatment options
Therapy of the underlying carcinoma
Serial paracentesis
Diuretics
Peritoneovenous shunts
(Intraperitoneal installation therapy)

quent chemotherapy; these measures may result in resorption of ascites. Similarly cytotoxic or endocrine therapy of breast carcinoma may stabilize disease, and control ascites. If a definitive therapy cannot be undertaken, then palliation is a priority.[9] While paracentesis may provide short-term palliation, consideration should be given to the acute consequences of intravascular fluid depletion following abrupt withdrawal of ascitic fluid, and chronic protein depletion, associated with repeated drainage, and risk of sepsis. Diuretic therapy using spironolactone also has a role to play.[10] A dose of 150 mg should be employed at the outset, with incremental rises if sustained weight loss does not result. Alternatively, therapy with frusamide may be considered.

For patients whose death is not apparently imminent, palliation of ascites can be undertaken by the insertion of a shunting device, without compromising protein status. Two types of shunt have been employed to this end, the LeVeen and Denver shunts.[11,12] Both consist of a distal catheter studded with perforations which is inserted in the peritoneal cavity. This drains into a valve chamber. The LeVeen shunt contains a silicone strut valve with a critical opening pressure of 3–5 cmH$_2$O, to prevent the backflow of blood into the tube. The Denver shunt consists of a mitral valve with the opposing flaps of the valve constructed asymmetrically, in a compressible pump chamber. The latter allows the application of manual pressure to increase the flow through the valve and help clear any obstruction caused by cell debris. The opening pressure of this valve is approximately 1 cmH$_2$O. The proximal end of the catheter is sited pre-operatively into the subclavian or external or internal jugular vein. During inspiration when intrathoracic pressure falls the fluid is effectively aspirated into the superior vena cava. The most important complications of this procedure relate to effects on cardiac and hepatic status peri-operatively. Sudden expansion of the intra-vascular fluid volume by a significant volume of a protein-rich peritoneal exudate can precipitate congestive cardiac failure in someone with limited cardiac reserve. Thus, pre-operative evaluation of cardiac status is important before proceeding to placement of the shunt. Additionally, post-operative hyper-bilirubinaemia may be seen. This is most often associated with multiple hepatic metastases and is caused by post-operative disseminated intravascular coagulation (DIC). While a degree of DIC is seen by laboratory testing in almost all patients following shunt insertion, in this particular subset of hyper-bilirubinaemic patients, a critical degree of clinical DIC may ensue, and may require aggressive treatment with platelets, fibrinogen, fresh frozen plasma and ε-aminocaproic acid, as necessary. Other complications of shunt insertion include sepsis, axillary vein thrombosis, dissemination of metastases, and renal failure. Long-term patency of peritoneovenous shunts in patients with malignant ascites varies from 60 to 80 per cent. Similarly long-term control of ascites is approximately 70 per cent. Median survival of patients following shunt placement is between 2 and 4 months.[13]

Therapy with intracavity instillation of chemotherapeutic agents and radio-active colloids has also been studied, based on the successful precedent set by these strategies in the treatment of pleural effusions. Uncontrolled studies suggest that the intraperitoneal instillation of bleomycin or quinacrine may be effective in 40–50 per cent of cases.

PITUITARY TUMOURS

Tumours in the sella turcica include a large number of lesions including cra-niopharyngiomas, teratomas, metastatic carcinomas and lymphomas. By far the majority however, are benign adenomas, some of which are hormone secreting. Since the focus of this chapter is on metabolic effects of tumours, this section will deal with the latter group only. Pituitary adenomas are benign epithelial tumours which consist of adenohypophyseal cells. They are often slow-growing tumours which expand and may distort the sella turcica. There is often invasion of the dura. The tinctorial characteristics of the cytoplasm using haematoxylin and eosin, and subsequently Mallory's stain has led to the practice of classifying these tumours as acidophilic (secrete growth hormone (GH) and/or prolactin), basophilic (secrete adenocorticotrophic hormone (ACTH), including thyro-trophic cell adenomas which secrete thyroid-stimulating hormone (TSH), and gonadotrophin-secreting adenomas which secrete follicle-stimulating hormone (FSH) and luteinizing hormone (LH)), and chromophobic (some prolactinomas, null-cell adenomas). The advent of immunocytochemistry for specific hormones, and the refinements obtainable with electron microscopy have allowed the classification of these tumours and the products they secrete to become much more refined, particularly in a research setting.

Clinical features

Clinically, pituitary tumours declare themselves by the products they secrete, and their local anatomical effect, either compromising visual pathways or com-promising the normal pituitary tissue resulting in functional hypopituitarism. Headache is a common presenting complaint, but it can vary in site and severity. The most commonly encountered visual field abnormality, associated with upward extension from the sella, is upper temporal field defects, or subsequently bitemporal hemianopia. While hypothalamic extension is rare and is most often seen with craniopharyngiomas, diabetes insipidus can occur, as can disturbances in sleep and eating patterns, with obesity. Lateral extension may result in lesion of the third, fourth or sixth cranial nerves. Hormonal changes, either due to secretion by the tumour, interference with the normal inhibitory control of prolactin secretion from the hypothalamus, or compromise of normal physio-logical reserve may all occur with pituitary tumours.

Prolactin-secreting tumours

Tumours that secrete prolactin cause galactorrhoea and amenorrhoea in women and impotence in males, and are associated with hypogonadotrophic hypogonad-ism. Galactorrhoea is not universal, and an inadequate luteal phase or an irregular menstrual cycle may occur, before the onset of amenorrhoea. Symp-toms of hypo-oestrogenism such as loss of libido may occur. Gynaecomastia is a rare presentation in male patients. The diagnosis is made by the demonstration of elevated basal prolactin levels.

Growth hormone-secreting tumours[14-17]

Growth hormone excess is manifest by the features of acromegaly, namely coarsening of the features with overgrowth of the hands, feet and jaw. Sometimes all facial bones are affected. An overbite may be evident. Hypertension and arthritis commonly occur. Patients frequently complain of increased sweating and headache. Many patients gain weight, while if the onset occurs before long bones are fused, gigantism may result. Since many GH-secreting tumours are also associated with prolactin excess, the features of hyperprolactinaemia may occur as well. Additionally diabetes mellitus occurs frequently in these patients. The diagnosis of growth hormone excess is made by the failure of growth hormone to suppress following the ingestion of 75 g of oral glucose. It is important that all aspects of potential hypopituitarism are investigated and followed when the diagnosis of acromegaly is made. Radiographic abnormalities occur in almost all patients and may be seen by CT or MRI imaging.

Cushing's disease

The term Cushing's syndrome refers to patients with glucocorticoid excess of any cause; Cushing's disease refers to pituitary-dependent ACTH excess. Clinical features include truncal obesity with moon face and buffalo hump. The thin arms and legs occur because of protein breakdown. Purple striae may be visible on the abdomen. Hypertension and glucose intolerance are common. Hirsutism and amenorrhoea may occur in female patients, while male patients may experience hypogonadism. Osteoporosis may occur in longstanding cases; if the tumour arises before puberty, growth arrest will be evident. Depression is the most common psychiatric abnormality seen.

Biochemical testing involves demonstrating that the patient is hypercortisolaemic, and that the elevated cortisol levels are relatively resistant to suppression (dexamethasone suppression test), compared with normals, while the plasma cortisol levels may show an exaggerated responsiveness to the administration of exogenous corticotrophin-releasing hormone. That the excess ACTH is derived from the pituitary gland may be demonstrated by petrosal sinus sampling, sometimes augmented by the concurrent administration of corticotrophin-releasing hormone. Levels of ACTH in the inferior petrosal sinuses may be shown to be elevated relative to a peripheral blood sample, taken concurrently. Radiographic abnormalities are less likely to occur in this group of patients, as more often these tumours are microadenomas.

Treatment

The treatment of pituitary tumours may need to be multifaceted. Three modalities are employed, local excision (hypophysectomy), radiotherapy and medical treatment. Prolactinomas may be treated with bromocriptine, a dopaminergic agonist.[18-21] This has been associated with a decrease in tumour size, resolution of visual field abnormalities, decrease in circulating prolactin levels, reduction of galactorrhoea and restoration of menstrual cyclicity. It is probably the preferred treatment for the prolactin-secreting microadenoma, but the prolactin-secreting macroadenoma more often comes to surgery. The macroadenoma of acromegaly is managed in the first instance by surgery. Radiotherapy is employed in the treatment of residual disease, but medical treatment with bromocriptine or somatostatin may also be indicated. Surgical management of Cushing's disease is the most likely to be efficacious;[22,23] if the tumour cannot be removed, adrenolytic therapy with ketoconazole, aminoglutethimide, trilostane, mitotane (o'p'DDD) or metyrapone may correct the hypercortisolaemia, the pernicious consequence of ACTH excess.

Careful follow-up of these patients for the sequelae of either recurrent/progressive tumour, or emergent hypopituitarism related to radiotherapy, is mandatory.

MEDULLARY CARCINOMA OF THYROID

Medullary carcinoma of thyroid (MCT), arises in the parafollicular area of C cells of the thyroid, cells which are responsible for the synthesis, storage and secretion of calcitonin.[24,28-30] Approximately three quarters of all cases arise sporadically, while a quarter are associated with multiple endocrine neoplasia type 2 (MEN-2).[24,25,27] The disease affects all patients with MEN-2. The disease presents in a younger age group in those patients with MEN-2, than in the sporadic form. The tumours are characterized by excessive production of calcitonin, which serves as a tumour marker for this disease. They frequently metastasize to local lymph nodes, and ultimately to lung, liver and bone. The only curative modality of treatment is surgery, although radiotherapy may confer some benefit. There is rarely a role for combination chemotherapy in the management of this tumour.

Pathology

MCT is typically a small, rounded tumour arising in the middle or upper lobes of the thyroid gland (Fig. 15.1). Histology shows solid nests of small round cells (these may occasionally have a follicular structure) with amyloid evident in the stroma of some tumours; these tumours are argentaffin-positive. Calcification occurs quite frequently in tumours. Immunocytochemistry most often shows positivity for calcitonin, but they may also stain for calcitonin gene-related product, chromogranin A, neuron-specific enolase, and synaptophysin. Hormones which may be secreted ectopically from these tumours include ACTH, somatostatin, bombesin, gastrin-releasing peptide, and substance P. The cells may also secrete biogenic amines, prostaglandins, histaminase and CEA.

When MCT occurs in MEN-2 the initial lesion is C-cell hyperplasia, and the recognition of this lesion should alert the pathologist to familial disease. The natural history in MEN-2 is to progress to malignant change. From the outset the lesions are multifocal, and involve both lobes, contrasting with sporadic disease.

Clinical features

Patients with this lesion may present with a thyroid nodule or goitre, a fixed cervical mass or cervical lymphadenopathy. Less commonly, their distinctive phenotype may alert the physician, or other endocrine features of the MEN-2 constellation may be present. Other symptoms may include diarrhoea which can

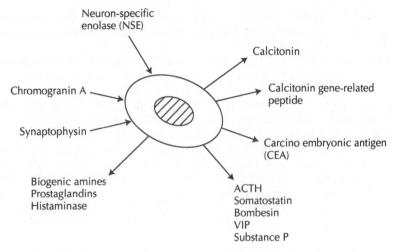

Fig. 15.1. Immunocytochemistry in medullary carcinoma of thyroid (MCT). MCT is recognized within thyroid tissue; it is rarely encapsulated. Cells may be rounded, polygonal or spindle-shaped; they rarely form follicles. Often they are contained within an amyloid stroma. There may be foci of calcification both in the primary tumour and in metastatic lesions. Medullary carcinomas of thyroid synthesize and secrete calcitonin and calcitonin gene-related peptide. Often they secrete other substances.

Immunocytochemistry may show positivity for the non-specific endocrine markers, neuron-specific enolase (NSE), chromogranin A and synaptophysin. Use of specific primary antibodies may show positive immunocytochemistry for other peptides or biogenic amines, as clinical features suggest.

be caused by calcitonin excess, and flushing associated with calcitonin gene-related peptide, or production of biogenic amines. Ectopic ACTH secretion with consequent Cushing's syndrome is a rare mode of clinical presentation. The asymptomatic patient may be detected as a result of screening in the context of known familial disease.

Calcitonin

Medullary carcinoma of thyroid secretes calcitonin, which serves as a marker of disease presence and response to therapy. Most patients with sporadic MCT have high basal plasma concentrations. However, some with familial MCT have normal concentrations. Provocative tests have been developed for family screening. The most sensitive seems to be stimulation of calcitonin secretion with either a calcium infusion or a response to pentagastrin injection.

Treatment

Total thyroidectomy with lymph node dissection is the treatment of choice if the disease is confined to the neck. Sometimes local involvement and invasion may indicate the need for radical neck resection. Post-operatively the patient should be treated with suppressive doses of L-thyroxine. Follow-up should include basal and pentagastrin-stimulated calcitonin concentrations. It is imperative that a phaeochromocytoma be ruled out in each patient found to have familial MCT prior to neck exploration. Prognosis seems to be worse in disease associated with MEN-2B when compared with sporadic lesions or those arising in association with MEN-2A; why is not known.

Patients with residual disease post-operatively have a variable prognosis, depending on the malignant potential of the tumour, which ultimately metastasizes to lung, liver and bone. Localization of residual disease may be aided by scintigraphy with ^{99m}Tc-dimercaptosuccinic acid. Chest X-ray may show a diffuse infiltrate. Computerized tomography of chest and abdomen, hepatic angiography and ultimately selective venous sampling with pentagastrin-stimulated calcitonin measurement may all play a role in the localization of further disease. Local disease may benefit from further surgery in the first instance, which is the preferred treatment modality. MCT is poorly sensitive to irradiation, and this should be reserved for clearly progressive disease or symptomatic local disease that is no longer amenable to surgery. The question of screening for MEN-2 should be addressed as outlined in Table 15.5.

NEUROENDOCRINE GASTROENTEROPANCREATIC TUMOURS

These tumours are rare and grow slowly. Most often they present with symptoms referable to the products they secrete, rather than disease bulk *per se*. They are classified on the basis of the products they secrete, although they can be non-secretory, or secrete a series of hormones, giving rise to mixed clinical syndromes. Most often, these occur in the pancreas, with the exception of carcinoid tumours. Most pancreatic endocrine tumours, while malignant, grow slowly. Patients may survive for many years, even in the presence of significant metastatic disease in the liver.

Histology

On simple haematoxylin and eosin staining, these tumours are composed of uniform round or polygonal cells with clear finely granular cytoplasm. Immu-

Table 15.5 Screening for familial medullary carcinoma of thyroid (MCT)

Family history

Histological review for C-cell hyperplasia, multifocal disease

Pentagastrin test: A bolus injection of 0.5 mg/kg is injected over 5 s. Blood should be sampled at 0, 2 and 5 min for measurement of immunoreactive calcitonin.

Calcium infusion: a 1 min injection of calcium 2 mg/kg/min is administered, and response at 0, 5, 10 and 15 min is assessed.

The two tests may be combined.

It seems likely that genetic studies for specific deletions on chromosome 10 will be the optimal screening in the future, particularly where a cohort of affected family members is available.

nocytochemical study with markers such as chromogranin A, synaptophysin or neuron-specific enolase will confirm their endocrine nature. The peptide(s) they synthesize may be demonstrated by immunocytochemistry, using specific antibodies. The hormones they make may be identified and formally assayed using specific radioimmunoassays.

Gastrin-secreting tumours

The Zollinger–Ellison syndrome (ZES) is peptic ulcer disease due to gastrin-secreting tumours either pancreatic, in the lymph nodes, stomach or duodenum. The diagnosis is made by demonstrating increased gastric acid secretion with simultaneously elevated gastrin levels. Consideration should be given to the differential diagnosis of elevated gastrin levels (see Table 15.6). Secretin infusions may cause augmented gastrin production in those patients whose basal values are equivocal. Satisfactory therapies are now available for the medical management of peptic ulcer disease, and the focus of attention is currently directed towards identifying and localizing gastrin-secreting tumours with a view to surgical resection if possible. Previously, surgical management of pancreatic tumour(s) was efficacious in less than 10 per cent of patients. This was in part due to the multifocal nature of these lesions, in part due to their established malignant nature at the time of surgery, combined with difficulty in their localization. More refined procedures have evolved for tumour localization including angiography and percutaneous transhepatic portal and pancreatic venography, with sampling for subsequent assay of gastrin levels. These procedures are causing a change in perspective. Medical treatment is now so efficacious in managing intractable ulcer disease, that the major threat to life is now delayed malignant invasion of the tumour. Since tumours are now being recognized earlier and better localized, current practice is consideration of primary resection. Chemotherapeutic options for patients with progressive malignant islet cell tumours include streptozotocin, 5-fluorouracil, doxorubicin, and latterly, somatostatin analogues. The successful use of human leucocyte interferon and hepatic artery embolization has been reported.

Insulin-secreting and other pancreatic tumours

Insulinomas are usually symptomatic, and the symptoms become more extreme the longer the diagnosis is unrecognized. Clinical presentation is with the symptoms of hypoglycaemia and catecholamine surge, namely, tremulousness, hunger, irritability, anxiety, dizziness, confusion, and rarely convulsions and coma. These symptoms tend to occur after a prolonged fast or following exertion and tend to be relieved by ingesting carbohydrate. Diagnosis is made by

Table 15.6 Potential causes of a raised gastrin level

Gastric achlorhydria (iatrogenic; use of ranitidine, omeprazole)
Atrophic gastritis
Pernicious anaemia
Hypercalcaemia
Renal failure

demonstration of inappropriate hyperinsulinaemia in the presence of hypogly-caemia. The standard provocation test is a 72 hour fast. The major differential diagnosis is with exogenous insulin administration (fictitious hypoglycaemia); on this account it is advocated that C-peptide and insulin concentrations be measured concurrently. Since the insulin is endogenously derived, C-peptide signifies this derivation as it is cosecreted. They should both be elevated in the presence of an insulinoma. In addition, disproportionate amounts or ratios of proinsulin to insulin may also be seen in this circumstance. Occasionally, suppression tests are used to distinguish physiologic from autonomous secretion. Suppression is assessed by measuring plasma concentrations of C-peptide fol-lowing the administration of exogenous insulin to produce hypoglycaemia The histological abnormality seen ranges from hyperplasia to frank carcinoma; nesidioblastosis has also been described. When the clinical and biochemical diagnosis of insulinoma is made, tumour localization procedures are performed, and attempts are made to determine whether or not the lesion is malignant. Current surgical practice is to perform a distal pancreatectomy, removing 80–90 per cent of the gland. This is because 90–100 per cent show multicentric involvement; between 5 and 15 per cent show malignant histological features at the time of surgery. The endocrine and exocrine sequelae of this surgery are much less than those of total pancreatectomy. Whether subtotal surgery is as effective as radical total pancreatectomy is unclear. Medical management of hyperinsulinism includes the provision of frequent meals, and the use of diaz-oxide. Chemotherapy with streptozotocin, or endocrine therapy with somatosta-tin is used in the management of metastatic disease.

Vipomas

Patients with tumours secreting vasoactive intestinal polypeptide (VIP) develop watery diarrhoea, hypokalaemia and achlorhydria, which is sometimes referred to as the Verner–Morrison syndrome. The diagnosis is established by document-ing elevated plasma VIP concentrations in the appropriate clinical setting. Therapy is guided by anatomic definition of the extent of disease.

Glucagonoma

This tumour of the alpha cells of the pancreas causes a clinical picture that includes angular stomatitis, cheilosis, necrolytic migratory erythema, weight loss and anaemia, with concurrent hyperglycaemia. Diagnosis is made by doc-umentation of hyperglucagonaemia. While surgery is the treatment of choice, the multifocal involvement and propensity to metastasize early, mean that it is only effective in 50 per cent of cases. Medical management of metastatic disease including the use of somatostatin analogue, streptozotocin, or 5-(3, 3-dimethyl-1-triazeno)imidazole-4-carboxamide (DTIC) has been partially successful in isolated incidences.

PPomas

Tumours secreting pancreatic polypeptide (PP) are found in a significant number of patients with MEN-1. They are clinically silent; their presence is confirmed biochemically.

PHAEOCHROMOCYTOMA

Phaeochromocytomas ('phaeos') are the most common tumours of neural crest origin developing in adult life.[31,32] The incidence is about 1 case per 100 000 population per annum, rising to 1 per 100 in patients with neurofibromatosis. Phaeos obey the rule of 10s, i.e. 10 per cent are bilateral, 10 per cent occur outside the adrenals, particularly along the sympathetic chain, but also sites such as the base of the bladder, and 10 per cent are malignant. Between 15 and 50 per cent of patients with MEN-2 are found to have phaeochromocytomas. They are also associated with von Hippel–Lindau, and Sturge–Weber syndromes.

Pathology

Phaeochromocytomas are usually benign adenomas composed of sheets of homogeneous cells with basophilic cytoplasm (Fig. 15.2). These cells stain brown with conventional stains, hence 'chromaffin'. It may be inferred that they contain catecholamines, which are reducing substances, by appearing gold with dichromate. They also contain a variety of neuropeptides. In patients with the MEN-2 syndrome, the pathologic spectrum of diffuse hyperplasia to large multilobular focal phaeochromocytomata is encountered. Disease is almost always bilateral; 24 per cent of patients have malignant phaeochromocytomas at the time of diagnosis. The diagnosis of malignancy in a phaeochromocytoma cannot readily be made histologically. It is most often made by the presence of metastatic disease.

The clinical presentation of the classical phaeochromocytoma is with headaches, palpitations, pallor, hypertension and postural hypotension and sweating; the hallmark of these is their paroxysmal nature. Other symptoms include tremor, anxiety, panic, nausea or vomiting and chest pain. The symptomatic episodes may be precipitated by exertion, e.g. sneezing, laughing, micturating. Tachycardias and congestive cardiac failure may signify extreme catecholamine excess. Attacks have been precipitated by the administration of certain drugs,

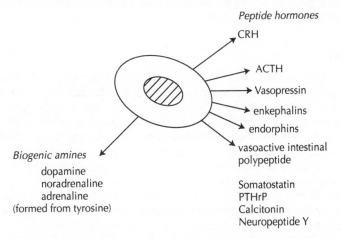

Fig. 15.2. A phaeochromocytoma cell, a small round cell, with basophilic cytoplasm, showing the range of biogenic amines and peptides which may be synthesized in such a cell.

e.g. anaesthetic agents, ACTH, glucagon, phenothiazines, beta-blockers, and tricyclic antidepressants. However, classic presentations are not necessarily the norm; for example only about 50 per cent of patients have sustained hypertension. Patients with MEN-2 often have asymptomatic disease.

Diagnosis

The myriad of clinical presentations make the diagnosis difficult, and consideration of it as a diagnosis in the presence of any of the above symptoms, or in the asymptomatic patient with MEN-2, is vital. It is essentially a diagnosis of a careful history including family history, rather than one of clinical examination. The diagnosis is established biochemically, and then the site of the lesion(s) is identified by imaging studies.

Biochemistry

Biochemical markers include urinary catecholamines, adrenaline and noradrenaline, and their metabolites, the metanephrines and vanillylmandelic acid. Plasma measurements of catecholamines have a role to play also. The urine should be collected in an acidified container; the patient should not concurrently be being treated with methyldopa, L-dopa, MAO inhibitors, chlorpromazine, reserpine or guanethidine, as this may invalidate results. Provocation tests in equivocal circumstances include the glucagon stimulation test, while in patients with marginally elevated catecholamines and sustained hypertension, when the disease needs to be ruled out, it is best performed by the clonidine suppression test.[33]

Imaging studies

CT or MRI will localize lesions greater than a centimetre in diameter;[34] [^{131}I]-metaiodobenzguanidine (MIBG) has specific uptake in some phaeochromocytomas, but this is less likely in malignant phaeochromocytomas.[35] Hepatic involvement should routinely be sought. Other common metastatic sites include bone, lymph nodes, and lung.

Treatment

The first priority of treatment is adequate alpha-blockade, and subsequently beta-blockade. Phenoxybenzamine is the drug of choice, and it is imperative that adequate alpha-blockade is achieved before the introduction of beta-blockade, generally with propranalol. (The converse leaves the patient at risk of unopposed alpha-mediated vasoconstriction which may prove fatal.) Treatment may be commenced with metyrosine. This drug, α-methyl-L-tyrosine is a competitive inhibitor of tyrosine hydroxylase, which catalyses the rate-limiting step in catecholamine biosynthesis.

Nitroprusside and plasma expanders should always be nearby during surgery. Surgery should involve total bilateral adrenalectomy, with a subsequent need for replacement glucocorticoid and mineralcorticoid in patients with MEN-2 or with known bilateral tumours. Some success has been achieved in the management of malignant phaeochromocytomas with combination chemotherapy involving cyclophosphamide, vincristine and dacarbazine, a regime originally shown to be efficacious in the management of neuroblastoma.[36] Success using [^{131}I]-iodomethylbenzguanidine has been achieved,[37] but failure of uptake in 40 per cent of malignant tumours limits its usefulness.

CARCINOID TUMOURS

Carcinoid tumours are neuroendocrine tumours that arise in cells with APUD (amine precursor uptake and decarboxylation) characteristics. They develop, generally, in the submucosa of the small intestine and the bronchi, although they may also arise in other diverse tissues.

While common, they are generally asymptomatic. When they enlarge, they tend to metastasize. When symptomatic, they may declare themselves by local effects, by the presence of metastatic disease, hepatomegaly and liver failure, or by their products of secretion, either 5-hydroxyindoles or ectopic production of peptide hormone.

Carcinoid syndrome is a rare syndrome (Table 15.7), occurring in that subset of carcinoid tumours which produce an excess of 5-hydroxyindoles, and that drain directly into the systemic circulation. Thus, patients with tumours of the bronchi and ovary may be associated with elevated plasma levels of 5-hydroxy-indole acetic acid, and may manifest carcinoid syndrome. However, patients with tumours of the small intestine do not have carcinoid syndrome unless they also have hepatic metastases to bypass metabolism by the liver and drain into the systemic circulation.

Carcinoid crisis may be triggered by various factors, including anaesthesia tumour handling, hepatic biopsy, hepatic artery embolization, or chemotherapy. It may be successfully treated with somatostatin analogue.

Pathology

Carcinoid tumours in the small intestine arise mainly within 60 cm of the ileocaecal valve. They may metastasize to local lymph nodes or more distally to liver and bone. They have variable histochemical and immunocytochemical staining, depending on their site of origin. Similarly, their propensity to secrete 5-hydroxyindoles and to secrete peptide hormones ectopically is associated with their site of origin, and embryonic derivation.

Table 15.7 Clinical features
of the carcinoid syndrome

Flushing
Diarrhoea
Right-sided valvular heart disease
Wheezing
Facial telangiectasis
Pellagra-like skin lesions

Clinical features

While they are commonly asymptomatic and only recognized at autopsy or coincidentally, they may also declare their presence by a local effect. Thus, tumours of the small intestine may be associated with obstruction, strangulation or perforation, while tumours of the bronchus may be associated with cough, hoarseness, haemoptysis, or breathlessness. Ovarian tumours may reveal themselves as a pelvic mass, or the patient may present with ectopic hormone secretion. A subset present with the features of the carcinoid syndrome. This subset represents a small minority of patients with carcinoid tumours. The main symptoms are flushing and diarrhoea. The flushing may be due to kinin release, at least in some patients. Kallikrein is found in carcinoids. Its release may be either spontaneous or stimulated by alcohol or catecholamines, and causes conversion of plasma kininogens to bradykinin. The diarrhoea tends to be secretory in type. Wheezing may occur, caused by transient bronchoconstriction. Patients who flush repeatedly may in time develop a cyanotic telangiectatic appearance which persists. The syndrome is also associated with fibrosis, particularly affecting the right side of the heart and causing tricuspid valve disease. Retroperitoneal fibrosis may also occur. Tryptophan is a precursor of nicotinic acid as well as of serotonin; thus in states of excessive activity of the 5-HT pathway, niacin-deficiency states may arise, manifest as pellagra. The presence of carcinoid syndrome in intestinal tumours normally indicates a significant tumour bulk, as intrahepatic metastases must be present to empty into the systemic circulation, and bypass the effect of intrahepatic metabolism. Similar metabolism on passage through the lung means that the left side of the heart tends to be spared fibrotic disease. Carcinoid crisis has been described as occurring in certain circumstances, including induction of anaesthesia, liver biopsy and following combination chemotherapy. It is manifest as extreme flushing, explosive diarrhoea, labile blood pressure and cardiac irregularities, including asystole. It has been successfully treated with the use of a somatostatin analogue.

Biochemistry (Fig. 15.3)

Tryptophan, an essential amino acid is first ring hydroxylated to form 5-hydroxy-tryptophan (5-HTP). This reaction is catalysed by the enzyme tryptophan hydroxylase and is the rate-limiting step in the biosynthesis of serotonin. Subsequently the enzyme aromatic amino acid decarboxylase is responsible for the decarboxylation of 5-HTP to yield 5-hydroxytryptamine, or serotonin (5-HT). This enzyme may be inhibited by methyldopa or carbidopa. The 5-HT is either stored in the neurosecretory granules of the tumour, or secreted into the vascular compartment. The remainder remains free in the plasma. Subsequent oxidative deamination to 5-hydroxyindole acetic acid (5-HIAA) inactivates the amine. This is catalysed by monoamine oxidase (MAO) and aldehyde dehydrogenase (AD). 5-HIAA is the major excretion product of indole metabolism in both normal subjects and in people with carcinoid syndrome.[37,38]

The normal excretion of 5-HIAA is <31.2 mmol/24 h. In patients with typical carcinoids, 99 per cent of their 5-hydroxyindole metabolism is excreted as 5-HIAA. Urinary 5-HIAA excretion is typically in the range 130–1300 mmol/24 h, generally exceeds 520 mmol/24 h and occasionally is as extreme as 2600 mmol/24 h.

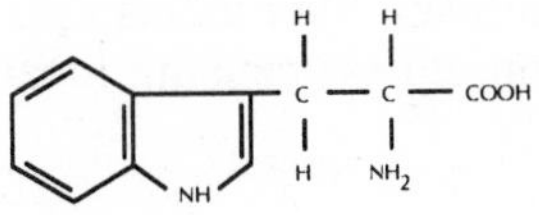

Tryptophan

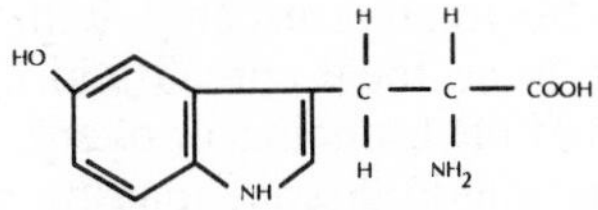

5-Hydroxytryptophan

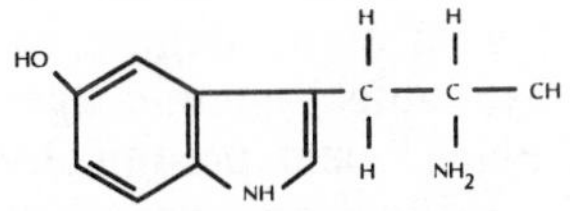

5-Hydroxytryptapamine or Serotonin

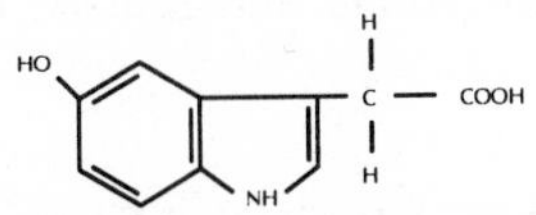

5-Hydroxyindole acetic acid

Fig. 15.3. Biochemistry of carcinoid tumours; synthesis and metabolism of serotonin. Tryptophan is the amino acid precursor of serotonin. Excessive synthesis of serotonin by tumour can cause pellagra, as the normal pathway to nicotinic acid biosynthesis is diverted. Tryptophan is first ring hydroxylated; subsequently the amino acid is decarboxylated to form 5-hydroxytryptamine or serotonin. The amine is ultimately oxidized and deaminated to form the inactive metabolite 5-hydroxyindole acetic acid (5-HIAA).

Clinical investigation

Biochemical

The most sensitive and specific indicator of serotonin and its metabolites is measurement of 24 h urinary 5-HIAA. A number of substances may interfere with the measurement of 5-HIAA, and appropriate precautions should be taken, both in specimen collection and assay.

Other investigations must be guided by clinical features and therapeutic intent. Patients who present with features suggestive of ectopic hormone secretion should be investigated as appropriate for the specific hormonal excess.

Tumour localization

Anatomical demarcation of tumour is guided by therapeutic intent. Thus, ovarian carcinoids and bronchial carcinoids may be cured by surgical excision for which purposes anatomical definition is important. Definition of a small intestinal lesion in the presence of significant liver metastases is futile and thus anatomical location of the primary lesion, unless causing local pathology, is not indicated.

Therapy

Therapeutic options may be curative or palliative. Circumscribed tumours of the small intestine which may be totally resected will, in general, be cured by surgery, particularly if there is no local spread and they are less than 5 cm in diameter. Similarly, tumours of the bronchus or ovary, if totally resected, may be cured. Significant hepatic metastatic disease may be helped by hepatic embolization, or resection of an involved lobe. While not curative, such a manoeuvre is certainly palliative. The recent use of somatostatin analogues has been particularly effective in the management of the symptoms of carcinoid syndrome,[39,40] although it is also associated with some degree of disease regression. It is currently the most effective available systemic agent. Other options include the use of alpha-interferon (IFNα)[41] and prednisolone. This has been shown to be particularly beneficial for midgut tumours. Systemic chemotherapy, with streptozocin and 5-fluorouracil can be effective,[42] particularly in the management of foregut tumours. Measures for symptomatic management include the use of antidiarrhoeal agents, histamine antagonists, and 5-hydroxytryptamine receptor antagonists.

MULTIPLE ENDOCRINE NEOPLASIA

Multiple endocrine neoplasia type 1 (MEN-1, Wermer's syndrome, multiple endocrine adenomatosis type 1) describes a syndrome of inherited endocrine disorders characterized by the presence of two or more of pituitary, pancreatic islet and parathyroid tumours. Less frequently, other tumours are also associated including carcinoid tumours, adrenal cortical tumours, thyroid and lipomatous tumours.

Multiple endocrine neoplasia type 2 (MEN-2, Sipple syndrome, multiple endocrine adenomatosis type 2) involves two or more of medullary carcinoma of thyroid, phaeochromocytomas and parathyroid tumour. The subclassification into types A and B is based on a phenotypic distinction which has been recognized. Type A has a normal phenotype; type B has a specific phenotype manifest as eye or oral (tongue, lips or mucus membranes) ganglioneuromata, a Marfanoid habitus, skeletal abnormalities, prominent corneal nerves, and a lesser tendency to have parathyroid disease. The designation type 2C recognizes a subgroup who have medullary carcinoma of thyroid only.

The genetic lesions for MEN-1 and MEN-2 have been mapped to two separate chromosomes. Multiple endocrine neoplasia may arise sporadically or be inherited in an autosomal dominant fashion. There is variable penetrance in the development of each tumour, both within and among affected families. The chromosomal mutation in MEN-1 has been mapped to chromosome 11, while the locus of abnormality in MEN-2 has been assigned to chromosome 10. These are the inherited endocrine diseases. They have a spectrum of clinical presentation from asymptomatic to symptomatic; the histological profile may be similarly variable. Thus a spectrum of histology ranging from hyperplastic to multifocal adenomatosis to overt neoplasia may be seen in the affected glands. Their diagnosis mandates that family screening become part of the management of this disorder.

MEN-1

The clinical manifestations depend on the tumour sites and their products of secretion. MEN-1 becomes manifest after the first decade with most patients developing symptoms in the third (women) and fourth (men) decades.

Parathyroid disease in MEN-1

This is the most frequent manifestation of MEN-1, and the most common reason for the disease coming to the attention of physicians. The pathological features are those of diffuse or asymmetric hyperplasia, with all four glands being involved, although perhaps not all to the same degree.

Symptoms related to hyperparathyroidism are the presenting symptoms in 9–30 per cent of patients with MEN-1. The symptoms are no different from those in patients with primary hyperparathyroidism, namely polyuria, polydipsia, constipation, altered mentation, colic related to nephrolithiasis, pancreatitis, bone pain and occasionally pathological fracture. Biochemical screening demonstrates hypercalcaemia; indices of bone metabolism and renal function may be secondarily affected. X-rays of the hand may show subperiosteal erosions, or changes of osteitis fibrosa cystica may be observed. If an elevated plasma parathyroid hormone concentration is found at the time calcium is elevated, assuming a specific assay and normal renal function, the diagnosis is confirmed.

Whether or not surgery is indicated in this group of patients is controversial. Surgery is certainly indicated if deteriorating renal function, or progressive bone destruction are problems. The impact of hypercalcaemia on systemic well-being is very difficult to assess, and surgery for this indication alone is harder to justify. Hypercalcaemia exacerbates hypergastrinaemia. Thus the presence of hyperparathyroidism may make Zollinger–Ellison syndrome (ZES) difficult to manage in patients with both disorders. Refractory ZES may in itself constitute an indication for parathyroid surgery.

The current preferred surgical practice is to perform a subtotal parathyroidectomy, removing three and a half glands, and leaving a residual 30–50 mg of parathyroid tissue. If surgery is excessive, functional hypoparathyroidism results. Alternately, if inadequate amounts of tissue are removed, hyperparathyroidism continues. It is becoming accepted practice to transplant the residual tissue subcutaneously to the non-dominant forearm. It may thus be more readily accessed if further surgery is needed to manage hyperparathyroidism subsequently. The other option is cryopreservation of this tissue, so that it may subsequently be implanted if functional hypoparathyroidism results.

MEN-2A and 2B

The incidence of involvement of the principal organ at diagnosis is: medullary carcinoma of thyroid (MCT) 100 per cent, phaeochromocytoma 20–40 per cent and parathyroid hyperplasia 17–60 per cent in patients with 2A disease;

parathyroid disease is rarely detected in 2B. Once again there appears to be a spectrum of progression of pathological involvement. Thus, C-cell hyperplasia precedes medullary carcinoma of thyroid, adrenal medullary hyperplasia precedes phaeochromocytoma, and occult parathyroid hyperplasia has been reported. The most frequent cause of death in this group of patients is either metastatic spread from medullary carcinoma of thyroid or phaeochromocytoma.

Parathyroid disease in MEN-2

There is evidence of parathyroid involvement in 20–60 per cent of patients at diagnosis of 2A disease; 84 per cent have hyperplasia and some 16 per cent have frank adenomata. Type 2B disease rarely has some microscopic abnormality. Symptoms are uncommon; when they do occur, they are similar to those experienced by patients with primary hyperparathyroidism. The diagnosis is made by the demonstration of simultaneously elevated plasma calcium and parathyroid hormone concentrations in patients with other evidence of MEN-2; the parathyroid disease may be occult in the earliest stages. The indications for surgery and subsequent treatment are as for MEN-1. Since the disease is more likely to be clinically occult, intervention may not be required.

ECTOPIC HORMONE SECRETION

Tumours produce signs and symptoms in the patient by the bulk of their presence, their compromise of normal function, their local invasion and infiltration, with ensuing physiological compromise, and similarly where the disease has metastasized. Tumours may also, however, produce signs and symptoms remote from the site or sites of tumour involvement. These are collectively termed 'paraneoplastic syndromes'. Hormone synthesis by a non-endocrine tumour, often termed ectopic hormone production, is one of the best characterized paraneoplastic syndromes (Table 15.8). More recently there has been characterization of other tumour-derived proteins such as cytokines and growth factors. Paraneoplastic syndromes may also be caused by proteins whose production is stimulated by the presence of tumour, e.g. the production of cachectin or tumour necrosis factor by monocytes, and the elicitation by tumour provocation of antibodies which ultimately have been shown to mediate the neurological paraneoplastic states, including Eaton–Lambert syndrome.

There are two schools of thought as to why tissues which have previously not been known to secrete hormones do so when they become neoplastic. The first would argue that some feature of the neoplastic cell removes the restraining portion of the regulatory element for that gene. Thus, inhibitory control of hormone output is no longer operant, and the hormone can be freely synthesized and secreted. Since at conception the first cell is pluripotential, the process of differentiation leads to functional specialization with loss of those functions which are not necessary to the organ in which the differentiated cell finds itself. The neoplastic cell, however, may be so dedifferentiated that the regulatory control of hormone secretion may not yet have been downregulated, and thus is being expressed, the second theory of hormone secretion.

Table 15.8 Hormones arising from tumours derived from tissue not classically associated with their secretion

Hormones	Associated tumours
Adrenocorticotrophic hormone, lipotrophin, melanocyte-stimulating hormone, endorphin, encephalin, other pro-opiomelanocortin fragments	Small cell carcinoma of lung Adenocarcinoma of lung Bronchial carcinoid Thymic carcinoid Medullary thyroid carcinoma Islet cell carcinoma of pancreas Phaeochromocytoma Gut, prostate, neurogenic and parotid tumours
Atrial natiuretic peptide	Small cell carcinoma of lung
Argenine vasopressin	Small cell carcinoma of lung Pancreatic carcinoma Breast carcinoma Thymic tumour
Calcitonin	Small cell carcinoma of lung Pulmonary carcinoid tumour
Calcitonin gene-related peptide	Small cell carcinoma of lung Pancreatic endocrine tumour
Corticotrophin-releasing hormone	Small cell carcinoma of lung Bronchial carcinoid
Erythropoietin	Uterine fibroma Cerebellar haemangioblastoma Hepatocellular carcinoma Phaeochromocytoma Ovarian tumour
Gastrin-releasing peptide	Small cell carcinoma of lung Medullary carcinoma of thyroid
Glucagon	Non beta islet cell tumour Anaplastic lung carcinoma Renal carcinoma
Growth hormone	Lung carcinoma Gastric carcinoma
Growth hormone-releasing hormone	Pancreatic islet cell tumour Phaeochromocytoma
Human chorionic gonadotrophin	Large cell lung carcinoma Gastric carcinoma
Colorectal carcinoma	Islet cell tumour Pancreatic adenocarcinoma Breast carcinoma Prostate carcinoma Melanoma Hepatoma/hepatoblastoma Carcinoid of lung or gut

Table 15.8 Continued

Hormones	Associated tumours
Human placental lactogen	Large cell carcinoma of lung
Insulin-like growth factor 2 and non-suppressible insulin-like protein	Mesodermal and mesenchymal tumour
Neurotensin	Pancreatic endocrine tumour Carcinoid tumour
Parathyroid hormone-related protein (PTHrP)	Squamous cell carcinoma of head and neck, oesophagus, cervix and lung Large cell carcinoma of lung Renal carcinoma Multiple myeloma Histeocytic lymphoma
Prolactin	Anaplastic lung carcinoma Small cell lung carcinoma Renal cell carcinoma
Renin	Renal adenocarcinoma Adenocarcinoma of pancreas Small cell carcinoma of lung Adenocarcinoma of lung Ovarian carcinoma Adrenocortical carcinoma
Somatostatin	Small cell carcinoma of lung Duodenal somatostatinoma Extra-adrenal paraganglionoma Phaeochromocytoma Medullary carcinoma of thyroid
Vasoactive intestinal polypeptide	Bronchial carcinoid tumour Ganglioneuroblastoma Phaeochromocytoma Non beta islet cell tumour Carcinoma of lung

Reproduced in part from Sherwood LM. Paraneoplastic endocrine disorders. In: deGroot LJ ed. *Endocrinology*, vol. 3. Philadelphia: WB Saunders, 1989, with permission.

Characteristics of ectopic hormone secretion

Ectopic hormone secretion may be considered as having specific characteristics. The hormone is secreted from a site not classically associated with its production or secretion. The hormone may be identifed in neoplastic tissue at a greater concentration than in normal tissue. The hormone may be measured in the venous outflow from the tumour at a greater concentration than within the general circulation. The cell of origin was capable at some time in its development, if only transiently, of secreting the hormone in question (if one subscribes to the latter theory of the pathogenesis of ectopic hormone secretion). Messenger RNA coding for the specific hormone may be demonstrable within the tumour tissue. The genes responsible for ectopic hormone production are transcribed normally in tumour cells from the conventional promoter. The synthesized and secreted hormone may not undergo appropriate post-translational processing. Thus, it may be secreted as the preprohormone, the prohormone or the hormone itself, with or without normal or abnormal glycosylation. Alternatively, it may undergo aberrant cleavage, so that peptide fragments are found in the circulation which are not usually present, and which may or may not be biologically active. The extent of hormone synthesis and secretion greatly exceeds both physiological levels, and the pathophysiological levels resulting from hyperplasia or tumour of the endocrine tissue normally responsible for its production. The latter tends to retain some sensitivity to stimulation and suppressing signals, albeit at a different threshold, which contrasts with ectopic secretion. In general, ectopic hormone secretion tends to be autonomous, and not to be furthur stimulated by known physiological secretagogues. Ectopic hormone secretion tends not to recognize feedback suppression by target organ hormone. More than one hormone may be cosecreted ectopically from neoplastic tissue, and the relative patterns of secretion may change. Treatment of the neoplasia is associated with remission of ectopic hormone secretion. (Appropriate treatment of the tumour may require treating the hormone excess independently.) Relapse of the tumour may be associated with recurrence of ectopic hormone secretion.

The structure of the gene

The genetic code, the blueprint containing all the information for the growth and development of a person, is contained within DNA (deoxyribonucleic acid), which condenses to form chromosomes (46 in the human), which can be visualized in the nucleus of a cell by light microscopy (Figure 15.4). At the molecular level, DNA consists of two linear sugar phosphate backbones from which chemical units, the nucleotide bases, adenine, guanine, cytosine and thymine, project at right angles. Hydrogen bonds form between the complementary base pairs (adenine with thymine, cytosine with guanine) of each strand, forming a stable double-stranded molecule which twists into an antiparallel double helix. The complementarity of the double strand forms the basis of DNA replication, as each strand can act as a template for daughter strands.

The amino acid sequence of every protein is coded by triplets of base pairs, called codons, which are arranged in a linear sequence. A sequence of codons represents the primary structure of a protein within a gene. When this gene is expressed, a unidimensional linear code is translated into the three-dimensional molecular structure of a protein.

Each gene consists of a series of exons and introns. The exons are those parts of the gene represented in the final mRNA (messenger ribonucleic acid, the mobile copy of DNA which carries genetic information from the nucleus to the cytosol), while the introns do not code for proteins but contain gene regulatory elements. For an ordered sequence of cell/tissue and subsequently organ growth and differentiation and function, gene expression must occur in an ordered sequence. Sequences located adjacent to the gene, *cis*-acting elements, bind sequence-specific regulatory proteins called *trans*-acting factors, and in this way govern the ordered manner of gene expression.

For a gene to be expressed and result in a peptide, the genetic information

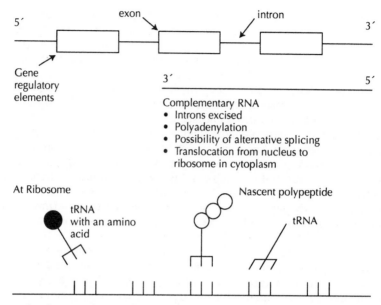

At the ribosome, the mRNA is translated into a polypeptide of amino acids

Fig. 15.4. The structure of a gene.

needs to be mobilized in a way that can leave the nucleus, and cross to the cytosol where the machinery exists to synthesize proteins. This is brought about by the transcription of DNA into a single complementary strand of RNA. This RNA contains a direct copy of the gene, including the introns. The introns must be removed and the exons joined together, a process known as splicing, before translation can occur. As a result the RNA consists of an open reading frame of codons that can be directly translated into a protein. Adenine residues are added to the 3' end of the RNA (poly-A tail); this polyadenylation stabilizes the molecule which is now mature mRNA. Certain mRNAs may be expressed and then spliced in different ways to yield mRNAs of differing lengths, a process termed alternative splicing.

The mRNA then passes out of the nucleus to ribosomes within the cytosol, where translation occurs. Ribosomes, which consist of RNA and protein, function as the protein factory of the cell. The mRNA strand passes through the ribosome, base by base and is 'read'. Molecules of transfer RNA (tRNA), which link anticodons, base triplets complementary to codons, to specific amino acids, are aligned along the mRNA. Simultaneously, each newly inserted amino acid residue is linked by a peptide bond between its amine group and the carboxyl group of its predecessor in the growing chain of amino acids forming a protein. Translation terminates when a termination codon, for which there are no tRNAs, is reached. Furthur modifications to the protein may occur in the endoplasmic reticulum and Golgi apparatus where the leader sequence is cleaved and proteins may undergo glycosylation.

Ectopic secretion of PTHrP (parathyroid hormone-related peptide)

We have chosen to illustrate some of the principles described above by consideration of the ectopic synthesis and secretion of PTHrP. Since this hormone has only recently been isolated, its molecular sequence cloned, and specific immunoassays become available, much of its physiology and pathophysiology remains to be clarified. Nonetheless it illustrates some of the complex issues associated with ectopic hormone secretion (Fig. 15.5).

PTHrP is a 141 amino acid peptide which is responsible for a large proportion of cases of humeral hypercalcaemia of malignancy. Eight of the thirteen amino-terminal amino acids are identical to those found in PTH itself, and it appears to act on the PTH receptor. There is evidence for its production in both the fetal parathyroid and in the lactating breast, raising the possibility that it has a physiological role in these two contexts. A carboxy-terminal fragment of PTHrP may act independently as an inhibitor of osteoclastic bone resorption.

The sequence predicted by cDNA cloning revealed, in the first instance, a mature protein consisting of 141 amino acids, with a leader sequence comprising 36 amino acids. Clones were also isolated which indicated that alternate splicing could also result in the production of mature PTHrP proteins of 139 or 173 amino acid residues in length.[43–47] The PTHrP molecule contains potential amidation sites at residues 86 and 95. There are also many potential proteolytic cleavage sites, particularly a predominantly basic sequence between residues 87 and 108. It is tempting to speculate that these sites raise the possibility of tissue-specific processing of PTHrP, resulting in peptides of variable biological activities.

The gene for PTHrP has proven to be very complex.[48–51] Multiple mRNAs have been discovered which are divergent at both the 3' and 5' ends. The PTHrP gene contains nine exons. Exons 5 and 6, which code for the prepro molecule and the majority of the coding region, do not exhibit variability in mRNA transcripts. Exon 6 comprises the majority of the coding region for the mature protein, up to residue 139, where a splice site is located. Readthrough of exon 6 into 7 results in the introduction of a termination signal producing a protein product of 139 amino acids in length, whereas inclusion of exons 8 and 9 by alternate mRNA splicing, results in protein products of 173 and 141 amino acids respectively. These alternate splice products leading to proteins with variable carboxyl-termini had been predicted earlier by the cDNA cloning data. In addition to the variable 3' exonic regions, production of multiple mRNA species

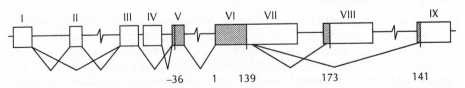

Fig. 15.5. Genomic organization of human preproparathyroid hormone-related protein (PTHrP) gene. The coding and untranslated regions are indicated by the closed and open boxes, respectively. Alternate splice products lead to proteins with variable C-termini. The variability in the 5' region represents the variety of promoter sequences possible.

Table 15.9   Sites of tissue-specific gene expression of PTHrP

Keratinocytes

Endocrine tissues
   Pancreatic islets
   Parathyroid gland
   Pituitary gland
   Adrenals
   Ovary
   Testis

Central nervous system
   Cerebral cortex
   Hippocampus
   Cerebellar cortex

Lactating breast

by the action of alternate 5' promoters is evident, congruent with the divergent clones noted during cDNA cloning. It may prove that the different promoters are used in a tissue-specific manner also. It is evident that there is potential for great heterogeneity in mRNAs for PTHrP, and this has indeed been the experience in studies of tumour and tissue mRNA for PTHrP (Table 15.9).

Sequence analysis of PTHrP in four species, rat, mouse, chicken and human, shows extraordinary degrees of sequence conservation across the species. This strongly supports a pivotal role for this protein through the evolutionary process.

The regulation of transcription of PTHrP is little characterized as yet.[52] Treatment with 1,25-dihydroxyvitamin D_3 or glucocorticoid has resulted in the suppression of PTHrP secretion in tissue culture studies, and transfection studies. Increased cAMP secretion is associated with increased PTHrP secretion. Recently evidence has become available that oestrogen has a role in the regulation of PTHrP transcription, which has potentially fascinating implications.

BIOCHEMICAL ABNORMALITIES COMMONLY SEEN IN CANCER PATIENTS

Calcium metabolism

Calcium, a divalent cation has multiple physiological roles, which may broadly be considered as structural or metabolic.[53] Its structural role is maintenance of skeletal integrity; failure results in osteopenia, with resultant predisposition to fracture. The metabolic actions of calcium are more numerous and complex. The extracellular concentration of calcium ions influences the threshold for nerve action potentials, a high calcium raising the threshold, while a low calcium lowers the threshold. The extracellular calcium ion concentration appears also to alter the gating of sodium and potassium channels. Calcium has a vital role in the mediation of intracellular events. The depolarization of nerve or muscle cells, or the binding of a hormone ligand or cytokine to its receptor on the surface of responsive cells produces an increase in the cytosolic calcium concentration. This results from the influx of calcium through plasma membrane channels or the release of calcium from the endoplasmic reticulum. For the latter to take place, receptor-activated hydrolysis of inositol phospholipids in the plasma membrane has to occur, with consequent release of inositol triphosphate into the cytosol. This binds to a receptor on the endoplasmic reticulum leading to the release of calcium into the cytoplasm. Cell functions are then influenced directly, e.g. the regulation of enzymes such as protein kinase C, or indirectly through the calcium receptor protein calmodulin. These pathways are vital for muscle contraction, neuroendocrine secretion and action, and the mechanisms of cell metabolism and growth.

The total body calcium is approximately 1 kg, 99 per cent of which is found in the skeleton. The ionized concentration of calcium, approximately 50 per cent of that which is circulating, is physiologically important and closely modulated.

Physiology of calcium regulation

Normal bone is a tissue with a constant turnover, i.e. it is resorbed and remodelled constantly (Fig. 15.6). In healthy bone, these two processes are coupled, and the amount of bone being resorbed is equal to the amount being accreted, thus maintaining a dynamic equilibrium. The process of bone break-down starts with the arrival of the osteoclast, a cell derived from the monocyte/macrophage lineage. This is a multinucleated giant cell which attaches by a 'suction cup' of integrins to a consensus sequence of collagen. Here the lysosomal proteases and acids are secreted which mediate resorption. The number

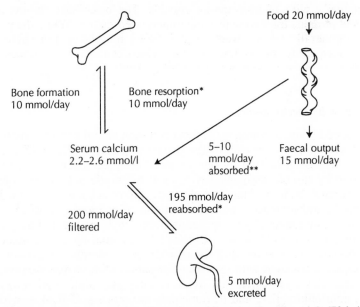

Fig. 15.6.   Representative calcium fluxes (mmol/day) in a healthy adult (70 kg). The major site of action of parathyroid hormone (PTH)* and 1,25-dihydroxyvitamin D$_3$** are indicated.

Table 15.10   Factors that affect bone formation or breakdown

	Increase	*Decrease*
Systemic bone formation	Fluoride Parathyroid hormone (intermittent) Prostaglandins (continuous)	Corticosteroids Parathyroid hormone
Local bone formation	TGF β Bone morphogenetic proteins IGFs	
Systemic bone resorption	Parathyroid hormone (continuous) PTHrP 1,25 dihydroxyvitamin D_3 Thyroxine	Calcitonin Oestrogen
Local bone resorption	IL-1 IL-6 IL-11 TNF α TNF β M-CSF	TGF β IFN γ IL-4

and activity of osteoclasts is controlled by both parathyroid hormone and 1,25-dihydroxyvitamin D_3.

Subsequently the surface which has been resorbed is lined by osteoblasts which elaborate a matrix composed of 90 per cent of type 1 collagen, but also osteocalcin, fibronectin and other proteins. This matrix is subsequently mineralized, principally with hydroxyapatite crystals. The osteoblast matures to an osteocyte, and remains trapped within the mineralized matrix. While the process of resorption generally takes a week, it may take 3 months or more before the new bone is adequately mineralized. Factors which can affect the processes of bone formation or bone breakdown are listed in Table 15.10.

Pathogenesis of hypercalcaemia

Tumour-induced hypercalcaemia is the most common complication of malignant disease, and occurs in 10 per cent of the patient population (Table 15.11). The pathogenesis may be mediated by one or more of three mechanisms, namely direct invasion by tumour associated with local osteolytic activity (e.g. breast, melanoma, adrenal, kidney, lung and thyroid), increased humorally mediated bone resorption, and increased tubular resorption of calcium (Table 15.12). In haematological malignancy, hypercalcaemia occurs in 30 per cent of all patients with myeloma, as well as those with Burkitt's lymphoma, retrovirus-associated T-cell lymphoma, leukaemia and lymphosarcoma. Rarely, haematological malignancies are associated with increased formation of 1,25-dihydroxyvitamin D_3, which mediates hypercalcaemia by enhancing gastrointestinal resorption. Principally, interleukins IL-1 and IL-6 mediate the process. If IL-4 is involved, alkaline phosphatase is rarely elevated, as it inhibits new bone formation. In solid tumours associated with humoral hypercalcaemia, this is most commonly

Table 15.11 Tumours most commonly
associated with hypercalcaemia

Lung (squamous) carcinoma	35%
Breast carcinoma	25%
Haematological malignancy	14%
Squamous carcinoma of head and neck	6%
Genitourinary tumours	6%
Others	15%

Table 15.12 Tumours associated with humoral
hypercalcaemia of malignancy

Squamous cell carcinoma of lung
Renal cortical carcinoma
Squamous cell carcinoma of skin and oesophagus
Pancreatic tumours
Ovarian tumours
Large bowel carcinomas
Phaeochromocytoma

mediated by parathyroid hormone-related protein (PTHrP).[54,55] This peptide is elaborated by the tumour, and may circulate in one of three isoforms, consisting of 139 amino acids, 141 amino acids or 171 amino acids, respectively. The biological activity of the peptide resides in the first 1–34 amino acids. This hormone mediates the hypercalcaemia by both increasing bony resorption, and enhancing renal tubular reabsorption of calcium. It binds to the PTH receptor, and mimics its physiological action.

Clinical presentation of hypercalcaemia

Tumours most likely to be associated with PTHrP excess are listed in Table 15.11. PTHrP excess mediates hypercalcaemia which has a generalized effect on cellular Na^+,K^+-ATPase, causing hyperpolarization, and thus increased refractoriness of cell membranes. This effect is particularly noticeable in cells of the central nervous system and cardiac muscle, causing the CNS effects of confusion, delirium, drowsiness and ultimately coma, while the neuromuscular effects cause constipation (Table 15.13). Hypercalcaemia also interferes with the effect of antidiuretic hormone (ADH) on the distal convoluted tubules and collecting ducts of the kidney, thus causing a syndrome akin to diabetes insipidus, with resulting polyuria, polydipsia, dehydration and prerenal azotemia.

Treatment of hypercalcaemia

The goals of treatment for hypercalcaemia are to correct the symptoms and signs, to normalize the serum calcium and to subsequently maintain normocalcaemia. The most important principle of treatment is rehydration, and the patient who presents with hypercalcaemia should be rehydrated with IV saline quite

Table 15.13 Symptoms and signs of hypercalcaemia

Gastrointestinal
Anorexia
Nausea
Vomiting
Constipation
Symptoms of peptic ulceration
Symptoms of pancreatitis

Renal
Polyuria
Polydipsia

Central nervous system
Difficulty in concentration and mood changes, mainly depression
Vagueness and fatiguability
Confusion
Obtundation
Coma

Cardiovascular
ECG abnormalities: QT shortening, tenting of the T waves, first-degree heart block
Predisposition to digitalis toxicity

briskly. As much as 5–10 l of saline may be required, and rehydration may need to be supervised with central venous pressure measurements.

Calcitonin is the treatment that would be expected to have the most immediate effect in the short term, but its duration of effectiveness is very short lived. The mainstay of treatment has come to be intravenous pamidronate.[56] This may take as long as 48 hours to produce a discernible effect but it gives a reliable response in 80 per cent of people. Bisphosphonates inhibit bony resorption. They inhibit the formation of osteoclasts from their progenitors, inhibit the action of mature osteoclasts on bone, and may also inhibit the capacity of osteoclasts to bind to mineralized surfaces. As a group they are stable analogues of pyrophosphate. The effect will last for a number of weeks. Oral bisphosphonates are also available, but bisphosphonates are much less efficacious when administered orally.

Mithramycin is a cytotoxic drug which inhibits DNA-dependent RNA synthesis.[57] It is effective in treating hypercalcaemia as it inhibits osteoclast-mediated bony resorption and osteoclast formation. However, it has high toxicity, causing hepatocellular damage, impairment of renal function, and it may cause a bleeding diathesis. Its use is probably best reserved for the subset of patients who do not respond well to pamidronate. Calcitonin and corticosteroids are useful in the treatment of patients with impaired renal function, particularly in the management of haematological malignancies.

Purine metabolism and urate nephropathy

The purine nucleotides, AMP (adenylic acid), IMP (inosinic acid) and GMP (guanylic acid), are the end-products of purine biosynthesis. They can either be synthesized directly from the purine bases, e.g. guanine to GMP, hypoxanthine

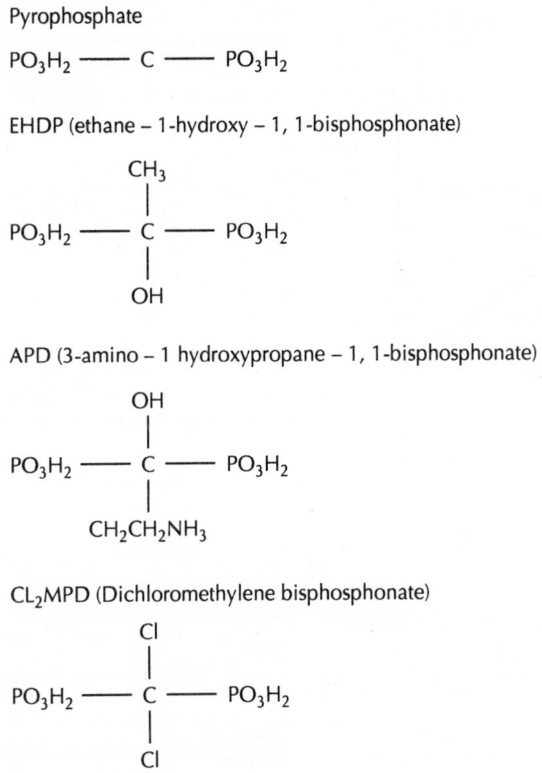

Pyrophosphate

$$PO_3H_2 \text{---} C \text{---} PO_3H_2$$

EHDP (ethane – 1-hydroxy – 1, 1-bisphosphonate)

$$PO_3H_2 \text{---} \underset{\underset{OH}{|}}{\overset{\overset{CH_3}{|}}{C}} \text{---} PO_3H_2$$

APD (3-amino – 1 hydroxypropane – 1, 1-bisphosphonate)

$$PO_3H_2 \text{---} \underset{\underset{CH_2CH_2NH_3}{|}}{\overset{\overset{OH}{|}}{C}} \text{---} PO_3H_2$$

CL$_2$MPD (Dichloromethylene bisphosphonate)

$$PO_3H_2 \text{---} \underset{\underset{Cl}{|}}{\overset{\overset{Cl}{|}}{C}} \text{---} PO_3H_2$$

Fig. 15.7. Clinical structure of bisphosphonates.

to IMP, and adenine to AMP, or they can be synthesized from non-purine precursors, progressing through a series of steps to IMP, the common intermediate nucleotide. IMP can be converted to either GMP or AMP (Fig. 15.8). Subsequently the nucleotides are utilized for the synthesis of nucleic acids, ATP, cyclic AMP, cyclic GMP and other cofactors.

The various purine components are degraded to the purine nucleotide monophosphates. GMP is degraded via guanosine, guanine and xanthine to uric acid. IMP is degraded through inosine, hypoxanthine and xanthine to uric acid. AMP can be deaminated to yield IMP, or it may be converted via adenosine to inosine.

Normal serum urate concentrations range between 0.24 and 0.48 mmol/l. At physiological pH uric acid exists as a monovalent sodium salt. Serum is saturated with monosodium urate at a concentration of 0.42 mmol/l but higher levels may remain stable as a supersaturated solution for a long period of time. The total body content of uric acid is normally about 200 mmol. Two thirds of this pool turns over every day. The kidney is responsible for the excretion of two thirds of the pool, while the remainder is metabolized in the gastrointestinal tract, where uric acid is further metabolized by bacterial flora to yield CO_2 and ammonia. In the nephron, the functional unit of the kidney, uric acid is filtered, undergoes proximal tubular reabsorption, active tubular secretion, and post-secretory reabsorption. The final uric acid secretion can be modified in various

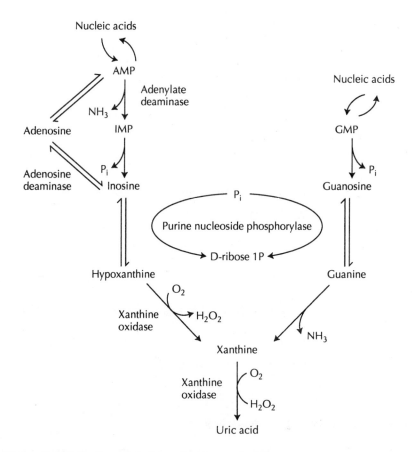

Fig. 15.8. Routes for the metabolism of purine nucleotides.

ways. Increased renal perfusion, brought about by expansion of the extracellular fluid can promote uric acid clearance, while dehydation will do the opposite. Metabolic acidosis will limit uric acid clearance; the mechanism is thought to be direct competition for active tubular secretion.

Urinary pH is critical in determining the solubility of uric acid. At pH 5.5 or less, uric acid is present in its free acidic form, whereas at a higher pH more uric acid is present as urate. This change in ionization has direct effects on solubility, being 20 mmol/l for the salt and 1.1 mmol/l for the acid. In the distal portion of the nephron, the high urinary concentration of uric acid and the low pH may lead to supersaturation of urine with uric acid crystals. Allopurinol, a drug which inhibits the conversion of hypoxanthine and xanthine to uric acid, is clinically useful in patients with pathological hyperuricaemia, since the xanthines are much more soluble in an aqueous medium, and will not precipitate out as crystals if present in excess.

In practical terms, patients with oncological disease are prone to hyperuricaemia because of rapid cell turnover, or acute tumour cell lysis.[58-61] While sporadic cases of uric acid nephropathy have been reported as occurring *de novo*, most cases arise following the institution of an effective treatment. The uric acid load presented to the kidney depends on the growth rate of the tumour, the tumour burden, and the sensitivity of the tumour to the treatment. (Drugs such as folate acid antagonists interfere with purine metabolism prior to the formation of uric acid; their use is therefore not associated with uric acid excess.) The haematological malignancies most commonly associated with hyperuricaemia and consequent hyperuricosuria are acute lymphoblastic leukaemia (ALL), acute myelocytic leukaemia (AML), some high-grade lymphomas and chronic myeloid leukaemia (CML). Patients with multiple myeloma are at risk of renal failure for a variety of reasons, including hyperuricosuria. Patients with myelofibrosis and polycythaemia rubra vera also carry a degree of risk. The only solid tumours associated with hyperuricaemia are rapidly growing bulky tumours such as testicular teratomas.

Uric acid nephropathy is clinically manifest as oliguric or anuric renal failure. The symptoms are those attributable to uraemia. Flank pain due to colic or haematuria may occur. Since uric acid may be very elevated in renal failure, the diagnosis can only be inferred in the appropriate clinical context. Urinalysis may reveal the presence of uric acid crystals, and the urinary concentration of uric acid may exceed 25 mmol/l. Ultrasound of the kidneys may show a dilated renal pelvis.

Prevention and treatment

It should now be possible to anticipate and prevent most cases of urate nephropathy in patients at risk. Vigorous hydration is critical to ensure adequate renal perfusion, thus augmenting uric acid secretion. General recommendations are 3–4 l of fluid over 24 hours, maintaining a urinary output of 100 ml/h. Urinary pH should be maintained above 7.0 to maximize the solubility of uric acid. Metabolic acidosis should be corrected before treatments which promote tumour destruction are instituted, if possible. Formal alkalinization of the urine may be induced by the use of sodium bicarbonate infusions (50–100 mEq of $NaHCO_3$ added to each litre of IV fluid) or the use of carboxyanhydrase inhibitors such as acetazolamide. Use of the latter is contraindicated in the presence of metabolic acidosis, however.

The mainstay in the management of hyperuricaemia and hyperuricosuria in oncology has been the use of allopurinol. This drug and its major metabolite act by inhibiting xanthine oxidase, the enzyme which catalyses the conversion of xanthine and hypoxanthine to uric acid. When this enzyme is inhibited, production of the more soluble xanthines is favoured while production of uric acid, and its subsequent crystallization out of solution, is prevented. The usual starting dose is 300 mg daily, and it is generally administered for at least 48 hours before the introduction of combination chemotherapy. In the presence of hyperuricaemia, however, 500 mg twice daily may be used. The effect is cumulative over the first 14 days. Dosage should be reduced in the presence of renal failure, as the drug is renally excreted. Side-effects include fever, gastrointestinal upset and, rarely, toxic epidermal necrolysis. It should be noted that the biological activity of azothiaprine, 6-mercaptopurine and cyclophosphamide is increased if co-administered with allopurinol, and relevant dose adjustments should be made.

The half-life of warfarin is also prolonged if administered with allopurinol, and the INR may need to be restabilized.

If uric acid nephropathy is established, the treatment of choice is haemodialysis.

Hyponatraemia

Syndrome of inappropriate antidiuretic hormone secretion (SIADH)

As originally defined, the syndrome includes: (1) hyponatraemia and hypotonicity of body fluids, with a urine which is relatively hypertonic to the plasma; (2) excessive natriuresis, despite prevalent hyponatraemia; (3) normal renal and adrenal function; (4) absent dehydration, hypertension, azotaemia, oedema, with suppressed plasma renin activity; (5) improvement in both hyponatraemia and natriuresis following fluid deprivation.

Pathogenesis of SIADH

Arginine vasopressin (AVP, commonly shortened to vasopressin, VP) is a nonapeptide composed of six amino acids in a ring attached to a side-chain of three amino acids. It is synthesized in the supraoptic and paraventricular nuclei of the hypothalamus. The axons of the neurons in these nuclei extend through the pituitary stalk to the posterior pituitary. Vasopressin migrates down the axons as part of a precursor protein and is stored as secretory granules within the nerve terminals of the posterior pituitary. The hormone is released by exocytosis into the bloodstream. Vasopressin or antidiuretic hormone (ADH) functions to conserve water; its release is coordinated with the activity of the thirst centre which regulates fluid intake. AVP acts on vasopressin receptors in the cells of the distal convoluted tubules and collecting ducts of the nephron. By rendering these cells permeable to water, it promotes the passage of water from the (hypotonic) luminal fluid to the hyperosmotic medullary interstitium. Thus, this water is not lost in dilute urine, but maintained within the body.

Under normal circumstances, AVP release is controlled by 'osmoreceptors' within the hypothalamus. Both the production and release of AVP are enhanced when the osmoreceptors are stimulated. This occurs when there is a change in plasma solute concentration to which the osmoreceptor cellular membrane is impermeable, causing a change in volume of the osmoreceptor cells. This results in the generation of electrical activity in these neurons which stimulates AVP release. While changes in plasma tonicity are the major stimulus to AVP release in the normal state, hypovolaemia may also indirectly stimulate the release of AVP, even to the point of overriding osmotic inhibition of AVP release. In the euvolaemic patient, with normal renal and adrenal function, AVP secretion is 'inappropriate' if plasma osmolality is not tending towards hypertonicity (Table 15.14).

Prevention and treatment of SIADH

Being aware of the risk of SIADH in patients with lung cancer, even in the presence of a normal sodium concentration, is vital. Forty-one per cent of patients with lung cancer have elevated AVP levels. If one just considers

Table 15.14 Syndrome of inappropriate antidiuretic hormone secretion (SIADH)

Endogenous ADH secretion

Trauma

Pulmonary disease
  Pneumonia
  Cavitation (TB, abscess, aspergillosis)
  Cystic fibrosis
  Acute respiratory failure
  Chronic obstructive pulmonary disease
  Pneumothorax
  Positive pressure ventilation

Central nervous system disease
  Trauma: subdural haematoma, subarachnoid haemorrhage
  Infections: meningitis, encephalitis, brain abscess
  Guillain–Barré syndrome
  Cerebral thrombosis, cavernous sinus thrombosis
  Primary brain tumour
  Brain metastases
  Acute intermittent porphyria
  Seizures
  Wernicke's encephalopathy

Endocrine disease
  Addison's disease
  Myxoedema
  Hypopituitarism

Drug-related
  Vasopressin
  Vinca alkaloids
  Cisplatin
  Cyclophosphamide, high-dose melphalan
  Morphine
  Thiazides
  Sulphonylureas
  Phenothiazines
  Tricyclic antidepressants
  Carbamazepine
  Clofibrate
  Nicotine
  Ethanol

Ectopic ADH secretion
  Small cell lung cancer
  Carcinoids of foregut origin
  Hodgkin's and non-Hodgkin's lymphomas
  Leukaemia
  Ewing's sarcoma
  Thymoma
  Mesothelioma
  Neuroblastoma
  Nasopharyngeal carcinoma
  Pancreatic, duodenal ureteric or prostatic carcinoma

Table 15.15 Prevention and treatment of SIADH

Treat primary tumour or withdraw causative drugs
Fluid deprivation to 0.5 l/day
Consider frusemide and repletion of the urinary Na output with 3% NaCl
Demeclocycline
Lithium

patients with small cell lung cancer, 9 per cent of patients will have the clinical syndrome of hyponatraemia, 32–44 per cent will have increased AVP levels by radioimmunoassay, even if they are not hyponatraemic, and 53–68 per cent of patients will have the syndrome precipitated by water loading. The avoidance of hypotonic fluids in these patients is judicious.

If the syndrome does develop in patients with known lung cancer, it is also important to consider the other conditions which may cause it in this group of patients, e.g. use of morphine, vincristine or cyclophosphamide, pulmonary infections and intracranial disease, either infective or neoplastic. In general, however, the syndrome arises due to the lung cancer, and remits if the disease remits, but recurs in the presence of relapse.

The most effective treatment of the established syndrome is fluid restriction, to between 500 and 1000 ml/day depending on the severity (Table 15.15). The situation is more complex now as to what constitutes the best treatment of the most severely affected (serum sodium <120 mmol/l), in the presence of neuro-logical symptoms, lethargy, obtundation and coma. Traditional teaching has held that induction of diuresis with furosemide 1 mg/kg, quantitation of urinary sodium excretion, and repletion of the excreted sodium as 3 per cent saline was the most appropriate management. However, the occurrence of central pontine myelinolysis (CPM) in those patients most rapidly corrected has been noted.[58–62] The syndrome is manifest one to several days after treatment by the development of pseudobulbar palsy, quadriparesis, and mutism and ultimate death. CT or MRI evidence of the lesion in the pons may be demonstrated, but the presence of demyelination in other sites has also been noted. Occasion-ally, the pathology may only be evident after death. In view of this risk, it seems prudent to correct the hyponatraemia slowly.

REFERENCES

1. Nixon DW, Heymsfield SB, Cohen AE *et al.* Protein calorie undernutrition in hospitalised cancer patients. *American Journal of Medicine* 1980; **68**: 683–90.
2. DeWys WD. Weight loss and nutritional abnormalities in cancer patients: incidence, severity and significance. In: Calman KC, Fearon KCH eds. *Nutritional support for the cancer patient.* London: WB Saunders, 1986: 251–61.
3. Calman KC. *British Journal of Hospital Medicine* 1982; **26**: 28–34.
4. Dempsy DT, Feurer ID, Knox LX, Crosby LO, Buzby GP, Mullen JL. Energy expenditure in malnourished gastrointestinal cancer patients. *Cancer* 1984; **53**: 1265–73.
5. Waterhouse C, Kemperman JH. Carbohydrate metabolism in subjects with cancer. *Cancer Research* 1971; **31**: 1273–8.

6. Hyltander A *et al*. Elevated energy expenditure in cancer patients with solid tumours. *European Journal of Cancer* 1991; **27**: 9–15.

7. Loprinzi CL *et al*. Phase III evaluation of four doses of megestrol acetate as therapy for patients with cancer anorexia and/or cachexia. *Journal of Clinical Oncology* 1993; **12**: 762–7.

8. Coates G, Bush RS, Aspin N. A study of ascites using lymphoscintigraphy with ^{99m}Tc-sulphur colloid. *Radiology* 1973; **107**: 577–83.

9. Lacey JH, Wieman TJ, Shively EH. Management of malignant ascites. *Surgery, Gynecology and Obstetrics* 1984; **159**: 397–412.

10. Greenway B, Johnson PJ, Williams R. Control of malignant ascites with spironolactone. *British Journal of Surgery* 1982; **69**: 441–2.

11. LeVeen HH, Wapnick S, Grosberg S, Kinney MJ. Further experience with peritoneovenous shunt for ascites. *Annals of Surgery* 1976; **184**: 574–9.

12. Lund RH, Newkirk JB. Peritoneovenous shunting system for surgical management of ascites. *Contemporary Surgery* 1979; **14**: 31–45.

13. Vo NM *et al*. Complications of peritoneovenous shunting for malignant ascites. A collective review. *Connecticut Medicine* 1981; **45**: 1–4.

14. Melmed S, Braunstein GD, Chang RJ, Becker DP. Pituitary tumors secreting growth hormone and prolactin. *Annals of Internal Medicine* 1986; **105**: 238–53.

15. Frohman LA. Therapeutic options in acromegaly. *Journal of Clinical Endocrinology and Metabolism* 1991; **72**: 1175–81.

16. Chiodini PG, Cozzi R, Dallabonzana D *et al*. Medical treatment of acromegaly with SMS201-995, a somatostatin analog: a comparison with bromocriptine. *Journal of Clinical Endocrinology and Metabolism* 1987; **64**: 447–53.

17. Eastman RC, Gorden P, Roth J. Conventional supervoltage irradiation is an effective treatment for acromegaly. *Journal of Clinical Endocrinology and Metabolism* 1979; **48**: 931–40.

18. Blackwell RE. Diagnosis and management of prolactinomas. *Fertility and Sterility* 1985; **43**: 5–16.

19. Vance ML, Thorner MO. Prolactinomas. *Endocrinology and Metabolism Clinics of North America* 1987; **16**: 129–55.

20. Nabarro JDN. Pituitary prolactinomas. *Clinical Endocrinology* 1982; **17**: 129–55.

21. Molitch ME, Elton RL, Blackwell RE *et al*. Bromocriptine as primary therapy for prolactin-secreting macroadenomas: results of a prospective multicenter study. *Journal of Clinical Endocrinology and Metabolism* 1985; **60**: 698–705.

22. Boggan JE, Tyrell JB, Wilson CB. Transsphenoidal microsurgical management of Cushing's disease. Report of 100 cases. *Journal of Neurosurgery* 1983; **59**: 195–200.

23. Krieger DT. Medical treatment of Cushing's disease. In: Tolis G, Labrie F, Martin JB, Naftolin F eds. *Clinical neuroendocrinology: a pathophysiological approach*. New York: Raven Press, 1979: 423–7.

24. Mathew CGP, Chin KS, Easton DF *et al*. A linked genetic marker for multiple endocrine neoplasia type 2A on chromosome 10. *Nature* 1989; **328**: 528–30.

25. Sobol H, Salvetti A, Bonnardel C, Lenoir GM. Screening multiple endocrine neoplasia type 2A families using DNA markers. *Lancet* 1988; **1**: 62–3.

26. Sikri KL, Varndell IM, Hamid QA *et al*. Medullary carcinoma of the thyroid. An immunocytochemical and histochemical study of 25 cases using 8 separate markers. *Cancer* 1985; **56**: 2481–91.

27. Ponder BAJ *et al*. Risk estimation and screening of families of patients with medullary thyroid carcinoma. *Lancet* 1988; **i**: 397–400.

28. Saad MF, Ordonez NG, Rashid RK *et al*. Medullary carcinoma of thyroid. A study of the clinical features and prognostic factors in 161 patients. *Medicine* 1984; **63**: 319–42.

29. Samaan NA, Yang KP, Schultz PN, Hickey RC. Diagnosis, management, and

pathogenetic studies in medullary thyroid carcinoma. *Henry Ford Hospital Medical Journal* 1989; **37**: 132–7.

30. Samaan NA, Schultz PN, Hickey RC. Medullary thyroid carcinoma: prognosis of familial versus sporadic disease and the role of radiotherapy. *Journal of Clinical Endocrinology and Metabolism* 1988; **67**: 801–5.

31. Ross EJ, Griffith DNW. The clinical presentation of phaeochromocytoma. *Quarterly Journal of Medicine* 1989; **71**: 485–96.

32. Sheps SJ, Jiang NS, Klee GG, van Heerden JA. Recent developments in the diagnosis and treatment of pheochromocytoma. *Mayo Clinic Proceedings* 1990; **65**: 88–95.

33. Grossman E, Goldstein DS, Hoffman A, Keiser HR. Glucagon and clonidine testing in the diagnosis of pheochromocytoma. *Hypertension* 1991; **17**: 733–41.

34. Doppman JL, Reinig JW, Dwyer AJ *et al*. Differentiation of adrenal masses by magnetic resonance imaging. *Surgery* 1987; **102**: 1018–26.

35. Krempf M, Lumbroso J, Mornex R *et al*. Use of m[^{131}I]iodobenzylguanidine in the treatment of malignant pheochromocytoma. *Journal of Clinical Endocrinology and Metabolism* 1991; **72**: 455–61.

36. Averbuch SD, Steakley CS, Young RC *et al*. Malignant phaeochromocytoma: effective treatment with a combination of cyclophosphamide, vincristine and dacarbazine *Annals of Internal Medicine* 1988; **109**: 267–73.

37. Pernow B, Waldenstrom J. Determination of 5-hydroxytryptamine, 5-hydroxyindoleacetic acid and histamine in 33 cases of carcinoid tumor (argentaffinoma). *American Journal of Medicine* 1957; **23**: 16–25.

38. Feldman JM, Lee EM. Serotonin content of foods: effect on urinary excretion of 5-hydroxyindoleacetic acid. *American Journal of Clinical Nutrition* 1985; **42**: 639–43.

39. Kvols LK, Martin JK, Marsh HM *et al*. Rapid reversal of carcinoid crisis with a somatostatin analogue. *New England Journal of Medicine* 1985; **313**: 1229–30.

40. Vinik AI, Thompson M, Eckhauser F *et al*. Clinical features of carcinoid syndrome and the use of somatostatin analogue in its management. *Acta Oncologica* 1989; **28**: 389–402.

41. Moertel CG, Rubin J, Kvols LK. Therapy of metastatic carcinoid tumour and the malignant carcinoid syndrome with recombinant leucocyte A interferon. *Journal of Clinical Oncology* 1989; **7**: 865–8.

42. Moertel CG, Kvols LK, O'Connell M, Rubin J. Treatment of neuroendocrine carcinomas with combination etoposide and cisplatin: evidence of major therapeutic activity in ananplastic variants of these neoplasms. *Cancer* 1991; **68**: 227–32.

43. Moseley KM, Kubota M, Diefenbach-Jagger H *et al*. Parathyroid hormone-related protein purified from a human cancer cell line. *Proceedings of the National Academy of Sciences of the USA* 1987; **84**: 5048–52.

44. Suva LJ, Winslow GA, Wettehall REH *et al*. A parathyroid hormone-related protein implicated in malignant hypercalcaemia: cloning and expression. *Science* 1987; **237**: 893–6.

45. Mangin M, Webb AC, Dreyer BE *et al*. Identification of a cDNA encoding a parathyroid hormone-like peptide from a human tumor associated with humoral hypercalcaemia of malignancy. *Proceedings of the National Academy of Sciences of the USA* 1988; **85**: 597–601.

46. Thiede M, Strewler GJ, Nissenson RA, Rosenblatt M, Rodan GA. Human renal carcinoma expresses two messages encoding a parathyroid hormone-like peptide : evidence for the alternative splicing of a single copy gene. *Proceedings of the National Academy of Sciences of the USA* 1988; **85**: 4605–9.

47. Mangin M, Ikeda K, Dreyer BE, Milstone L, Broadus AE. Two distinct tumor-derived parathyroid hormone-like peptides result from alternative ribonucleic acid processing. *Molecular Endocrinology* 1988; **2**: 1049–55.

48. Yasuda T, Banville D, Hendy GN, Goltzman D. Characterization of the human

parathyroid hormone-like peptide gene. *Journal of Biological Chemistry* 1989; **264**: 7720–5.

49. Suda LJ, Mather LA, Gillespie MT *et al.* Structure of the 5' flanking region of the gene encoding human parathyroid hormone-related protein (hPTHrP). *Gene* 1989; **77**: 95–105.

50. Mangin M, Ikeda K, Dreyer BE, Broadus AE. Isolation and characterization of the human parathyroid hormone-like peptide gene. *Proceedings of the National Academy of Sciences of the USA* 1989; **86**: 2408–12.

51. Mangin M, Ikeda K, Dreyer BE, Broadus AE. Identification of an upstream promoter of the human parathyroid hormone-like peptide gene. *Molecular Endocrinology* 1990; **4**: 851–8.

52. Ikeda K, Lu C, Weir EC, Mangin M, Broadus AE. Transcriptional regulation of the parathyroid hormone-related peptide gene by glucocorticoids and vitamin D in a human C-cell line. *Journal of Biological Chemistry* 1989; **264**: 15743–6.

53. Mundy GR. General concepts of calcium homeostasis. In: *Calcium homeostasis: hypercalcaemia and hypocalcaemia*, 2nd edn. London: Martin Dunitz, 1990: 1–16.

54. Yates AJP, Gutierrez GE, Smollens P *et al.* Effects of a synthetic peptide of a parathyroid hormone-related protein on calcium homeostasis, renal tubular calcium reabsorption and bone metabolism. *Journal of Clinical Investigation* 1988; **81**: 932–8.

55. Heath DA, Senior PV, Varley JM, Beck F. Parathyroid hormone-related protein in tumors associated with hypercalcaemia. *Lancet* 1990; **335**: 66–9.

56. Siris ES, Sherman WH, Baquiran DC *et al.* Effect of dichloromethylene diphosphonate on skeletal mobilization of calcium in multiple myeloma. *New England Journal of Medicine* 1980; **302**: 310–15.

57. Ralston SH, Gardner MD, Dryburgh FJ *et al.* Treatment of severe hypercalcaemia with mithramycin and aminohydroxypropylidene. *Lancet* 1988; **ii**: 277.

58. Kelley WN, Palella TD. Gout and other disorders of purine metabolism. In: *Harrison's principles of internal medicine*, 11th edn., New York: McGraw-Hill, 1987: 1623–32.

59. Seegmiller JE, Laster L, Howell RR. Biochemistry of uric acid and its relationship to gout. *New England Journal of Medicine* 1963; **268**: 712–16.

60. Tsokos GC, Balow JE, Spiegel RJ *et al.* Renal and metabolic complications of undifferentiated and lymphoblastic lymphomas. *Medicine* 1981; **60**: 218–29.

61. Krakoff IH, Meyer RL. Prevention of hyperuricaemia in leukemia and lymphoma. *Journal of the American Medical Association* 1965; **193**: 1–6.

62. Sterns RH. The treatment of hyponatremia: first do no harm. *American Journal of Medicine* 1990; **88**: 557–60.

63. Sterns RH, Riggs JE, Schochet SS Jr. Osmotic demyelination syndrome following correction of hyponatremia. *New England Journal of Medicine* 1986; **314**: 1535–42.

64. Tien R, Arieff AI, Kucharczyk W, Wasik A, Kucharczyk J. Hyponatremic encephalopathy: is central pontine myelinolysis a component? *American Journal of Medicine* 1992; **92**: 513–22.

65. Arieff AI. Hyponatremia, convulsions, respiratory arrest, and permanent brain damage after elective surgery in healthy women. *New England Journal of Medicine* 1986; **314**: 1529–35.

66. Cluitmans FHM, Meinders AE. Management of severe hyponatremia; rapid or slow correction? *American Journal of Medicine* 1990; **88**: 161–6.

Index

Page numbers printed in **bold** type refer to figures; those in *italic* to tables